Human–Computer Interaction Series

For further volumes:
http://www.springer.com/series/6033

HCI is a multidisciplinary field focused on human aspects of the development of computer technology. As computer-based technology becomes increasingly pervasive—not just in developed countries, but worldwide—the need to take a human-centered approach in the design and development of this technology becomes ever more important. For roughly 30 years now, researchers and practitioners in computational and behavioral sciences have worked to identify theory and practice that influences the direction of these technologies, and this diverse work makes up the field of human–computer interaction. Broadly speaking it includes the study of what technology might be able to do for people and how people might interact with the technology. The HCI series publishes books that advance the science and technology of developing systems which are both effective and satisfying for people in a wide variety of contexts. Titles focus on theoretical perspectives (such as formal approaches drawn from a variety of behavioral sciences), practical approaches (such as the techniques for effectively integrating user needs in system development), and social issues (such as the determinants of utility, usability and acceptability).

Titles published within the Human–Computer Interaction Series are included in Thomson Reuters' Book Citation Index, The DBLP Computer Science Bibliography and The HCI Bibliography.

Stephen H. Fairclough · Kiel Gilleade
Editors

Advances in Physiological Computing

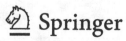
Springer

Editors
Stephen H. Fairclough
Kiel Gilleade
School of Natural Sciences and Psychology
Liverpool John Moores University
Liverpool, Merseyside
UK

ISSN 1571-5035
ISBN 978-1-4471-6993-2   ISBN 978-1-4471-6392-3   (eBook)
DOI 10.1007/978-1-4471-6392-3
Springer London Heidelberg New York Dordrecht

Printed on acid-free paper

Springer is part of Springer Science+Business Media (www.springer.com)

Foreword

Teleman's physiological and biochemical status was monitored constantly during the mission through a specially tailored system of instruments blended together to form the Physiological Control and Monitoring System (PCMS). At the start of the mission, an intravenous catheter was inserted in the superior vena cava vein through a plug implanted surgically in his shoulder. A glass electrode was brought into intimate contact with his bloodstream at this nearest acceptable point to the heart. Through the electrode a series of minute pulses, set up by an electrochemical reaction with his blood, informed the computer continually of his body status. The computer was programmed to receive inputs directly from various parts of the aircraft's controlling instrumentation that, coupled with the *in vivo* status reports, determined the time and dosage of the drugs he received.

From Joe Poyer's science fiction novel *North Cape* (p. 31).

This collection, "Advances in Physiological Computing," constitutes the most significant milestone thus far on an idea track that stretches back through the vision posed by Allanson and Fairclough's "A research agenda for physiological computing" (2004) and the body of work cited there to the genius of Wiener, Walter, and Ashby. My own leg of this relay was inspired by several whose work is little known, but whose contributions merit commending to present-day workers in this field.

Kenneth Gaarder was one of the three organizers of the 1969 Santa Monica meeting where the new technique of biofeedback was defined and named (Moss 1999), and coauthor of "Clinical biofeedback: A procedural manual" (1967), formatted in the style of Ashby's "Design for a Brain" (1954). Ken was an early mentor who urged this writer to apply control systems theory to the biofeedback enterprise, an entreaty that eventually found expression in empirical investigations of biocybernetic adaptation (Pope et al. 1995).

An important source of inspiration for the adaptive automation system described in the 1995 paper was John Reising's concept of a "symbionic" cockpit system that senses the physiological and mental state of the pilot and responds accordingly (Reising and Moss 1986), a concept that presaged the DARPA Augmented Cognition program. The resulting biocybernetic system at NASA Langley Research Center (LaRC) was the culmination of a series of developments that began with the publication of an agenda for research in pilot mental state assessment (Pope and Bowles 1982). A workshop was sponsored in 1987 (Comstock 1988) to assess the state of the art in "mental state estimation."

A paper (Reising and Moss 1986) published the previous year prior to the workshop had inspired planning at LaRC toward the design of a biocybernetic system applicable to the problem of mental disengagement in automated system operation. Itself inspired by a technology described in a 1969 science fiction novel by Poyer, the paper predicted the "symbionic" cockpit of 2010: "Nevertheless, it is certain that the pilot's 'plant dynamics' will be monitored in real time and that the data will be used to dynamically allocate tasks between the pilot and the electronic crewmember" (Reising and Moss 1986). This cockpit is yet to be realized; nevertheless, today's physiological computing researchers are creating science and technology that will one day enable symbiotic cyborg capabilities.

The immediate inspiration for the work reported in our 1995 paper was the work of a biofeedback research pioneer, Thomas Mulholland, on "Biofeedback as Scientific Method" (1977). Tom, too, imagined that the biofeedback process could be conceptualized with feedback control principles, and went further to show how biofeedback could be adapted to embody a scientific method. It continues to be an ambition of mine to extend Tom's ideas further, mapping more concepts from feedback control theory onto the biocybernetic loop.

One aspect of Tom's approach bears highlighting because it represents an instance of what appears to be a thread of creative shifts in perspective that appear in the physiological computing field. That aspect involved demonstrating that the temporal patterning of alpha activity, in the loop with light stimulation, exhibited the contrasting behavior expected for a feedback control system under positive (deviation amplifying) versus negative (deviation reducing) feedback conditions. This result was taken as evidence of a feedforward path (functional relationship) between light stimulation and alpha production (Mulholland 1977). What has been done here is to make profitable use of an otherwise unwanted phenomenon—system instability under positive feedback. In other words, turning a behavior usually to be avoided into a benefit. Similarly, Fairclough finds a use for "undesirable" positive feedback, suggesting interspersing positive feedback in games with negative feedback to provide periods of skill "stretching" among periods of skill consolidation (Fairclough 2008).

Fairclough argues also that brain–computer interfaces (BCI) are ideally suited to "extraordinary abilities" types of game mechanics because they are "limited in terms of degrees of control, less than 100 % accurate and require specific training"—again turning shortcomings into a "feature" (Fairclough 2008). Likewise, the problem of movement disruption of physiological sensing motivated a new method of modulating one player's game controller using the physiological signals of another, collaborating player who is physically inactive, thus enhancing the social interaction experience of electronic gameplay (Pope and Stephens 2012).

The physiologically modulated videogame concept has evolved from the failure of the closed loop biocybernetic method to achieve its intended purpose as an assessment procedure designed to determine the requirements for operator involvement that promote effective operator awareness states (Pope et al. 1995). Testing with the system revealed that, given enough practice, a subject may learn how to deliberately control automation to the level at which they prefer to work by regulating their EEG, thereby rendering the subject's responses unusable for the method's intended purpose. The assessment procedure then functions as a training protocol in that the subject is rewarded for producing the EEG pattern that reflects an increasing level of engagement by having the automated system share more of the work. If the original flight simulator is replaced with a video game, the system becomes a way to deliver biofeedback training that motivates trainees to partici- pate in and adhere to the training process, transforming a failure into an idea for a new technology. As Gilleade et al. (2005) note, "...if through practice, the player becomes proficient in controlling their natural physiological responses; the awareness of volitional control makes the game become a biofeedback game once again."

The novel character of physiological computing seems to nurture the imagi- nation and foster ingenuity in such ways. It is exhilarating to witness the inven- tiveness abundant in the physiological computing field and the meaningful application of analysis tools that are being brought to bear on the fascinating challenges of blending physiology with machines. Seeing that exploitation of tools is reminiscent of the experience of discovering in psychology graduate school what all those arcane engineering tools learned in college were actually good for. I expect to witness more examples of conceptual and technological innovation as this field advances, crystallized here by this timely volume. Its editors' writings have already helped me to get my bearings amid the concepts of cybernetics, biofeedback, and biocybernetic adaptation, orienting my perspective on even my own work. I look forward to furthering that educational process with the present volume.

Hampton, VA, December 2013   Alan Pope

References

Ashby WR (1954) Design for a brain. Wiley, New York

Allanson J, Fairclough SH (2004) A research agenda for physiological computing, Interacting with Computers. 16:857–878

Comstock JR (1988) Mental State Estimation 1987. NASA Conference Publication 2504

Fairclough SH (2008) BCI and physiological computing: similarities, differences and intuitive control, Paper presented at the Workshop on BCI and Computer Games: CHI'08

Gaarder KR, Montgomery PS (1977) Clinical biofeedback: a procedural manual. Williams and Wilkins, Baltimore, pp. 177–191

Gilleade K, Dix A, Allanson J (2005) Affective videogames and modes of affective gaming: assist me, challenge me, emote me. In: Proceedings of Digital Games Research Association (DiGRA) Conference, Vancouver, Canada, June 2005, pp. 16–20

Moss D (ed) (1999) Humanistic and transpersonal psychology: a historical and biographical sourcebook. Greenwood Publishing, Westport, CT, 154–155

Mulholland T (1977) Biofeedback as scientific method. In Schwartz G, Beatty J (eds) Biofeedback: theory and research. Academic Press, New York, 9–28

Pope AT, Bowles RL (1982) A program for assessing pilot mental state in flight simulators. American institute of aeronautics and astronautics paper No. 82–0257, January 1982

Pope AT, Bogart EH, Bartolome DS (1995) Biocybernetic system validates index of operator engagement in automated task. Biol Psychol 40:187–195

Pope AT, Stephens CL (2012) Interpersonal biocybernetics: connecting through social psychophysiology, ICMI 2012, Santa Monica, California, 22–26 October, 2012

Poyer J (1969) North cape. Sphere Books Limited, London

Reising JM, Moss RW (1986) 2010: The symbionic cockpit. Aerospace and electronic systems magazine. IEEE 1(1) pp 24–27, Jan 1986

Contents

Contributors

Daniel Afergan Tufts University, Medford, MA, USA, e-mail: afergan@cs.tufts.edu

Esubalew Bekele Vanderbilt University, 518 Olin hall, 2400 Highland Ave, Nashville, TN 37212, USA, e-mail: bekele@vanderbilt.edu

Jonas Brönstrup Team PhyPA, Berlin Institute of Technology, MAR 3-2, 10587 Berlin, Germany, e-mail: jonas.broenstrup@gmail.com

Andreas Bulling Perceptual User Interfaces, Max Planck Institute for Informatics, Campus E1.4, 66123 Saarbrücken, Germany, e-mail: bulling@mpi-inf.mpg.de

Elke Daemen Philips Research Europe, Eindhoven, The Netherlands

Gert-Jan de Vries Philips Research Europe, Eindhoven, The Netherlands

Chelsea Dobbins School of Computing and Mathematical Sciences, Liverpool John Moores University, Byrom Street, Liverpool L3 3AF, UK, e-mail: C.M.Dobbins@ljmu.ac.uk

Stephen H. Fairclough School of Natural Sciences and Psychology, Liverpool John Moores University, Liverpool, UK, e-mail: s.h.fairclough@ljmu.ac.uk

Paul Fergus School of Computing and Mathematical Sciences, Liverpool John Moores University, Byrom Street, Liverpool L3 3AF, UK

Kiel Gilleade School of Natural Sciences and Psychology, Liverpool John Moores University, Liverpool, UK, e-mail: gilleade@gmail.com

Robert J. K. Jacob Tufts University, Medford, MA, USA, e-mail: jacob@cs.tufts.edu

Joris Janssen Philips Research Europe, Eindhoven, The Netherlands

Alexander J. Karran School of Natural Science and Psychology, Liverpool John Moores University, Liverpool, UK, e-mail: a.j.karran@ljmu.ac.uk

Ute Kreplin School of Natural Science and Psychology, Liverpool John Moores University, Liverpool, UK, e-mail: U.Kreplin@2011.ljmu.ac.uk

Laurens R. Krol Team PhyPA, Berlin Institute of Technology, MAR 3-2, 10587 Berlin, Germany, e-mail: lrkrol@mailbox.tu-berlin.de

Francine Lalooses Tufts University, Medford, MA, USA, e-mail: francine. lalooses@tufts.edu

David Llewellyn-Jones School of Computing and Mathematical Sciences, Liverpool John Moores University, Byrom Street, Liverpool L3 3AF, UK

Romy Lorenz Team PhyPA, Berlin Institute of Technology, MAR 3-2, 10587 Berlin, Germany, e-mail: lorenz.romy@googlemail.com

Päivi Majaranta School of Information Sciences, University of Tampere, 33014 Tampere, Finland, e-mail: paivi.majaranta@uta.fi

Madjid Merabti School of Computing and Mathematical Sciences, Liverpool John Moores University, Byrom Street, Liverpool L3 3AF, UK

Domen Novak Sensory-Motor Systems Lab, ETH Zurich, Tannenstrasse 1, 8092 Zurich, Switzerland, e-mail: domen.novak@hest.ethz.ch

Martin Ouwerkerk Philips Research Europe, Eindhoven, The Netherlands

Evan M. Peck Tufts University, Medford, MA, USA, e-mail: evan.peck@ tufts.edu

Alan T. Pope NASA Langley Research Center, Hampton, VA 23681, USA, e-mail: alan.t.pope@nasa.gov

Nilanjan Sarkar Vanderbilt University, 518 Olin hall, 2400 Highland Ave, Nashville, TN 37212, USA

Chad L. Stephens NASA Langley Research Center, Hampton, VA 23681, USA, e-mail: chad.l.stephens@nasa.gov

William van Beek Philips Research Europe, Eindhoven, The Netherlands

Joyce Westerink Philips Research Europe, Eindhoven, The Netherlands

Beste F. Yuksel Tufts University, Medford, MA, USA, e-mail: beste.yuksel@ tufts.edu

Thorsten O. Zander Team PhyPA, Berlin Institute of Technology, MAR 3-2, 10587 Berlin, Germany, e-mail: tzander@gmail.com

Introduction

Physiological computing is the term used to describe any technological system where human physiology is directly monitored and transformed into a control input. It represents the logical endpoint of convergence between the human nervous system and its silicon-based counterparts. This category of technology endeavors to render input control as intuitive as a simple volitional act, such as raising one arm or moving forward. The capacity of sensor-based systems to monitor the brain and body yields a dynamic representation of the cognition, emotions, and motivations of the user. Tapping this implicit model of the user extends the adaptive repertoire of technology, creating a dialog between body and computer and shaping the interaction in a generative sense. The act of monitoring via sensor technology inevitably generates data that can be quantified, visualized, inspected, and shared. Users can acquaint themselves with a digital self that provides a quantified perspective on exercise, sleeping patterns, and changes in mood.

The current collection has been developed to provide a broad overview across this emerging area of research. The strong interdisciplinary character of physiological computing research encapsulates significant breadth of knowledge, from neuroscience to engineering. For those of us working in this field, particularly in multidisciplinary teams, one benefit of this research is the potential for psychologists to work alongside computer scientists and engineers on a common problem. But this interdisciplinary approach can create problems as research across the continuum of physiological computing systems, from brain-control interfaces to telemedicine, fractures into system-based communities working on very specific topics. To an extent, this development is both inevitable and necessary. However, research on physiological computing systems, whether the target system is concerned with input control, adaptation, or monitoring, has many more similarities than differences. All systems involve: sensor technology and the measurement of physiology in the field, biomedical signal processing, and classification. These areas are core to most categories in the current volume and almost every active researcher has engaged with this area in order to create new types of interactive experience. One focus of the current collection is to emphasize common ground between the range of physiological computing applications.

We have arranged the collection to reflect a progression from pervasive areas to specific categories of application. Our opening contribution on meaningful interaction is an attempt to engage with one of the least-explored topics in this field—namely the process of inference that arises whenever a user interacts with a physiological computing interface. As stated earlier, there are a number of common concerns across physiological computing systems such as sensor design, signal processing, and classification. These fundamental issues are covered by Novak in the second chapter of this volume on engineering issues.

The next two chapters are both concerned with the use of physiological activity as a form of input control. The prominence of brain–computer interfaces (BCI) has perhaps overshadowed developments in the area of eye tracking as an alternative form of input control. The use of eye tracking as a form of human–computer interaction is an overlooked form of physiological computing and so the chapter by Majaranta and Bulling is a welcome addition to the current volume. These authors provide an introduction to the technologies, research, and issues for eye tracking in a naturalistic environment. The chapter by Zander and colleagues on BCI provides a novel perspective on this category of system. The traditional form of BCI is based upon recognition of an volitional intention (to move the cursor to the left or right) or a stimulus (letter or number) that the user wishes to select. By contrast, Zander and colleagues focus on passive BCI—a form of interaction where the wishes of the user are conveyed implicitly to the system without the need to actively formulate a volitional intention.

It is accurate to say that biofeedback is the grandparent of all physiological computing technology. It was the biofeedback approach that first used technology to create a closed-loop design to teach human participants the necessary skills for autonomic self-regulation. The connection between biofeedback and the biocybernetic loop at the heart of all physiological computing systems is discussed in detail by Pope and colleagues in their chapter. These authors provide an overview of biofeedback as a clinical intervention, which provides the basis for research into adaptive gaming technologies where the act of self-regulation is integrated directly into gameplay for both individuals and groups.

Monitoring brain activity for physiological computing has traditionally been achieved using EEG-based measurement, but there are other available alternatives. Peck and colleagues provide an overview of their work on functional near-infrared spectography (fNIRS) as a means of monitoring mental workload. fNIRS is a technology that is slowly making the transition from a laboratory-based method to an approach that can be used in the field. The monitoring of spontaneous changes in psychological states, such as increased mental workload or anxiety, can be used to inform the adaptation of technology. The net effect of this innovation is for software to adapt in a manner that is both timely and intuitive. This type of "intelligent" adaptation is particularly important for human–robot interaction as there is an increased requirement for robotic systems to demonstrate social awareness from the perspective of their human users. Bekele and Sarkar describe their research on the use of psychophysiological classification to enhance human–

robot interaction; their work includes an intriguing case study involving an interaction between a robot and individuals on the autistic spectrum.

Some of the pioneers of physiological computing performed their original research in the context of affective computing. The development of new application domains has shifted the emphasis from the detection of traditional emotional categories (e.g., happiness, fear, disgust) to those nuanced states that incorporate elements of both emotion and cognition. The chapter by Karran and Kreplin describes a program of research to investigate the detection of interest in the context of cultural heritage. This work is challenging in several respects, the psychological research underpinning the concept of interest is sparse, and the detection of psychophysiological change in response to media presentation creates a lot of noise and relatively little signal. This chapter captures the tension between a desire to explore new application domains and the real-world obstacles to system accuracy and usage. This theme is revisited by Westerlink and her colleagues at Philips Research Europe who describe the creation of a bracelet designed to measure anxiety. This chapter provides an industrial perspective on the development of a physiological computing device. The goal of this device is to provide the user with insight into one's own health and wellbeing and this therapeutic strand of physiological computing is the focus of the final chapter by Dobbins and her colleagues. Monitoring the physiology of an individual on a 24/7 basis will inevitably produce huge amount of data that may be adopted for the creation of digital memories. This is a form of life logging where the pervasiveness of physiological data is exploited and tagged in order to form memory cues, especially for those elderly users who are living with cognitive impairment.

One goal of this collection is to define the field of physiological computing with respect to the breadth of applications involving physiological data. Physiological computing is an exciting area for research because it provides a speculative vision of how we may interact with technology in the future. It also speaks of the increasing convergence between wearable sensors and wearable computing systems. But we have a long way to go, especially as those methods and measures developed under laboratory conditions must be transformed into robust and reliable data to inform working systems in the field. In that sense, this collection provides a perspective on the range and potential of physiological computing as a work-in-progress.

Liverpool, December 2013   Stephen H. Fairclough
                                                                              Kiel Gilleade

Chapter 1
Meaningful Interaction with Physiological Computing

Stephen H. Fairclough and Kiel Gilleade

Abstract Physiological data can be used as input to a computerised system. There are many types of interaction that can be facilitated by this form of input ranging from intentional control to implicit software adaptation. This type of interaction directly with the brain and body represent a new paradigm in human–computer interaction and this chapter will discuss how meaning is associated with data interpretation and changes at the interface. The chapter will categorise the different systems physiological input allows and discuss how interaction with the system can be made meaningful for the user.

Introduction

The general mode of human interaction with computing systems has remained unchanged for the last 30 years. We communicate our intentions overtly to the computer via peripheral devices such as the keyboard and mouse. The advent of tablet computers and gesture recognition presents a challenge to traditional methods of input control but the basic interaction paradigm remains unchanged. There are other alternative paradigms under development that allow the user to communicate with a computer without any need for overt forms of input control. Brain–computer interfaces (BCI) are designed to read actions and intentions directly from the cortex of the brain by translating signals into actions at the interface (Tan and Nijholt 2010; Allison et al. 2012). Thereby replacing the physical based motion involved in traditional input controls by monitoring the source of the perceptual-motor chain in the brain. The same logic applies to those

S. H. Fairclough (✉) · K. Gilleade
School of Natural Sciences and Psychology, Liverpool John Moores University, England, UK
e-mail: s.h.fairclough@ljmu.ac.uk

K. Gilleade
e-mail: gilleade@gmail.com

S. H. Fairclough and K. Gilleade (eds.), *Advances in Physiological Computing*,
Human–Computer Interaction Series, DOI: 10.1007/978-1-4471-6392-3_1,
© Springer-Verlag London 2014

systems that translate eye movements into cursor control at the interface (San Agustin et al. 2009), where directed gaze is a proxy for motor control.

The development of BCI and eye control systems represents an alternative form of input control that is directive and intentional, just like pointing and clicking with a mouse. In these cases, the mode of input control is novel but the mechanics of human–computer interaction (HCI) remain essentially unchanged. There is another form of human–computer communication where the form of HCI is novel and the mechanics of the interaction are neither deliberate or volitional in any conventional sense. In this case, the nervous system of the user is monitored during the HCI and the resulting data is used to characterise the cognitive, emotional or motivational status of the user, these data provide a dynamic representation of the psychological status of the individual, which is relayed to the system in order to inform a real-time process of software adaptation (Fairclough 2009). This method of "wiretapping" the psychophysiology of the individual may have profound implications for the future of HCI. Previous research into affective computing (Kapoor et al. 2007) and adaptive automation (Wilson and Russell 2007) have demonstrated how physiological data can be used to trigger software adaptation that is timely and intuitive. Hence, a frustrated user receives help in order to avoid an escalation of anger (Klein et al. 2002), the autopilot on an aircraft cockpit is activated in time to alleviate high mental workload experienced by the pilot (Kaber et al. 2005), and the computer game makes an upward adjustment of difficulty to challenge a bored gamer (Gilleade et al. 2005). These biocybernetic control systems (Pope et al. 1995) rely on implicit monitoring of the psychophysiological status of the user and can be used to promote desirable psychological states and/or to mitigate those negative emotions or hazardous states of awareness (Prinzel 2002) that could be detrimental to the health and safety of the individual.

One innovation of biocybernetic control is the ability for software to adapt to the individual in a highly personalised way. Hence, the physiological computing system is capable of dynamic adaptation in order to tailor the interaction to a particular person or a particular usage scenario. Biocybernetic control is also capable of taking an initiative and adapting the interface in order to shape the experience of the human according to a predefined agenda, i.e. to mitigate frustration or promote positive affect. The capacity of adaptive software to operate upon the human represents a fundamental change in how people and computers work together, as the autonomy of the technological system is enhanced and human–computer interaction is shifted toward a dyad that may be more accurately characterised as 'teamwork' between user and computer (Klein et al. 2004).

Categories of Physiological Computing System

Physiological computing systems fall into two broad groupings. The first are designed to extend the body schema, i.e. the representation of the body used to guide perceptual-motor tasks that are targeted and volitional. These functions are guided by intentionality, when we want to reach out to touch an icon or click a link to go to a particular web page. For routine activities, such as picking up a coffee cup or opening a door, the body schema guides action at an unconscious level. The body schema rests upon a sense of agency, of being the initiator or source of a movement or action (Gallagher 2005). The second category of physiological computing system is concerned with self-perception of those dynamic processes that occur within the body and contribute to an awareness of a psychological state. *This body image has been defined as "a complex set of intentional states and dispositions... in which the intentional object is one's own body"* (p. 24) (Gallagher 2005). With respect to physiological computing applications, augmentation of the body image is achieved by monitoring spontaneous changes in physiology and adapting the interface in response to a dynamic representation of the body image. In addition, as we are using physiological measures to represent psychological processes, the intentional object extends beyond the physical body to those interoceptive pathways (Craig 2003) that inform self-awareness across a number of psychological states. This 'wiretapping' approach may be used to capture a range of physiological data, such as: physical activity (running, walking) as well as psychological processes, such as increased mental workload or frustration, and markers of health e.g. a hypertensive user monitoring blood pressure. This type of physiological computing system facilitates the perception of self by providing an additional channel of quantitative feedback to the user.

There are three distinct categories of physiological computing system Fairclough 2011): input control, biocybernetic adaptation and ambulatory monitoring. As stated earlier, our conventional mode of HCI involves expanding the body schema. This psychomotor control loop is the basis for interaction with a keyboard/mouse, touchscreen or gesture-based control. The physiological computing approach can be applied to this type of input control interaction by capturing activity related to the psychomotor control loop originating from either the cortex or sites of motor output. Electrooculography (EOG) refers to the measurement of the muscles that control vertical and horizontal eye movements. Eye movement can be used to control a cursor moving in two-dimensional space and intentional eye blinks used as a selection mechanism (see Majaranta and Bulling in the current volume). These interfaces have been developed for users with physical disability, but it is plausible that healthy users can also benefit from this kind of input control. BCIs offer an alternative mode of input control. Rather than tapping the final stage of the psychomotor loop, most BCIs are designed to capture electrocortical activity at source: the intention that precedes movement, the spark of activation in response to a particular item, the localisation of visual attention. BCIs offer a highly novel form of hands-free interaction capable of communicating with standard screen-based technologies as well as specialised devices such as prostheses. Like muscle controlled interfaces, BCIs function as an alternative form of input control designed to emulate the functional vocabulary of standard devices, such as the keyboard and mouse. All forms of BCI are treated as alternative modes of input control that operate within the human–computer interaction paradigm, in other words, they allow the user to communicate intentional actions via a command interface. Therefore, issues like novelty, ease of use, communication bandwidth and speed of information transfer are important influences on user acceptance.

The third category of physiological computing is called biocybernetic adaptation. These systems monitor spontaneous activity from the brain and the body in order to capture psychological states relating to performance and wellbeing. These states include psychophysiological signatures of emotions, such as anger, frustration or fear; in this respect these systems overlap with affective computing technology (Picard 1997). Changes in cognition related to mental workload may be also measured via involuntary patterns of psychophysiology (see Peck et al. in current volume). For certain categories of computer software, such as games or auto-tutoring systems, we may be interested in changes in both cognition and emotion, i.e. when someone is mentally overloaded (too much information, not enough time), they also may experience anxiety or anger. This type of biocybernetic adaptation encompasses a wide array of software applications, from the control of adaptive automation to human–robot interaction (see Sarkar in current volume). Regardless of precise context, biocybernetic systems are fundamentally designed to deliver software adaptations that will be perceived as timely, intuitive and 'intelligent' by the user.

The biocybernetic category of physiological computing systems relies on passive monitoring of psychophysiology. The user behaves in a naturalistic fashion and spontaneous physiological responses are recorded and relayed to a monitoring system. This surveillance function of physiological computing systems is most prominent in the final category that we have called ambulatory monitoring. It is reasonable to assume that all three categories of physiological computing system will rely on lightweight and unobtrusive 'wearable' sensors. In some cases, the user may only connect to the system when they are working within a particular context or using a specific piece of software. Other users may wear sensor apparatus during every waking hour, some may even have implanted sensors capable of transmitting data for every second of every day. The flow of physiological data from person to system is the lifeblood of all systems already described, these data drive the algorithms used to facilitate computer control or software adaptation, but they may be recorded for other purposes. One obvious group of candidates for continuous physiological monitoring are those people with chronic health problems who are being treated as out-patients. Basic autonomic functions, such as heart rate, blood pressure and respiration patterns, could be recorded wirelessly and made available to qualified medical staff who wish to monitor those individuals outside of a medical facility. Alternatively, a social network of carers, close friends and family members may be granted access to real-time data feeds from patients for purposes of monitoring or reassurance. This is the concept of "body blogging" where physiological data is made available in a public or private web domain for the purpose of medical monitoring or social networking (Gilleade and Fairclough 2010). This approach to physiological monitoring could also be useful to an individual engaged in a life-logging or self-tracking project. The big difference between the ambulatory monitoring approach and BCI/biocybernetic adaptation is that the purpose of the physiological data in the former is feedback and data visualisation, for the individual and other connected people, and unlike the later does not necessitate real-time adaptive control.

The three categories of physiological computing systems are intended to represent a continuum rather than a hard distinction between different types of system. It is anticipated that modes of physiological computing control will be used in combination with conventional modes of input control (mouse, keyboard, console, gestures). It is easy to imagine an integrated system where BCI working alongside conventional input control. The introduction of biocybernetic adaptation is complimentary to conventional input control because it may be used for the adaptation of settings and special commands (Fairclough 2008); hence, a user could interact with a virtual character via keyboard/mouse who responds to their emotional state with a repertoire of affective inflections and expressions. The key point is that physiological computing is intended to enhance conventional modes of HCI, not to replace them.

The conceptual framework of a biofeedback loop is effectively the parent of all physiological computing systems. Crucial biofeedback concepts, such as fidelity of feedback, real-time control and enhanced self-regulation, are relevant to all four categories of physiological computing. This common ground creates huge potential for convergence and mash-ups between the different types of physiological computing system.

Meaningful Interaction

If the purpose of physiological computing is to extend the body schema and the body image, the challenge for system design is how to connect the intentions and experiences of the user with the interface in a meaningful way. Physiological computing systems are based upon a direct connection between activity in the central nervous system and events at the interface. This biocybernetic loop (Pope et al. 1995) transforms raw physiological data into a semantic classification (e.g. move up/down, angry, excited), which is converted into an adaptive response from the system. Interaction with a physiological computing system is perceived as meaningful by users when events at the interface conform to their expectations or experiences.

The process of analysis within the biocybernetic loop is analogous to an act of translation. In the book God and Golem Inc, Wiener (1964) described a hypothetical system capable of translating English into Russian and back into English; he argued that the degree of similarity between the original document and English text translated from the Russian provided an index of system efficiency, i.e. how well does a re-representation match an original representation. The same analogy may be adopted to understand the inherent complexities of the biocybernetic control loop. In this case, we have a number of systems where intention or experience, as perceived phenomenologically by the person, are converted into physiological data, which are subsequently decoded into an event at the user interface. The first obstacle to meaningful interaction is basically metaphysical; the experience of an intention or psychological state is rich and nuanced compared to an operationalisation of that intention/state via psychophysiological data. This discrepancy has been accurately articulated by Hayes (1999) as the gap between "the plentitude of experience compared to the sparseness of abstraction" (p. 99). Given that a degree of simplification is an essential starting point for representation within the biocybernetic loop, the next challenge is to accurately classify incoming data according to the internal lexicon of the system. If a BCI is designed to recognise two axes of movement (e.g. up/down, left/right), it is important for an intention to move upwards to the right is recognised as such by the system. For biocybernetic adaptation, the identification of a target state (e.g. anger) from a range of other emotional states (e.g. excitement, fear, boredom) should coincide with bodily changes that are consistent with the experience of anger, e.g. increased cardiovascular reactivity and respiration rate. Unlike other categories, the goal of ambulatory monitoring is to represent data records directly to the user or to another user. In this case, the challenge is one of representation and visualisation, to render data meaningful and digestible for the user. The final barrier to meaningful interaction concerns the response from the system at the interface. For BCI, correct identification of the intended direction of movement must be translated into analogous cursor movement. The correct selection of appropriate response for input control is relatively straightforward in comparison with biocybernetic adaptation. The latter may respond in several ways to the identification of a specific user state; in the case of frustration for example, the system could offer help information or automate on behalf of the user or play calming music. If the interaction is to be meaningful for the user, it is important that a system response resonates with experience in some way, to either acknowledge that experience or provide an intervention designed to mitigate negative experience (or promote positive experience).

The following sections will consider the issues surrounding meaningful interaction with respect to three categories of physiological computing: input control (muscle interfaces and BCI), biocybernetic adaptation and ambulatory monitoring (body blogging).

Meaningful Interaction with Input Control

The most significant challenge for systems, such as BCI and muscle control, is utilising physiological signals for input control is matching the speed and intuitive ease of traditional input devices; in addition, the standards of user acceptance in this field has been arguably raised in recent years with the advent of gesture-based input. Given that competition in terms of speed and accuracy from traditional modes of input control is so strong, the designer must consider the motivations of the healthy user and the context of usage when he decides to incorporate eye-based control or BCI (Allison et al. 2007a) into the system. For example, BCI or gaze-control may be used to supplement existing modes of input control, such as gesture recognition or point-and-click devices. We may imagine a system where gestures are used to locate a specific area of the screen and the BCI is deployed to trigger an event or command. Similarly, eye-based tracking may be used to direct a cursor within a document and keyboard or voice input used to edit or add text. We should also consider activities where the hands of the user are fully occupied, e.g. drivers, pilots, surgeons, gamers. It has been argued that "hands-busy" tasks lead to "induced disability" (Allison et al. 2007a) where healthy users have limitations on communication bandwidth that approximate those restrictions experienced by users with physical disabilities. In the "hands-busy" cases, BCI and eye-tracking represent an additional input channel to restore communication bandwidth. Another advantage of these technologies (compared to overt gesture recognition) is that they may be used privately in a public space. At the time of writing, BCI technologies (e.g. peripherals) are being marketed to gamers and entertainment software. This focus plays to a particular strength of BCI for healthy users, namely the novelty of the experience and satisfaction associated with mastery of this particular mode of input control in a competitive context.

In order for input control via physiological computing to be meaningful for a user, we must consider the motivational context for system use. In the case of hybrid systems (where BCI is used in conjunction with gesture or keyboards), use of BCI or equivalent is meaningful to the user to the extent to which it "fits" with alternative modes of input control.

The use of physiological signals as a proxy for input control occurs in two different situations. Certain types of BCI (Allison et al. 2007b) are operated by exposing the user to specific categories of stimulation at the interface and the response from the electroencephalogram (EEG) determines whether a selection is made. For example, one system (Krusienski et al. 2008) exposes the user to an array of letters that flash in sequence, the amplitude of the P300 evoked response potential (ERP) to each flashing letter determines whether the letter is selected, i.e. higher amplitude P300 response is related to greater processing, which serves as a proxy for intention. There is also a BCI protocol structured around Steady State Visual Evoked Potentials (SSVEPs); in this case, discrete areas on the screen are programmed to flicker at a specific frequency. These 'target' frequencies may be identified in the EEG data record at the visual cortex and the synchrony between the EEG and target frequencies used as a proxy for selection. Both cases adopt a similar strategy based upon experimental protocols whereby the user is exposed to 'probe' stimuli and the response of the EEG to these probes is the aspect of data analysis that determines response selection. From the perspective of the user, the only directive is to attend to that letter or area of the screen that is of interest, hence it is essential that the system successfully matches attention with the desired selection in order to imbue interaction with meaning for the user. The other dimension to this interaction is temporal synchrony. If the user attends to a particular point on the screen, in the case of a SSVEP-based BCI, how much time is required before the system makes a response? The correct identification of a desired command or selection represents the semantics of input control, but minimal time lag is equally important to ensure a sense of connection with the interface. The importance of the temporal dimension is particularly important when input control represents a continuous response, such as cursor movement in two-dimensional space, as opposed to the selection of discrete commands, i.e. using eye movement as a mode of cursor control. There are other categories of BCI that do not rely on external stimulation to trigger input control, these systems rely on motor imagery to produce distinct EEG patterns in the somatosensory cortex, which may be matched to discrete commands at the interface (Ramoser et al. 2000). For example, the user may be requested to think about the right hand or left hand or to imagine making specific categories of movement with each limb. This mode of input control originates from internal stimulation and capability of the user with respect to mental imagery. In terms of meaningful interaction, the same criteria of speed and accuracy are essential; the user looks to the system for a timely confirmation that mental imagery has been achieved, i.e. if I think of my right hand, I expect to see the button on the right side of the screen to activate.

The simplest case of input control via physiology is the use of eye tracking technology to enable cursor control. This system converts vertical and horizontal eye movement into x and y coordinates that are translated into cursor movement on the screen. In this case, the sense of connection between the actions/intentions of the user and event on screen is created when the cursor successfully mirrors the movement of the eyes as experienced by the user. The only real threats to continuity come from involuntary distraction (e.g. gaze being automatically oriented to an event outside the screen) and accuracy of second-order tracking. This latter factor is characterised as a sensitivity gradient, which describes the ratio of eye movement to cursor movement on the screen and may cause slow movement towards or overshooting of the desired target.

As described earlier, BCI systems that operate on the basis of external stimulation or a trigger event are based upon voluntary acts of attention. The meaning of the interaction is derived from the accuracy of selection, or more specifically, the relationship between intention and selection. When the BCI is constructed around imagined movement or orienting attention to a specific part of the body, the sense of connection between mental activity and events at the interface is achieved via accurate and sensitive input control. In this sense, the mechanics of connecting imaginary movement to input control are similar to the recognition of overt gestures. One major distinction between actual and imagined movement is the presence of individual differences with respect to the latter. The inability of some people to produce consistent patterns in the EEG during motor imagery may account for the phenomenon of 'BCI illiteracy' (Kubler and Muller 2007). In this case, the sense of connection between user and system is undermined by variability inherent in self-regulation and the EEG signal. However, there is evidence that people can improve motor imagery and BCI communication via training in a neurofeedback regime (Hwang et al. 2009). It has also been suggested that playing certain types of videogame may lead to improved BCI control (Lotte et al. 2013) through stimulation of related cognitive processes e.g. mental rotation tasks.

The basic problem of BCI as input control for healthy users is that it remains relatively slow and inaccurate compared to the available alternatives. One response to this limitation is to select usage cases where a slow or inaccurate response are intuitive from the perspective of the user. It has been argued that computer games represent one test case where these limitations may be acceptable to the user (Nijholt et al. 2009). If we imagine a game where the player may enhance his chance to win by activating a special ability (e.g. flying), which confers great advantage but is also temperamental, this may add another dimension to game play (Fairclough 2008). This particular case exemplifies how matching the limitations of physiological computing to the usage case and expectations of the user may generate meaningful interaction.

Meaningful Interaction with Biocybernetic Adaptation

A biocybernetic adaptive system passively monitors psychophysiological changes in a user in order to inform real-time system adaptations. Physiological data is autonomously collected as the user performs a task, the biocybernetic system subsequently uses this information to activate software adaptation if certain triggering conditions are met. Biocybernetic systems operate outside the direct, intentional control of the user. These systems function on a control loop that is associated with a target state, therefore the system has a specific agenda (e.g. to achieve a specific target state in terms of human performance or psychological state) and is designed to influence the psychophysiology of the human operators in order to establish/sustain a target state. One of the earliest biocybernetic adaptive systems was developed by NASA for use in flight simulators (Pope et al. 1995); the psychophysiology of the pilot (spontaneous EEG) was monitored in order to manage the status of an auto-pilot facility during flight time. The agenda of the system was to sustain the level of alertness of the pilot at an optimal level via manipulation of the auto-pilot status i.e. alertness tended to decline during auto-pilot activation and to increase when the pilot manually controlled the craft.

Biocybernetic systems are designed to adapt the operating environment in order to optimise user experience. For example, computer games represent a category of technology that are designed for a particular skill set that may not accurately reflect the skill set of the individual player (Gilleade and Dix 2004). There are a multiple measures of cognitive workload e.g. frontal theta (Klimesch 1999), which can be used to infer the experience of difficulty during game play. A biocybernetic system can utilise these measures to dynamically adjust the level of difficulty in order to match the ability level of the player in real-time. Another popular agenda for this type of system is the mitigation of negative affective states, such as frustration, during computer use. This agenda has roots in the field of affective computing (Picard 1997) whereby computers are designed to understand their user's affective state and regulate undesirable states, in this case, the biocybernetic loop is designed for the personalisation and optimisation of player states (Pope and

Palsson 2001; Gilleade and Allanson 2003; Rani et al. 2005). Other biocybernetic agendas have been proposed for adapting gaming experiences (Gilleade et al. 2005) and information dissemination in social situations (Peck et al. 2011).

Biocybernetic adaptation operates in the background of the user experience, only intervening in the HCI when triggering conditions are met, as such the facilitation of a meaningful interaction can be problematic. A biocybernetic system must achieve an agenda in a manner that satisfies both user expectation of that agenda (e.g. this computer is designed to help me when I get frustrated) and their assessment of their self (e.g. self-perception of frustration). This directive necessitates a tricky proposition of providing the correct adaptation for a specific usage scenario at the right time. If the system fails to fulfil this requirement, biocybernetic adaption has the potential to cause enormous disruption to the user experience.

The design of a biocybernetic system that delivers adaptations that are both timely and intuitive is a complex challenge. Implementing an agenda for the system requires the selection of appropriate physiological measures for the task environment, deciding which type and magnitude of physiological change will trigger an adaptation and what type of adaptation will be triggered with respect to the frequency of intervention and magnitude of change. There are no ideal solutions or generic design rules for meaningful interaction at the present time; the desired effect of the system will differ according to the task, agenda and user. The most pressing issue in biocybernetic system design is accurate diagnosis of the user state based upon the psycho-physiological inference (Cacioppo and Tassinary 1990). Interpreting psychophysiology using real-time analysis in a physiological computing paradigm is problematic as measures can be easily influenced by a range of confounds e.g. movement; therefore, the system is unlikely to be working with a perfect (one-to-one) representation of psychological state. When the biocybernetic loop decides to manipulate the system state there is no guarantee that the resulting intervention will be appropriate and deemed meaningful by the user. If the adaptation is overt and obvious to the user, any conflict between the assumed and actual user state are obvious. For example, if a system is designed to intervene when the user becomes frustrated, e.g. appearance of a virtual agent asking "Would you like assistance?" and does so in the absence of frustration as perceived by the user, it is liable to both annoy the user (ironically creating the emotional state it set out to avoid) and negatively affect the perceptions of biocybernetic control as a technological advancement. By comparison, conflict during covert adaptation, e.g. making minor cumulatively or indirect environmental changes, are unlikely to be perceived by the user, provided that the trajectory of the adaptations over a long time frame is in the correct direction. Implementing a meaningful interaction with biocybernetic control is a design trade-off between sustaining a connection between user experience and the system response and the ability of the system to push user experience in the desired direction. A case study in the design of a biocybernetic loop has been provided by Fairclough and Gilleade (2012) that outlines a process-based approach to these problems.

Meaningful Interaction with Body Blogging

Physiological data provides intimate information about a person with respect to affective, cognitive and physical states. As physiological sensors have become affordable, the general public has the opportunity to quantify, visualise and log their own physiological processes and share these data with family and friends or medical professionals. There is a trend towards automating the data collection process and to integrate the resulting data into Internet applications for a personalised physiological log, e.g. tracking fitness performance. Sharing this information with others provides opportunities to improve health and lifestyle choices, e.g. evaluation of fitness performance by experts. For example, a pedometer can be used to track an individual's daily physical activity in order to generate a database; once uploaded to the Internet, this data may be reviewed by other individuals who can provide feedback to both inform and motivate the user, e.g. Philips Direct Life (Philips 2011). This process of collecting and sharing physiological data is known as Body Blogging (Gilleade and Fairclough 2010) and is defined as the act of logging physiological data using web technology.

Body blogs can be applied in a wide range of domains including the tracking of psychological/physical health, sports performance and self-quantification. In work by Ståhl et al. (2008), physiological information was incorporated into a digital diary. Operating through a mobile phone, the system not only collected a user's normal phone activity e.g. SMS, but it also collected skin conductance and motion data. These data were used to create what is known as an affective diary which could be used by a diarist to view both their subjective experience of their day (via phone activity) and the physical sensations that co-occurred with them. This visualisation allows the diarist to access a more complete picture of their experiences and learn how they may be affected by their environment, e.g. identifying stress triggers, as well as being used for memory recall. While physiological information can potentially be a powerful tool for the purposes of introspective, presenting information in an informative manner that conveys meaning can be problematic. As noted during the development of the affective diary (Lindström et al. 2006), the authors felt visualising physiological information as a standard time series graph would risk creating a disconnect between the data and the diarist. In other words the diarist wouldn't be able to associate their experiences with the format in which the data was presented. During user trials (Ståhl et al. 2008), these data were presented as a series of amorphous body postures, with activity represented by posture and skin conductance by colour. While this interface was designed to resonate with the experience of the person, user opinions were divided on the matter and depended much on users being able to connect their subjective experience with the data representations (e.g. during the trial one user, not being able to understand the data representations being provided by the system, exported the raw physiological data to another program to interpret them). This can be difficult to facilitate as such connections are made on an individual basis.

Body blogs are not simply meant for introspective purposes, e.g. personal reviews of past activity, but provide avenues for in-depth analysis e.g. identify health problems from real-world physiological data, and recommendations for behaviour modification e.g. expert analysis of current sports performance. A variety of interested stakeholders can access the data facilitating new application paradigms using the Internet as a platform for data sharing. For example, in an experiment with public bodying blogging, The Body Blogger (Gilleade and Fairclough 2010), a single user's real-time physiological information was streamed continuously for over a year across a range of online websites e.g. Twitter, allowing the public to informally interpret the physiological and psychological state of the data's owner (Gilleade 2010). Interested stakeholders ranged from the owner, friends of the owner and the public at large. Depending on the stakeholder each accessed the data with a different agenda and found a different meaning from the dataset. The data owner learned how their physiology responded to different life events which are not normally observed e.g. impact of a major holiday on physical health (Gilleade 2011), and friends learned to remotely interpret affective states e.g. work stress (Gilleade 2010). In addition, as physiological data can be interpreted differently within different contexts of measurement, a singular physiological measure can have multiple applications; data collected by a wearable electrocardiogram monitor can be used to provide medical information about the individual's heart performance to a cardiologist and fitness information to a personal trainer.

A body blog must be capable of processing and presenting large data sets in a meaningful way for a variety of interested stakeholders. For example, heartbeat rate sampled over the course of a few minutes or hours can be appropriately presented as a time series graph. From the graph, stakeholders obtain an understanding of how heart activity is affected over time e.g. during sports performance. This begs a question regarding the representation of this kind of data over the course of days, months or even years. This eventuality poses two related questions: (1) is there any meaningful information to be had from such vast data sets, and (2) how is this information to be represented or visualised? In the case of long-term heart activity, Fig. 1.1 illustrates how heart rate activity collected as part of The Body Blogger experiment was condensed into a heat map to allow stakeholders identify meta trends that occurred over the course of a month such as their sleep cycle (shaded blue) and evening exercise regime (shaded orange–yellow).

For each measure in a body blog, the designer must consider how to represent information in a manner that relates to the stakeholder, especially the data owner whose sense of self is embodied within that data. As illustrated during the development of the affective diary, this is a difficult process as the meaning the designer wishes to convey must also align with the expectations the user brings to the data. This is likely to be easier for more objective bodily states e.g. posture, where the user can readily confirm the interpretation of the data (e.g. the sensor reported me as standing up, and I remember standing up at this time, therefore the interpretation is correct). However for more subjective bodily states e.g. emotions, where the associated physiological signals are more open to interpretation, then the

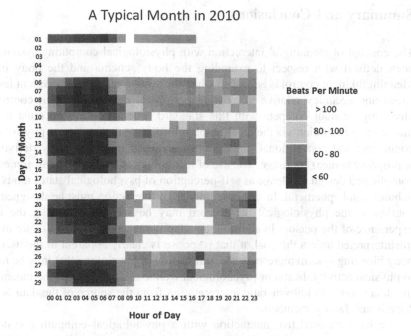

Fig. 1.1 Heat map of user's heartbeat rate over the course of a month

conveyance of meaning at the interface will be more difficult. In a biocybernetic system, poor psychophysiological inferences lead to poor adaptations and can thereby lead to user mistrust, similarly here, if the user is not able to associate their body blog data with their experiences there are more likely to be mistrustful of its interpretation. A potential way to build trust in body blogs would be to allow the user access to the different stages in creating a visualisation e.g. from raw signal to display, so they can create a dialog with the data and their own understanding of how these signals represent their own experiences.

The sharing of physiological data online raises a variety of privacy and ethical dilemmas (Gilleade and Lee 2011). The presentation and analysis of physiological data has been predominately the domain of health and fitness professionals. When these data are provided to new stakeholders, it is likely that they will require training in order to interpret this information. For example an individual sharing medical information online such as blood pressure opens the data for interpretation by medical amateurs. This may lead to an informal misdiagnosis causing the individual and their data's followers undue stress. Therefore in such instances a meaningful interface is not just about conveying relevant information, but to convey that data at a suitable level for the given audience and application context (Gilleade and Lee 2011).

Summary and Conclusions

The concept of meaningful interaction with physiological computing systems has been defined with respect to extending the body schema and the body image. Meaningful input control is enhanced when the system offers an equivalent level of speed and accuracy relative to existing peripheral devices. If input control via physiology cannot compete with this standard, interaction design must accommodate this limitation via the creation of hybrid systems (i.e. where physiological computing and conventional input control are used together) or by deriving an appropriate context for usage. The use of technology to extend body awareness is a complicated design challenge as self-perception of psychological states tends to be nebulous and ephemeral. In this case, modes of interaction must be designed with caution as the physiological data record may be seen to contradict the direct experience of the person. In addition, an adaptive response from software may be misinterpreted unless the goal of that response is clearly apparent to the user. The body blogging system represents a quantification of physiology that may be related to physical activity, health or psychological wellbeing. In this case, the meaning of the data is open to idiosyncratic interpretation from the source of the data or their friends and family members.

We have claimed that interaction with a physiological computing system is rendered meaningful when events at the interface conform to the expectations or experience of the user. This is logical but we believe it is also crucial to the adoption of this technology. The primary barriers to acceptance of physiological computing system are: (1) usage is perceived to be synonymous with an invasion of privacy (2) an emphasis on physiological data is seen to be potentially threatening as methods and measures are associated with medical procedures, and (3) biocybernetic adaptation represents a new mode of HCI where the computer has a greater degree of autonomy. Most nascent technologies are viewed with a mixture of apprehension and suspicion (often with good reason) and it is likely that the requirement for physiological monitoring will increase the trepidation of the user in this particular case. It is intended that meaningful interaction should promote greater understanding of this technology by enhancing a sense of connection between person and machine. This connection may be achieved by promoting the bootstrapping potential of the technology as tool to increase communication bandwidth (with other people as well as computers) and to enhance the self-awareness of the individual. It is especially important for users to understand the meaning of physiological interactions in order to develop a sense of trust in the technology. With respect to the latter, lessons may be learned from human factors work on trust in automation (Lee and See 2004). The user trusts a system when they understand the mechanism by which the system produces its behaviour. This analytic mode of trust development may be contrasted with an analogic route where systems are trusted based upon membership of a particular group or context, i.e. I've read great reviews about this BCI system, therefore I am positively disposed towards it.

The development of trust is particularly important in the case of biocybernetic adaptation. These systems possess a degree of autonomy and for a user faced with the novelty of a semi-autonomous system, a degree of vulnerability is to be expected on the part of the user. The design of meaningful interaction will enhance understanding in order to promote trust in the technology. Sustained exposure to meaningful interaction allows the user to make broad inferences about the connection between body and machine in order to reduce apprehension and uncertainty. In short, meaningful interaction is a means of maintaining the primacy of the user as we learn to communicate with a new category of technology via the body and the brain.

References

Allison B, Graimann B, Graser A (2007a) Why use a BCI if you are healthy? In: ACE workshop—Brainplay'07: brain–computer interfaces and games, Salzburg

Allison BZ, Wolpaw EW, Wolpaw JR (2007b) Brain–computer interface systems: progress and prospects. Expert Rev Med Devices 4:463–474

Allison BZ, Dunne S, Leeb R, Millan J, Nijholt A (2012) Towards practical brain–computer interfaces: bridging the gap from research to real-world applications. Springer, New York

Cacioppo JT, Tassinary LG (1990) Inferring psychological significance from physiological signals. Am Psychol 45:16–28

Craig AD (2003) Interoception: the sense of the physiological condition of the body. Curr Opin Neurobiol 13(4):500–505

Fairclough SH (2008) BCI and physiological computing: similarities, differences and intuitive control. In: Workshop on BCI and computer games: CHI'08, Florence

Fairclough SH (2009) Fundamentals of physiological computing. Interact Comput 21:133–145

Fairclough SH (2011) Physiological computing: interfacing with the human nervous system. In: Ouwerkerk M (ed) Sensing emotions in context. Springer, New York

Fairclough SH, Gilleade K (2012) Construction of the biocybernetic loop: a case study. In: Proceedings of the 14th ACM international conference on multimodal interaction, ACM, Santa Monica

Gallagher S (2005) How the body shapes the mind. Oxford University Press, Oxford

Gilleade K, Allanson J (2003) A toolkit to explore affective interface adaptation in videogames. In: Stephanidis C, Jacko J (eds) HCI International 2003, vol 2. Lawernce Erlbaum Associates, Crete, pp 370–374

Gilleade KM, Dix A (2004) Using frustration in the design of adaptive videogames. In: Proceedings of the 2004 ACM SIGCHI international conference on advances in computer entertainment technology

Gilleade K, Dix A, Allanson J (2005) Affective videogames and modes of affective gaming: assist me, challenge me, emote me. In: DiGRA 2005, Vancouver

Gilleade K, Fairclough SH (2010) Physiology as XP—Bodyblogging to Victory. In: BioS-Play workshop at fun and games 2010, Leuven, Belgium

Gilleade K (2010) The body blogger—physiology in a public space. Presentation at quantified self London. http://vimeo.com/16649098. Accessed 03 Feb 2012

Gilleade K (2011) Lessons from a year of heart rate data. Presentation at quantified self Europe. http://quantifiedself.com/conference/Amsterdam-2011. Accessed 03 Feb 2012

Gilleade K, Lee K (2011) Issues inherent in controlling the interpretation of the physiological cloud. In: CHI 2011 workshop on brain and body interfaces: designing for meaningful interaction, Vancouver

Haynes NK (1999) How we became post human: virtual bodies in cybernetics, literature and informatics. University of Chicago Press, Chicago

Hwang H-J, Kwon K, Chang-Hawang I (2009) Neurofeedback-based motor imagery training for brain-computer interface (BCI). J Neurosci Methods 179:150–156

Kaber DB, Wright MC, Prinzel LJ, Clamann MP (2005) Adaptive automation of human–machine system information processing functions. Hum Factors 47:730–741

Kapoor A, Burleson W, Picard RW (2007) Automatic prediction of frustration. Int J Hum Comput Stud 65:724–736

Klein J, Moon Y, Picard RW (2002) This computer responds to user frustration: theory, design and results. Interact Comput 14:119–140

Klein G, Woods DD, Bradshaw JM, Hoffman RR, Feltovich PJ (2004) Ten challenges for making automation a "team player" in joint human–agent activity. IEEE Intell Syst 19(6):91–95

Klimesch W (1999) EEG alpha and theta oscillations reflect cognitive and memory performance: a review and analysis. Brain Res Rev 29:169–195

Krusienski DJ, Sellers EW, McFarland DJ, Vaughan TM, Wolpaw J (2008) Towards enhanced P300 speller performance. J Neurosci Methods 167:15–21

Kubler A, Muller K-R (2007) An introduction to brain-computer interfacing. In: Dornhedge G, del R Millan J, Hinterberger T, McFarland DJ, Muller K-R (eds) Towards brain–computer interfacing. MIT Press, Cambridge, pp 1–25

Lindström M, Ståhl A, Höök K et al. (2006) Affective diary: designing for bodily expressiveness and self-reflection. In: CHI '06 extended abstracts on human factors in computing systems. ACM, New York, pp 1037–1042

Lee JD, See KA (2004) Trust in automation: designing for appropriate reliance. Hum Factors 46:50–80

Lotte F, Larrue F, Mühl C (2013) Flaws in current human training protocols for spontaneous brain–computer interfaces: lessons learned from instructional design. Frontiers in Hum Neurosci. doi:10.3389/fnhum.2013.00568

Nijholt A, Plass-Oude Bos D, Reuderink B (2009) Turning shortcomings into challenges: brain–computer interfaces for games. Entertain Comput 1:85–94

Peck E, Lalooses F, Chauncey K (2011) Framing meaningful adaption in a social context. In: CHI 2011 workshop on brain and body interfaces: designing for meaningful interaction, Vancouver

Philips Direct Life (2011) http://www.directlife.philips.com. Accessed 12 Jan 2011

Picard RW (1997) Affective computing. The MIT Press, Cambridge

Pope AT, Bogart EH, Bartolome DS (1995) Biocybernetic system evaluates indices of operator engagement in automated task. Biol Psychol 40:187–195

Pope AT, Palsson OS (2001) Helping video games "rewire our minds". In: Playing by the rules. University of Chicago Cultural Policy Center, Chicago

Prinzel LJ (2002) Research on hazardous states of awareness and physiological factors in aerospace operations. NASA, Hampton

Ramoser H, Muller-Gerking J, Pfurtscheller G (2000) Optimal spatial filtering of single trial EEG during imagined hand movement. IEEE Trans Rehabil Eng 8:441–446

Rani P, Sarkar N, Lui C (2005) Maintaining optimal challenge in computer games through real-time physiological feedback. In: 11th human–computer interaction international, Las Vegas, 2005

San Agustin J, Skovsgaard H, Paulin Hansen J, Witzner Hansen D (2009) Low-cost gaze interaction: ready to deliver the promises. In: Human factors in computing systems (CHI), ACM

Ståhl A, Höök K, Svensson M et al (2008) Experiencing the affective diary. Pers Ubiquit Comput 13:365–378. doi:10.1007/s00779-008-0202-7

Tan DS, Nijholt A (2010) Brain–computer interfaces. Springer, New York

Wiener N (1964) God and golem inc. MIT Press, Cambridge

Wilson GF, Russell CA (2007) Performance enhancement in an uninhabited air vehicle task using psychophysiologically determined adaptive aiding. Hum Factors 49:1005–1018

Chapter 2
Engineering Issues in Physiological Computing

Domen Novak

Abstract Prototypes of physiological computing systems have appeared in countless fields, but few have made the leap from research to widespread use. This is due to several practical problems that can be roughly divided into four major categories: hardware, signal processing, psychophysiological inference, and feedback loop design. This chapter explores these issues from an engineering point of view, discussing major weaknesses and suggesting directions for potential solutions. Specifically, some of the topics covered are: unobtrusiveness and robustness of the hardware, real-time signal processing capability, different approaches to design and validation of a psychophysiological classifier, and the desired complexity of the feedback rules. The chapter also briefly discusses the challenge of finding an appropriate practical application for physiological computing, then ends with a summary of recommendations for future research.

Introduction

Prototypes of physiological computing systems have appeared in countless fields, from critical applications such as stress and fatigue monitoring to home entertainment solutions such as physiology-based music selectors. However, despite the wealth of publications and fascinating prototypes, few physiological computing systems have made the jump from research to widespread use. We may wonder why this is so: is there no need for them or are they not yet ready for consumers?

While there is certainly a need for computers that could recognize and adapt to human psychological states, several practical problems have prevented physiological computing from achieving widespread use. In the author's personal experience, these issues are frequently raised by both engineers and potential

D. Novak (✉)
Sensory-Motor Systems Lab, ETH Zurich, Tannenstrasse 1, 8092 Zurich, Switzerland
e-mail: domen.novak@hest.ethz.ch

S. H. Fairclough and K. Gilleade (eds.), *Advances in Physiological Computing*,   17
Human–Computer Interaction Series, DOI: 10.1007/978-1-4471-6392-3_2,
© Springer-Verlag London 2014

end-users, but do not yet have reliable solutions. They can be roughly divided into four major categories corresponding to the main components of a physiological computing system. In such a system, physiological data is first recorded by a sensor or range of sensors in next section. The raw data is then processed using algorithms that remove artefacts and extract potentially relevant features (Signal processing). A set of inference rules is used to convert the processed physiological data into an estimate of the user's psychological state (Inferring psychological states). Finally, the system acts on the inferred user state (Feedback loop) and the process begins again with a new recording.

This chapter explores engineering issues related to each of the above four components of a physiological computing system. It is not intended to cover all existing concerns, but to point out and describe some of the major problems that people may be unaware of as well as suggest directions for potential solutions. Since many people involved in physiological computing are either psychologists or computer scientists, we felt that an engineering perspective could be beneficial. This perspective attempts to be broad, progressing from electrical and mechanical engineering (hardware) to computer engineering and computer science (signal processing and machine learning) with a particular emphasis on evaluation and validation of all components. After covering the main specific topics, Finding the appropriate application explores the general challenge of finding an appropriate practical application for physiological computing. Finally, the last section summarizes the main issues and presents some recommendations for future research in the field.

Hardware

Physiological measurement equipment is the basic building block of physiological computing, and low-quality measurements invalidate the entire system. All sensors thus need to be carefully calibrated and validated. Commercial solutions are generally well-validated in laboratory conditions, but are geared toward researchers and often inappropriate for widespread use. As an alternative, ambulatory systems have been developed to measure physiological data in varied conditions such as walking and driving. The common feature of such systems is that they sacrifice accuracy in favour of increased unobtrusiveness. A, by now slightly outdated, list of ambulatory hardware was compiled by Ebner-Priemer and Kubiak (2007).

The Trade-Off Between Unobtrusiveness and Accuracy

The main weakness of research-grade physiological sensors is their obtrusiveness, as complex setups and controlled conditions are required to achieve good results. As an example, consider electroencephalography (EEG), which requires the subject to wear a cap with electrodes. For proper measurement, the head needs to be measured and the cap needs to be properly applied to ensure proper electrode positioning. As it is often not clear which electrode sites are the most informative, researchers commonly use as many electrodes as possible. Furthermore, electrode gel is generally applied to improve signal quality and the electrooculogram (EOG) is measured to remove ocular artifacts from the EEG. The preparation time for an EEG measurement is thus around 30 min when using a cap with ~15 signal electrodes, a reference, ground, and EOG electrodes. Few people are willing to spend so much time applying a cap and ruining the appearance of their hair unless absolutely necessary.

If we wish to make the whole experience faster and more pleasant for the user, a number of things can be changed: the number of electrodes can be reduced, dry electrodes with no gel can be used, and the EOG can be omitted. All of these approaches have been implemented in consumer hardware. Devices such as the Emotiv EPOC allow EEG to be measured unobtrusively and at a far lower cost, but with also an obviously lower accuracy (Duvinage et al. 2012). The question is then: how much accuracy must we sacrifice to obtain a consumer-friendly device?

Research-grade sensors are usually made for a variety of possible situations. Consumer solutions are likely to be application-specific and can be made very specialized (as noted by e.g. Brunner et al. 2011). Some sensors can be made contactless: for instance, temperature could be measured using infrared cameras. Others can be built into the user interface or the surrounding environment. Lin (2011), for example, built their sensors into the steering wheel of a car while Wilhelm et al. (2006) built them into clothing. These sensors have great potential, but need to be validated to ensure that factors such as intermittent contact with the skin do not invalidate the measurements. Furthermore, real-time capability needs to be ensured, as sensors such as those developed by Wilhelm et al. (2006) only allow data to be stored on a memory card and analyzed later. While this is fine for initial research, practical applications require the data to be either wirelessly transmitted to a central computer in real time or analyzed with e.g. microcontrollers placed near the sensors.

Validating Ambulatory Physiological Sensors

Major progress has already been made in the validation of ambulatory equipment, especially dry and wireless EEG systems. Three approaches have commonly been used:

- An ambulatory system is used, and the study evaluates whether its accuracy is sufficient for a particular application (e.g. Berka et al. 2004).
- An ambulatory system is used together with a reference laboratory system, and the study evaluates whether the two systems infer significantly different psychological information such as stress level (e.g. Estepp et al. 2010).

- An ambulatory system is used together with a reference system, and the study evaluates whether the two systems record significantly different raw physiological signals such as ECG (e.g. Chi et al. 2012).

The third option is by far the most general, as guaranteeing high-quality raw data guarantees usability of an ambulatory system in a variety of applications. It can, however, be problematic for physiological computing developers, as it can be very difficult to ensure that the ambulatory and reference system are measuring the same data. For instance, as electrodes from two sensors cannot be placed in the exactly same spots at the same time, it is impossible to measure the exactly same signals even using identical sensors (Chi et al. 2012). Nonetheless, it has been shown that it is possible to measure raw EEG (Chi et al. 2012), respiration (Grossman, Wilhelm and Brutsche 2010) and ECG (Chi, Jung and Cauwenberghs 2010) using ambulatory sensors with practically the same accuracy as using laboratory hardware. Of course, this has only been demonstrated for some particular models of hardware.

Since validating the quality of raw data from ambulatory sensors is technically demanding, it would be optimally left to the manufacturer, who would publish evaluations of ambulatory hardware as compared to a reference, similarly to how traceability is performed in metrology. The evaluations would ideally be done in both ideal operating conditions (which, for an ambulatory system, are still worse than laboratory conditions) and poor operating conditions (e.g. many motion artefacts). With such hardware validation, physiological computing could utilize ambulatory systems without worrying about their performance.

When such data is not easily accessible, developers can nonetheless use ambulatory systems and compare the obtained information (extracted features or inferred psychological states) to either a reference device used in the same conditions or results obtained by other studies in similar situations. Such comparisons are useful not only to ensure acceptable accuracy, but also to ensure that a device is measuring the quantity it should measure. For instance, if stress in a task is correlated with physical activity, a poorly designed ambulatory sensor may actually measure motion artefacts and successfully infer increased stress from them despite not actually measuring any physiological processes.

Robustness

Many commercial sensors (ambulatory or not) are not at all robust. They are adversely affected by factors such as movement, temperature, humidity etc. These factors do not prevent the sensor from outputting a value; rather, they affect the output value either directly (e.g. motion artefacts cause electrode movement and thus incorrect readings of skin conductance) or indirectly via human physiology (e.g. increased environmental temperature causes sweating, increasing skin conductance for nonpsychological reasons). While indirect effects are not the fault of hardware, sensors do need to be made more robust to direct effects.

The primary problem are motion artefacts, which shift electrodes on the skin and cause incorrect readings. Even if the subject is perfectly still, artefacts can occur due to movement of the cables between the electrodes and the analog-digital converter. This can partially be compensated for by signal processing (Signal Processing), but not always. The motion artefacts in the skin conductance signal, for instance, can be very difficult to distinguish from actual skin conductance changes. Motion artefacts in the electrocardiogram (ECG) can be noticed easily, but are still difficult to remove since their frequency range partially overlaps the frequency range of the ECG.

Ambulatory sensors may be the solution for at least some environmental factors, as they are specifically built for robustness in rough conditions. Even researchers who are only interested in laboratory studies could thus benefit from ambulatory sensors. Other factors, however, will likely remain a problem (e.g. sensor output can vary with operating temperature). In such cases, physiological computing experts should keep up to date with discoveries in fields such as metrology and biomedical engineering while remaining aware of sensors' shortcomings and potentially compensating for them using signal processing (Signal Processing).

Standardization and Measurement Guidelines

Though physiological sensors can be made very application-specific, a certain degree of standardization would nonetheless allow easier implementation of practical solutions as well as allow results to be more easily compared between studies. First, this could involve very simple components. For example, Brunner et al. (2011) suggested the standardization of connectors between EEG caps and signal amplifiers. Similar steps could be taken for other sensors, making it easier and cheaper to build a complete system.

In addition to standardizing the components themselves, measurement procedures could also be standardized. As an example, let's look at skin conductance measurements, where several attempts at standardization have been made with no major success. Scarpa Scerbo et al. (1992) showed that the highest skin conductance values are obtained when measuring at the distal phalanges of the fingers. Nonetheless, many studies still place electrodes on the medial phalanges, proximal phalanges or palm of the hand. Proper preparation of the skin is also uncertain: Boucsein (2011) summarizes various preparation strategies, with no clear advantage of any method. This becomes doubly important since some skin conductance sensors (such as the g.GSR from g.tec Medical Engineering GmbH, Austria) are not meant to be used with electrode gel. This makes it very difficult to compare results from different studies.

Standardization could even be extended from low-level issues of obtaining a good signal to high-level issues such as obtaining good psychophysiological information. Strict standardization cannot be expected at higher levels since different goals and conditions require different hardware and measurement procedures, but it should be possible to at least develop guidelines for particular goals. For instance, laboratory studies commonly use every available sensor to infer psychological states. Features are extracted from all the sensors, and machine learning algorithms are commonly used to determine which features are the most important (Novak et al. 2012). However, as the field moves toward downscaled and cheaper measurement solutions, it becomes necessary to know just which sensors are important in a given situation and which can be ignored. Researchers should thus, if possible, report which signals most contributed to psychophysiological inference. This can be done using the same machine learning methods used for psychophysiological inference. For instance, in our previous study, we used stepwise linear discriminant analysis to identify the features that had the largest effect on classification (Novak et al. 2011). Though we used a respiration sensor in the study, no respiration features had a large effect on classification, and a downscaled system for the same application could thus omit respiration altogether. Similarly, Wilson and Russell (2007) began their work on adaptive assistance using a full set of EEG electrodes, but later downscaled their system to five electrodes since they found them to be the most important.If researchers consistently report the most important features and sensors in their studies, a meta-analysis would be able to produce guidelines on which sensors to use in which situations (e.g. mental workload assessment in office tasks, fun assessment in physically demanding tasks), allowing application-specific sensors to be made simpler and cheaper with little loss in accuracy.

Signal Processing

The raw data collected from physiological sensors must generally be processed before it can be used for psychophysiological inference. In general, this process consists of filtering the signals to remove irrelevant low- and high-frequency information, removing any noise (due to e.g. motion) and calculating psychophysiologically relevant features from the cleaned signals (e.g. band power from the EEG). The required methods are fairly well-known and for the most part not limited to physiological computing: ECG processing is based on decades of clinical ECG analysis while EEG processing uses essentially the same methods for both physiological computing and active brain-computer interfaces. Nonetheless, some issues still need to be addressed.

Real-Time Noise Removal

Physiological computing systems must be able to quickly detect and respond to changes in the inferred psychophysiological state. While physiological quantities

Table 2.1 Measures of heart rate variability calculated from the ECG over a 2-minute rest period when a single additional heartbeat is erroneously detected due to noise

	no noise	at 50 %	at 20 %
SDNN (% of true value)	100.0	123.6	136.5
RMSSD (% of true value)	100.0	116.1	143.5
pNN50 (% of true value)	100.0	100.4	99.0
HF power (% of true value)	100.0	226.7	4156.2
LF power (% of true value)	100.0	153.5	1319.2
LF/HF ratio (% of true value)	100.0	67.7	31.8

The additional heartbeat is added either halfway between two real heartbeats (column 'at 50 %') or at 20 % of the interval between two real heartbeats (column 'at 20 %')

can be measured in real time, real-time processing is significantly more challenging. First of all, the raw data often contains noise that is not at all related to the measured physiological response. Examples include motion artefacts, speech artefacts in respiration signals, eye artefacts in the EEG, and so on. While some of these can be removed using simple bandpass filtering, this is not always possible. For instance, the frequency bands of the EEG, electrooculogram and electromyogram all partially overlap, so bandpass filtering does not remove all eye and motion artefacts from the EEG (Vaughan et al. 1996).

As an example of how noise can affect measurements, let's look at a 2-minute ECG recording from a 25-year-old healthy subject resting without performing any activity. As a very small change, an additional peak is added between two consecutive R-peaks in the signal, simulating an extra heartbeat erroneously detected due to an artefact. It is first added exactly halfway between the two R-peaks, then 20 % of the distance from the first peak to the second. Standardized measures of heart rate variability are computed according to recommendations of the Task Force of the European Society of Cardiology and the North American Society of Pacing and Electrophysiology (1996): standard deviation of NN intervals (SDNN), square root of the mean squared differences of successive NN intervals (RMSSD), percentage of differences of successive NN intervals greater than 50 ms (pNN50), total power in the high-frequency heart rate band (HF power), total power in the low-frequency heart rate band (LF power), and the ratio of LF and HF power. Results are shown in Table 2.1.

A single erroneously detected heartbeat can thus cause huge changes in calculated heart rate variability. Sufficiently large errors could be automatically detected even online. For instance, if no R-peak occurs for more than 2 seconds, this could automatically be declared an error by the preprocessing algorithm. More complex criteria have been evaluated for heart rate in a classic psychophysiological paper by Berntson et al. (1990). In a similar vein, during online feature extraction, it would be possible to set acceptable ranges for individual features. For instance, expected values of SDNN and RMSSD in a given population could be obtained from the literature, and any value outside this range would be automatically declared an error. A larger problem is presented by smaller errors (e.g. 30 %

increase), which may be incorrectly interpreted as a change in psychological state and cause inappropriate reactions by the computer.

Such small errors require more complex approaches to detect online. The first popular approach uses a secondary reference sensor that gauges the quality of the primary sensor's output. With EEG, for instance, it is common to detect noise due to eye movements by measuring the EOG. Signal processing algorithms can then remove noise from the EEG by using the EOG as a reference (Croft and Barry 2000). Similarly, motion artefacts can be detected using sensors such as accelerometers. A second popular approach uses processing methods such as principal or independent component analysis to remove artefacts without the need for an additional sensor. It has been successfully used to remove motion artefacts from ambulatory EEG (Gwin, Gramann, Makeig, and Ferris 2010) and ambulatory ECG (Wartzek et al. 2011) and thus has high potential, but has not yet seen widespread adoption in physiological computing.

As a final note, though modern real-time artefact removal algorithms are quite advanced, it is not unreasonable to expect occasional errors due to artefacts, and the physiological computing system should plan for this (for instance, by acting conservatively).

Feature Extraction

The features commonly extracted from physiological responses for the purpose of psychophysiological inference are relatively well-defined, with lists of common features available in the work of e.g. Kreibig (2010) for autonomic nervous system responses. Nonetheless, some problems remain. The chief problem again has to do with real-time use: how often should features be extracted and over what kind of time periods?

The frequency of feature extraction depends both on the needs of the study and the real-time processing capabilities. While the raw data must be recorded with a high sampling frequency, it is not necessary to calculate features with the same frequency if we only wish to perform psychophysiological inference every few minutes. It is also difficult with current hardware, as many physiological features (e.g. spectral analysis of heart rate or EEG) require significant computing power to calculate. In general, it seems most appropriate to perform feature extraction once per instance of psychophysiological inference.

This feature extraction should be performed over a time period ('window') spanning from a point in the past to the present moment. It is unclear, however, what the best length of the feature extraction window is. The upper bound is likely the time between instances of psychophysiological inference: since (we assume) an action is performed by the physiological computing system after each inference, measurements taken before the action should be irrelevant to the current state. Of course, we may wish to make the window even shorter. Immediately after an action is taken by the computer, the user is not in a steady state since he/she must get used to the effects of the action. We could thus only include data from the steady state. There are also some theoretical considerations; for instance, some heart rate variability features should only be extracted from a steady-state period of at least 2 min (Task Force of the European Society of Cardiology and the North American Society of Pacing and Electrophysiology 1996). Nonetheless, we also do not want to make the window too long, as the magnitude of physiological responses to a stimulus diminishes over time. Long windows may thus make it difficult to extract stimulus-related information from background noise. As some physiological signals respond more quickly to stimuli than others (EEG in less than a second, skin conductance in a few seconds, and skin temperature in up to a minute), different windows may be needed for different features.

Finally, regardless of real-time use, we should consider the definitions of the features themselves. Although most features are well-defined, some definitions seem somewhat arbitrary and stem from literature published before physiological computing ever got started. Consider, for example, the skin conductance signal. A common skin conductance feature is the number of skin conductance responses, which are defined as sufficiently large and rapid changes from the baseline value. A commonly used amplitude threshold for a skin conductance response is 0.05 microsiemens. But why this specific value? As Boucsein (2011) explains, this threshold originally largely depended on the skin conductance signal's expected range and amplification. Old recording devices with paper output did not use thresholds below 0.5 microsiemens, but values as low as 0.01 microsiemens have been suggested for modern sensors (Boucsein 2011). The 0.05 microsiemens value seems to be used today mainly because it is popular. However, given the myriad of possibilities regarding sensor placement, use of gel, sensor amplification, and filtering, all of which affect the range of the signal, it makes little sense to always use the same threshold. In fact, we may wonder whether counting the number of skin conductance responses itself may not be a relic. The practice originated in the time of recorders with paper output, when manual analysis was required, but in the era of personal computers it may be more sensible to use e.g. the central moments of the signal (i.e. variance, skewness or kurtosis).

The evaluation of different windows and the evaluation of potential new features are both better suited for basic psychophysiological research than for physiological computing, but an easy first step would be to identify a set of potential window lengths and/or new features, then calculate features on old data from several published studies and evaluate how well-correlated they are with psychological information.

Inferring Psychological States

Inferring the subject's psychological state from measured physiological responses represents a major challenge in physiological computing, and requires knowledge of both psychology and computer science. As stated by Cacioppo and Tassinary

(1990), connections between physiology and psychology are rarely one to one (a single psychological element affecting a single physiological response), but are more likely to be one-to-many (one psychological element affects many physiological responses) or many-to-one (many psychological elements affect one physiological response). Researchers have already raised the issue of whether physiological responses even contain enough psychological information to allow practical implementations of physiological computing (e.g. Fairclough 2009).

Engineers may be frustrated by the lack of standardized methods for the interpretation of psychophysiological responses. Asked about his dislike of physiological computing, a colleague with over a decade of engineering experience remarked:

> When I'm doing sensor fusion, I know that the Kalman filter is great. In control engineering, I always know the basic approaches to build on. But with psychophysiology, it seems like you start over with every new application.

To a degree, his concern is valid: due to the inherently subjective nature of psychophysiological responses, there can probably never be a 'standard' recipe for a physiological computing system. Nonetheless, at the moment it can be assumed that most physiological computing systems can share the same general structure and deal with the same issues. In their seminal work on psychophysiological inference, Picard et al. (2001) demonstrated several steps that have now become commonplace: feature extraction, dimension reduction and classification. A recent review (Novak et al. 2012) shows that most studies that perform data fusion with autonomic nervous system responses in psychophysiology still perform feature extraction and classification, with many incorporating dimension reduction. The used classifiers range from linear discriminant analysis to neural networks, but generally each study only uses a single static classifier (i.e. one that does not take temporal relations into account). Classification is usually performed on a prerecorded dataset that contains roughly equal numbers of physiological data examples from each possible class. While this approach is perfectly valid, it has several weaknesses.

Context-Awareness

Psychophysiological responses are affected by a huge number of confounding factors. Age, gender, disease, time of day, physical activity, external temperature, ingested substances (coffee, medicine…) and many other factors can completely obscure any physiological changes due to psychological factors. Laboratory studies generally try to control as many of these factors as possible, creating very artificial conditions that are not feasible in the real world (Wilhelm and Grossman 2010).

In real-world applications, we need to take into account both the nonpsychological context (temperature, physical activity…) as well as psychological context (situation-specific demands of enacting a given psychological state) of physiological responses in order to accurately interpret them (Kreibig 2010; Wilhelm and Grossman 2010). As an illustration of how problematic this can be, Picard et al. (2001) analyzed the psychophysiological responses of a single subject who expressed eight emotional states daily over 20 days. They were able to classify the eight emotions with an accuracy of 81 %. They then attempted to classify the measured emotions according to the day they were evoked and were able to classify the day with an accuracy of 83 %. It is therefore easier to determine the day on which an emotion was expressed than the type of emotion from physiology! This is even more startling since there were 8 possible emotions and 20 possible days, making day classification much more challenging in principle.

Picard et al. (2001) also found that the subject's daily mood (long-term psychological state) affects what emotion (short-term psychological state) can be expressed and to what degree. Kreibig (2010) thus emphasized the importance of separating moods from emotions, but Wilhelm and Grossman (2010) noted that it is very difficult to capture mood alterations with physiology in most studies.

Luckily, many confounding factors can be measured using various sensors. As reviewed by Wilhelm and Grossman (2010), it is possible to measure e.g. physical activity using accelerometers, speech using respiration sensors, food intake using electronic diaries or circadian rhythms using clocks. The measured confounding factors could thus be included and accounted for in a sufficiently complex psychophysiological inference algorithm. This is what we refer to as context-awareness. The end goal should be to establish reliability of inference across a range of representative test conditions, test environments and individual differences (Fairclough 2009).

Unfortunately, psychophysiological studies only rarely distinguish between different contexts (Wilhelm and Grossman 2010), a problem that has also been noted in affective computing fields such as speech and gesture recognition (Zeng et al. 2009). This is not because the idea itself is new; the psychophysiological inference algorithm of Picard et al. (2001) already included multiple measures that should correspond to physical activity and circadian rhythms. Context-awareness does seem to be gaining popularity, especially in fatigue studies. Ji et al. (2006) and Yang et al. (2008) both combined physiological measurements of fatigue with user conditions (e.g. sleep quality, workload) as well as environmental conditions (e.g. weather). Nonetheless, context-awareness is in its infancy, and should represent a major avenue of new physiological computing research. In the beginning, context could represent only an additional input feature to the psychophysiological inference algorithm, but more complex approaches should be possible later. For instance, the context could represent the prior probability for a probabilistic inference algorithm, or the system could switch between different inference algorithms depending on the context.

Dynamic and Ensemble Classification Algorithms

A recent review of data fusion algorithms using autonomic nervous system responses in physiological computing shows that most existing algorithms are static single-level classification algorithms (Novak et al. 2012). Essentially, features from the current time period are input into a single static classifier that outputs the inferred psychological state among a limited number of possibilities. Even ignoring context-awareness (Context-awareness), this is a relatively simple approach.

First of all, a single static classifier ignores the dynamic nature of physiological measurements and emotions by treating each measurement as independent of previous ones. However, current cognitive workload, for instance, is not independent of cognitive workload felt a few minutes ago, and current skin conductance is not independent of recent skin conductance. While most physiological features are averaged over a period of time (up to a few minutes), thus reducing temporal relations in the data, dynamic classifiers that take temporal relations into account could potentially increase accuracy. This is especially important since different physiological signals have different response times to stimuli, so information from different periods of time should be taken into account.

The most promising dynamic classifiers are dynamic Bayesian networks. Kalman filters, which are commonly used in general sensor fusion and have been shown to improve psychophysiological inference with autonomic nervous system responses by 'learning' about a subject over time (Koenig et al. 2011; Novak et al. 2011), are theoretically a simple dynamic Bayesian network, though not well-validated in physiological computing. More advanced dynamic Bayesian networks have been tested, some of them incorporating context-awareness (Ji et al. 2006; Lee and Chung 2012; Yang et al. 2008). Besides Bayesian networks, alternate dynamic classifiers include e.g. Long Short Term Memory recurrent neural networks (Wöllmer et al. 2011).

In addition to dynamic classifiers, one possibility that has remained relatively unexplored are ensemble classifiers: combining several classifiers (of the same type or different types) to obtain a final result. For instance, each measurement 'category' (autonomic nervous system, central nervous system, nonphysiological) could have its own classifier, and the outputs of the individual classifiers would then be combined to obtain the final result. This was performed, among others, by Chanel et al. (2009). Another possibility is the so-called decision cascading, where one classifier makes a rough first estimate and a second classifier then confirms or discards that estimate (e.g. Picot et al. 2012).

Both dynamic and ensemble classifiers could in principle improve inference accuracy, providing a more complex and intelligent inference algorithm. However, they are also likely to require a large amount of training data, which is not always available in physiological computing. They thus need to be properly compared to simple classifiers in order to evaluate their effectiveness.

Detecting Brief Critical States

Most psychophysiological inference algorithms assume that all psychological states are equally probable. This is often true in laboratory studies, but not in the real world. When trying to detect stress and fatigue during driving, for instance, the vast majority of the measured psychological states would involve normal driving, and a small number of brief high-stress or high-fatigue periods would need to be detected. This challenge was mentioned as early as Picard et al. (2001).

The same problem is well-known in gesture and speech recognition, where the majority of recordings consist of 'garbage' and actual events occur only briefly. Hidden Markov models, for instance, can try to deal with the problem using a 'garbage' model where one possible class is dedicated specifically to various types of meaningless measurements (Bernardin et al. 2005; Wilpon et al. 1990). For physiology, Kreibig (2010) suggested tackling the problem by first using unspecific physiological responses (which distinguish between neutral and nonneutral conditions) to detect periods of interest, then using specific physiological responses to determine the exact psychological state experienced—a type of ensemble classification. Wilhelm and Grossman (2010) similarly suggested using abrupt changes in physiology to detect nonneutral conditions. Nonetheless, the problem is currently unsolved and likely requires the development of new types of inference algorithms.

Inference Validation

Once we have created a system capable of inferring a person's psychological state, we need to test it and see if it works correctly. For this, it is necessary to compare inferred psychological states to another, reference measurement that we assume is correct. Possibilities include self-report questionnaires, observable behavior, or simply using standardized stimuli that are expected to always induce the same psychological state. All of these have their own weaknesses.

Self-report questionnaires measure conscious processes only, while physiological responses are based on both conscious and unconscious processes. Thus, conditions may arise when subjects are unaware of their psychological states despite observable physiological and behavioral indicators (Fairclough 2009; Kreibig 2010). This is especially likely in subjects who are not healthy young adults, such as severe stroke victims (Koenig et al. 2011). Analysis of observable behavior provides an alternative, but psychophysiological changes can occur in the absence of any corresponding expression of overt behavior (Fairclough 2009). Finally, induction of psychological states using standardized stimuli such as media or standard tasks is very context-specific and does not generalize well (Fairclough 2009). Frustration induced with an extremely difficult mental arithmetic task, for instance, may not evoke the same physiological responses as frustration due to a traffic jam. At this time, finding appropriate reference measurements is likely to remain an application-specific affair. Some engineers may actually be content not to separately validate the inference part and simply consider the system a success if it accomplishes its overall goal such as higher performance or user satisfaction.

Assuming that we find a reference measure, we can then calculate the accuracy of the psychophysiological inference: the percentage of times that the psychological state inferred by physiology is the same as the state inferred by the reference measurement. Accuracy remains the primary and often only quantitative way to validate psychophysiological inference (as reviewed by Novak et al. 2012). However, it is not always clear what the target accuracy in a certain setting should be. With active brain-computer interfaces, which are closely related to physiological computing, users were found to expect and accept approximately 75 % accuracy in recognition of four possible desired movements (Ware et al. 2010), but the finding is very application-specific.

In critical situations such as driver fatigue monitoring, physiological computing systems should be very accurate, as any mistake would either cause harm (potential problem not detected) or annoy the user (alarm or automated assistance engaged inappropriately). In casual applications such as computer games where the difficulty is regularly adjusted, accuracies of around 70 % for a two-class problem (increase/decrease difficulty) may be acceptable since the general trend would lead the player toward the optimal difficulty given enough time. On the other hand, such low accuracies would likely not be very useful since the same level of information can likely be obtained from simple performance measures. In any case, physiological measurements should always be compared to other (non-reference) measures to determine whether they can provide sufficient accuracy both on their own and when combined with other sources of information.

Of course, overall accuracy is not the only important factor in validation. Accuracy is frequently described using confusion matrices, which state how often each particular psychological state is misclassified as a different one (e.g. Healey and Picard 2005). This can help us better evaluate the practical usefulness of the classifier. For instance, if we have three possible levels of stress (low, medium and high), we may accept a classifier that regularly confuses low and medium stress, but always correctly detects high stress, as we would only wish to react to high stress. Other measures such as confidence values are also sometimes used together with accuracy (e.g. Picard et al. 2001), but not very frequently in physiological computing.

Finally, classification (which selects one psychological class out of many) is not the only possible method of psychophysiological inference. An admittedly less popular alternative is estimation, which uses methods such as linear regression or fuzzy logic (as reviewed by Novak et al. 2012) to output a continuous value of a particular psychological dimension (e.g. stress value 4.1 out of 10). This is intuitively useful when the goal of physiological computing is to adjust continuous variables such as the amount of lighting in a room or the speed of opponents in a computer game. However, the problem of estimation is that commonly accepted validation metrices practically do not exist in physiological computing. While it should be possible to determine, for instance, the mean squared error, variance, or bias of an estimator, this is rarely done in psychophysiological studies, and results are instead often described only qualitatively. An important exception is the work of Mandryk and Atkins (2007), who validate the accuracy of a fuzzy estimator using mean squared error and a questionnaire as the reference measure. Since estimation could represent a useful alternative to classification in specialized applications where we only wish to monitor one psychological dimension, this work could serve as the starting point for development of more advanced validation methods.

Feedback Loop

Once the psychological state of the user has been inferred, the physiological computing system must respond to undesirable user states, thus closing the biocybernetic feedback loop. Three broad categories of feedback exist: offering assistance to a frustrated user, adapting the level of challenge if the user is bored or discouraged by a task, or adding an emotional display to encourage positive and mitigate negative emotions (Gilleade et al. 2005). However, while the theory of physiological feedback is well-developed and many possible feedback stimuli have been identified, implementations have proven challenging. It appears to be unclear just when and how feedback should be provided in order to achieve the desired goals.

Feedback Complexity and Speed

We should first ask ourselves: in a given system, how many actions should the system have at its disposal to achieve the desired goals? A larger selection of possible actions could increase the potential precision and helpfulness of the system, as it could then respond to more specific issues or simply perform a variety of actions so that the user does not constantly experience the same feedback. However, it is questionable whether the specificity of psychophysiological inference is sufficient to allow more than a small number of user states to be reliably identified. Furthermore, adding more and more actions could make it harder to analyze the performance of the system, as it becomes unclear just which of many possible actions made a contribution to the user's psychological state. This is especially problematic since there is no guarantee that contributions are additive; performing two actions consecutively may have a wildly different effect than the sum of the effects of each individual action.

At the moment, a small number of discrete actions or a small number of continuous variables (e.g. game difficulty level) should be sufficient for physiological computing. If the developer of the system has time, it may be best to first analyze the response of the user to each individual action and then to likely combinations of actions, leading to the best possible understanding of the system.

Once we have defined the possible actions the system can take, it is also necessary to determine how often feedback should be provided. This depends on the physiological measurements used, the application, and the actions themselves. Firstly, different physiological signals have different stimulus response times, from less than a second for EEG to more than ten seconds for peripheral skin temperature. This sets the upper boundary for feedback frequency: once an action is taken by the system, its effect should become visible in the physiological response before a new action is taken.

The feedback frequency should also take into account the intrusiveness and explicitness of the individual actions (Fairclough 2009; Ju and Leifer 2008). Very explicit actions should be taken only occasionally, as they may otherwise upset the users. Consider the example of changing the difficulty of the game: if the difficulty changes every ten seconds, users may become annoyed at the inability to enjoy a stable game experience. Conversely, if the system offers assistance every ten seconds, users may become upset as attention is drawn to their poor performance. Implicit, unobtrusive actions such as changing the lighting of the room can be taken more often, but have two disadvantages. First, they may not be able to evoke large changes in the user's psychophysiological state since they are by definition weaker than explicit actions. Second, even if implicit actions can evoke changes, they may be difficult to both design and validate due to their unobtrusive nature. An example is the application of Ritter (2011), which aims to improve task performance by subtly changing the visual appearance of items on the screen. While improved performance is shown, the entire system is basically a 'black box' and it is very hard to determine just what factors led to improved performance.

User- and Situation-Specific Feedback Rules

We have already mentioned that each person's physiological responses are unique and that psychophysiological inference should take into account factors such as age and gender. Similarly, the feedback loop should also take each person's characteristics into account, as two people in the same situation will not necessarily respond to the same stimulus in the same way. As an example, studies of socially assistive robotics have shown that, in stroke rehabilitation, some users will perform best when a robot provides nurturing statements ("I know it's hard, but it's for your own good!") while others will perform best when the robot provides challenging statements ("Oh come on, you can do it!") (Tapus et al. 2008).

The feedback loop should also consider previously taken actions. On one hand, this would allow the physiological computing system to learn what actions 'work' (as suggested by Serbedzija and Fairclough 2012). On the other hand, it would also allow it to better gauge what the situation is like, thus identifying actions that should not be taken since a certain opposing action or a very similar (perhaps even the same) action was taken shortly beforehand.

Unfortunately, feedback in existing applications is generally limited to a handful of predefined rules independent of either user or situation (see Novak et al. 2012, for a review of feedback loops using autonomic nervous system responses). Exceptions do, however, already exist. One promising example is the work of Liu et al. (2008), where players need to throw baskets through a basketball hoop controlled by a robotic arm. The hoop is constantly moved in different directions according to the measured psychophysiological state. The movement rules themselves are gradually adapted as the robot tries different patterns and discovers the effect each pattern has on the current player's enjoyment of the game. This application shows the promise of context-awareness in physiological computing.

Since context-awareness is a major field of study in other fields, it should be possible to adapt many lessons on context-aware feedback for physiological computing. As the feedback rules themselves do not necessarily depend on how the user's psychological state is obtained, the same feedback rules could, for instance, be used with a system that infers cognitive workload from physiology and a system that infers cognitive workload from movement patterns. This perhaps makes the task easier than context-aware psychophysiological inference, where the effects of context on physiology are very specific. On the other hand, context-aware feedback rules may include a physiology-specific factor: the reliability of the psychophysiological inference itself. A physiological computing system could provide strong feedback when it is confident that the psychological state has been correctly identified while taking only minor actions or even explicitly querying the user when the inferred psychological state is uncertain. This was done by e.g. Gruebler et al. 2012, whose robot performs actions slowly when uncertain, giving the user more time to intervene. It could be a welcome approach to also partially dealing with psychophysiological inference issues, which are likely to remain problematic for quite some time.

Finding the Appropriate Application

In the previous four sections, we examined the main issues that physiological computing currently needs to address. While most of these will undoubtedly be dealt with in time, we should think about what applications would benefit from physiological computing in its current state. The purpose of this section is not to discourage research in applications with no immediate practical benefit, but rather to help researchers consider the presented topics in a more 'applied' manner.

It might seem almost trivial that any product will only be successful if it provides a useful service: improved performance, higher pleasure, or something else. But at the same time, it must be better at providing this service than alternative solutions. In physiological computing, it must essentially provide the computer with enough additional information to justify the added cost and the obtrusiveness of the sensors. Furthermore, this additional information should not be more easily obtained by other, nonphysiological means. End-users are usually very aware of this, leading to questions such as:

> But why would I want to wear a cap and gel on my head just for that?
>
> Why don't I just tell the computer what I want myself?

As an example, consider the physiology-guided music selector, which has been explored by numerous authors (the first being Healey et al. 1998). The premise is that the device selects an appropriate song for the listener based on the current psychological state, which is inferred from various physiological measurements (usually skin conductance and/or heart rate). However, we might ask whether an expensive music player with potentially unreliable inference of psychological state would really be preferable to a simple music player where we can select the playlist ourselves.

Similarly, numerous studies have shown prototypes of games or tasks where the difficulty can be dynamically adjusted using physiological measurements to provide a moderate challenge to the user. As with the music player, we can ask whether expensive, obtrusive and potentially unreliable sensors are preferable to either letting users change the difficulty themselves or having the system change difficulty based on some measure of task performance. For example, the Director of the Left 4 Dead video games by Valve Software is an artificial intelligence that dynamically adjusts the challenge posed by the game in response to the players' performance, which is assumed to be proportional to their emotional intensity (Booth 2009). Physiological computing would thus be more appropriate for tasks where performance measures do not exist or are not necessarily connected to psychological state (e.g. a task where the user is likely to maintain high performance while becoming excessively stressed).

Critical situations such as fatigue monitoring in vehicles may be the most promising application of physiological computing at the moment. The potential costs of failing to detect fatigue are high, making the investment reasonable. A vehicle is unlikely to be used by a large amount of people, so it would be possible to tailor the data fusion algorithms to each user. Physiological sensors built into the seat and steering equipment (e.g. Lin 2011) could reduce the obtrusiveness of the system, and sensors already existing in vehicles such as speedometers and clocks could provide context information. Less critical applications such as home entertainment are unlikely to see widespread use until physiological computing has been made less expensive, less intrusive, and better at performing psychophysiological inference. An expensive or obtrusive device will never be used by consumers, and an inaccurate one will serve more as a novelty than anything else.

Recommendations

Physiological computing currently faces many issues, which we roughly divided into four categories: hardware, signal processing, psychophysiological inference, and feedback design. At the moment, they are severe enough to hamper practical use of physiological computing in most applications, but they should not be thought of as insurmountable. A brief summary of practical steps that physiological computing experts and psychophysiologists in general can take today is as follows.

In hardware, the most important issue is the development and validation of ambulatory physiological sensors. It is crucial that the such systems are robust and properly validated with comparison to either laboratory hardware or previous literature. The field has advanced far enough that simply presenting a prototype is no longer sufficient; it should be proven to work so that future studies do not need to worry about low-level problems. At the same time, even researchers not working with ambulatory sensors can contribute by reporting which specific sensors and features were found to be most useful for a given situation. This would immensely assist hardware developers in 'pruning' unnecessary electrodes or sensors from ambulatory solutions. Finally, as hardware improves, manufacturers should consider greater standardization so that different devices can be used together more easily.

In signal processing, the most important issue is real-time artefact detection and removal. While offline methods are common, advanced online approaches have not yet seen widespread use in physiological computing. At the moment, physiological computing should adopt existing online approaches and test their effectiveness. A second important issue is the real-time extraction of features from raw data. Here, it may be beneficial to take data from several already published studies and explore different extraction methods (different window lengths, normalization approaches or even new features) to see how they affect psychophysiological inference.

Psychophysiological inference remains somewhat mired in the 'classic' laboratory approach of classifying different psychological state using a single static classifier with no regard for context or temporal trends. Especially context-awareness is a promising avenue of research that could provide useful knowledge not only for physiological computing but human-machine interaction in general. Continuous estimation of psychological dimensions should also be explored as an alternative to classification. Finally, there should be a major focus on algorithms that detect brief critical states, unlike the classic approach where all emotions are equally likely and the baseline is the only neutral state.

Feedback design is still in its infancy, and its practicality must be better explored. User experience studies are needed to determine just how complex feedback rules can be and how often feedback should be provided. At the moment, such studies could work with very basic feedback rules and evaluate not only how accurate the psychophysiological inference is, but also how satisfied the user is with the system. As more complex feedback rules are designed, studies could evaluate whether the complexity is beneficial to the user. In particular, user-specific and context-aware feedback rules could have a great effect on the performance of a feedback loop.

While the above challenges do not cover every issue in physiological computing, they can hopefully serve as an overview of the more technical side of the field. As they are gradually overcome, physiological computing will mature and spread into different facets of everyday life. But even in its current state, physiological computing could already gain acceptance in applications such as fatigue monitoring, helping to popularize the field and pave the way for the future.

References

Berka C, Levendowski DJ, Cvetinovic MM, Petrovic MM, Davis G, Lumicao MN et al (2004) Real-time analysis of EEG indexes of alertness, cognition, and memory acquired with a wireless EEG headset. Int J Hum-Comput Int 17:151–170

Bernardin K, Ogawara K, Ikeuchi K, Dillmann R (2005) A sensor fusion approach for recognizing continuous human grasping sequences using hidden Markov models. IEEE Trans Rob 21:425–430

Berntson GG, Quigley KS, Jang JF, Boysen ST (1990) An approach to artifact identification: application to heart period data. Psychophysiology 27:586–598

Booth M (2009). The AI Systems of Left 4 Dead. Artificial Intelligence and Interactive Digital Entertainment Conference at Stanford

Boucsein W (2011). Electrodermal Activity (2nd ed.)

Brunner P, Bianchi L, Guger C, Cincotti F, Schalk G (2011) Current trends in hardware and software for brain-computer interfaces (BCIs). J Neural Eng 8(2):025001

Cacioppo JT, Tassinary LG (1990) Inferring psychological significance from physiological signals. Am Psychol 45:16–28

Chanel G, Kierkels JJM, Soleymani M, Pun T (2009) Short-term emotion assessment in a recall paradigm. Int J Hum Comput Stud 67:607–627

Chi YM, Jung T, Cauwenberghs G (2010) Dry-contact and noncontact biopotential electrodes: methodological review. IEEE Rev Biomed Eng 3:106–119

Chi YM, Wang Y-T, Wang Y, Maier C, Jung T-P, Cauwenberghs G (2012) Dry and noncontact EEG sensors for mobile brain-computer interfaces. IEEE Trans Neural Syst Rehabil Eng 20:228–235

Croft RJ, Barry RJ (2000) Removal of ocular artifact from the EEG: a review. Neurophysiol Clin 30:5–19

Duvinage M, Castermans T, Dutoit T, Petieau M, Hoellinger T, De Saedeleer C, Seetharaman K, et al. (2012). A P300-based quantitative comparison between the emotiv Epoc headset and a medical EEG device. In: Proceedings of the 9th Iasted conference on biomedical engineering

Ebner-Priemer UW, Kubiak T (2007) Psychological and psychophysiological ambulatory monitoring. Eur J Psychol Assess 23:214–226

Estepp J, Monnin J, Christensen J, Wilson G (2010). Evaluation of a dry electrode system for electroencephalography: applications for psychophysiological cognitive workload assessment. In: Proceedings of the 2010 human factors and ergonomics society annual meeting, pp 210–214

Fairclough SH (2009) Fundamentals of physiological computing. Interact Comput 21:133–145

Gilleade, K., Dix, A., & Allanson, J. (2005). Affective videogames and modes of affective gaming: assist me, challenge me, emote me. In: Proceedings of DiGRA

Grossman P, Wilhelm FH, Brutsche M (2010) Accuracy of ventilatory measurement employing ambulatory inductive plethysmography during tasks of everyday life. Biol Psychol 84:121–128

Gruebler A, Berenz V, Suzuki K (2012) Emotionally assisted human-robot interaction using a wearable device for reading facial expressions. Adv Robot 26:37–41

Gwin JT, Gramann K, Makeig S, Ferris DP (2010) Removal of movement artifact from high-density EEG recorded during walking and running. J Neurophysiol 103:3526–3534

Healey JA, Picard RW (2005). Detecting stress during real-world driving tasks using physiological sensors. IEEE Transactions on Intelligent Transportation Systems, 6, 156–166

Healey JA, Picard RW, Dabek F (1998). A new affect-perceiving interface and its application to personalized music selection. In: Proceedings of the 1998 workshop on perceptual user interfaces. San Francisco, USA

Ji Q, Lan P, Looney C (2006) A probabilistic framework for modeling and real-time monitoring human fatigue. Sys Man Cybern Part A Syst Hum 36:862–875

Ju W, Leifer L (2008) The design of implicit interactions: Making interactive systems less obnoxious. Des Issues 24:72–84

Koenig A, Novak D, Omlin X, Pulfer M, Perreault E, Zimmerli L, Mihelj M et al (2011) Real-time closed-loop control of cognitive load in neurological patients during robot-assisted gait training. IEEE Trans Neural Syst Rehabil Eng 19:453–464

Kreibig SD (2010) Autonomic nervous system activity in emotion: a review. Biol Psychol 84:394–421

Lee B-G, Chung W-Y (2012) Driver alertness monitoring using fusion of facial features and bio-signals. IEEE Sens J 12:2416–2422

Lin Y (2011) A natural contact sensor paradigm for nonintrusive and real-time sensing of biosignals in human-machine interactions. IEEE Sens J 11:522–529

Liu C, Conn K, Sarkar N, Stone W (2008) Online affect detection and robot behavior adaptation for intervention of children with autism. IEEE Trans Rob 24:883–896

Mandryk RL, Atkins MS (2007) A fuzzy physiological approach for continuously modeling emotion during interaction with play technologies. Int J Hum Comput Stud 65:329–347

Novak D, Mihelj M, Munih M (2012) A survey of methods for data fusion and system adaptation using autonomic nervous system responses in physiological computing. Interact Comput 24:154–172

Novak D, Mihelj M, Ziherl J, Olenšek A, Munih M (2011) Psychophysiological measurements in a biocooperative feedback loop for upper extremity rehabilitation. IEEE Trans Neural Syst Rehabil Eng 19:400–410

Picard RW, Vyzas E, Healey J (2001) Toward machine emotional intelligence: Analysis of affective physiological state. IEEE Trans Pattern Anal Mach Intell 23:1175–1191

Picot A, Charbonnier S, Caplier A (2012) On-line detection of drowsiness using brain and visual information. IEEE Trans Syst Man Cybern Part A Syst Hum 42(3):764–775

Ritter W (2011) Benefits of subliminal feedback loops in human-computer interaction. Adv Hum-Comput Interact 2011:346492

Scarpa Scerbo A, Freedman LW, Raine A, Dawson ME, Venables PH (1992) A major effect of recording site on measurement of electrodermal activity. Psychophysiology 29:241–246

Serbedzija N, Fairclough SH (2012). Reflective pervasive systems. ACM Transactions on Autonomous and Adaptive Systems 7(1), article 12

Tapus A, Tapus C, Matarić M (2008) User—robot personality matching and assistive robot behavior adaptation for post-stroke rehabilitation therapy. Intel Serv Robot 1:169–183

Task Force of the European Society of Cardiology and the North American Society of Pacing and Electrophysiology (1996) Heart rate variability: standards of measurement, physiological interpretation, and clinical use. Eur Heart J 17:354–381

Vaughan TM, Wolpaw JR, Donchin E (1996) EEG-based communication: Prospects and problems. IEEE Trans Rehabil Eng 4:425–430

Ware MP, McCullagh PJ, McRoberts A, Lightbody G, Nugent C, McAllister G, Mulvenna MD et al. (2010). Contrasting levels of accuracy in command interaction sequences for a domestic brain-computer interface using SSVEP. 5th Cairo international biomedical engineering conference, pp 150–153

Wartzek T, Eilebrecht B, Lem J, Lindner H-J, Leonhardt S, Walter M (2011) ECG on the road: robust and unobtrusive estimation of heart rate. IEEE Trans Biomed Eng 58:3112–3120

Wilhelm FH, Grossman P (2010) Emotions beyond the laboratory: theoretical fundaments, study design, and analytic strategies for advanced ambulatory assessment. Biol Psychol 84:552–569

Wilhelm FH, Pfaltz MC, Grossman P (2006) Continuous electronic data capture of physiology, behavior and experience in real life: towards ecological momentary assessment of emotion. Interact Comput 18:171–186

Wilpon JG, Rabiner LR, Lee C-H, Goldman ER (1990) Automatic recognition of keywords in unconstrained speech using hidden Markov models. IEEE Trans Acoust Speech Signal Process 38:1870–1878

Wilson GF, Russell C (2007) Performance enhancement in an uninhabited air vehicle task using psychophysiologically determined adaptive aiding. Hum Factors 49:1005–1018

Wöllmer M, Blaschke C, Schindl T, Schuller B, Färber B, Mayer S, Trefflich B (2011) Online driver distraction detection using long short-term memory. IEEE Trans Intell Transp Syst 12:574–582

Yang G, Lin Y, Bhattacharya P (2008) Multimodality inferring of human cognitive states based on integration of neuro-fuzzy network and information fusion techniques. EURASIP J Adv Signal Process 2008:371621

Zeng Z, Pantic M, Roisman GI, Huang TS (2009) A survey of affect recognition methods: audio, visual, and spontaneous expressions. IEEE Trans Pattern Anal Mach Intell 38(1):39–58

Chapter 3
Eye Tracking and Eye-Based Human–Computer Interaction

Päivi Majaranta and Andreas Bulling

Abstract Eye tracking has a long history in medical and psychological research as a tool for recording and studying human visual behavior. Real-time gaze-based text entry can also be a powerful means of communication and control for people with physical disabilities. Following recent technological advances and the advent of affordable eye trackers, there is a growing interest in pervasive attention-aware systems and interfaces that have the potential to revolutionize mainstream human-technology interaction. In this chapter, we provide an introduction to the state-of-the art in eye tracking technology and gaze estimation. We discuss challenges involved in using a perceptual organ, the eye, as an input modality. Examples of real life applications are reviewed, together with design solutions derived from research results. We also discuss how to match the user requirements and key features of different eye tracking systems to find the best system for each task and application.

Introduction

The eye has a lot of communicative power. Eye contact and gaze direction are central and very important cues in human communication, for example, in regulating interaction and turn taking, establishing socio-emotional connection, or indicating the target of our visual interest (Kleinke 1986). The eye has also been said to be a mirror to the soul or window into the brain (Brigham et al. 2001; Ellis et al. 1998). Gaze behavior reflects cognitive processes and can give hints of our thinking and intentions. We often look at things before acting on them (Land and Furneaux 1997).

P. Majaranta (✉)
School of Information Sciences, University of Tampere, 33014 Tampere, Finland
e-mail: paivi.majaranta@uta.fi

A. Bulling
Perceptual User Interfaces, Max Planck Institute for Informatics, Campus E1.4,
66123 Saarbrücken, Germany
e-mail: bulling@mpi-inf.mpg.de

S. H. Fairclough and K. Gilleade (eds.), *Advances in Physiological Computing*,
Human–Computer Interaction Series, DOI: 10.1007/978-1-4471-6392-3_3,
© Springer-Verlag London 2014

Eye tracking refers to the process of tracking eye movements or the absolute point of gaze (POG)—referring to the point the user's gaze is focused at in the visual scene. Eye tracking is useful in a broad range of application areas, from psychological research and medical diagnostic to usability studies and interactive, gaze-controlled applications. This chapter is focused on the use of real-time data from human eye movements that can be exploited in the area of human-technology interaction. The aim is to provide a useful starting point for researchers, designers of interactive technology and assistive technology professionals wishing to gain deeper insight into gaze interaction.

Initially, eye movements were mainly studied by physiological introspection and observation. Basic eye movements were categorized and their duration estimated long before the eye tracking technology enabled precise measurement of eye movements. The first generation of eye tracking devices was highly invasive and uncomfortable. A breakthrough in eye tracking technology was the development of the first "non-invasive" eye tracking apparatus in the early 1900s (Wade and Tatler 2005), based on photography and light reflected from the cornea. It can be considered as the first ancestor of the current widely used video-based, corneal reflection eye tracking systems. The development of unobtrusive camera-based systems (Morimoto and Mimica 2005) and the increase of computing power enabled gathering of eye tracking data in real time, enabling the use of gaze as a control method for people with disabilities (Ten Kate et al. 1979; Friedman et al. 1982). Since then, eye tracking has been used in a wide range of application areas, some of which are reviewed later in this chapter.

Using the eye as an input method has benefits but also some considerable challenges. These challenges originate from eye physiology and from its perceptive nature. Below, we briefly introduce the basics of eye physiology and eye movements. The rest of the chapter concentrates on giving an overview of eye tracking technology and methods used to implement gaze interaction. We will also review related research and introduce example applications that should help the readers to understand the reasons behind the problem issues—and to design solutions that avoid the typical pitfalls. We will conclude this chapter with a summary and a discussion of potential future research directions for gaze-based interfaces.

Eye Physiology and Types of Eye Movement

To see an object in the real world, we have to fixate our gaze at it long enough for the brain's visual system to perceive it. Fixations are often defined as pauses of at least 100 ms, typically between 200 and 600 ms. During any one fixation, we only see a fairly narrow area of the visual scene with high acuity. To perceive the visual scene accurately, we need to constantly scan it with rapid eye movement, so-called saccades. Saccades are quick, ballistic jumps of 2° or longer that take about 30–120 ms each (Jacob 1995). In addition to saccadic movements, the eyes can

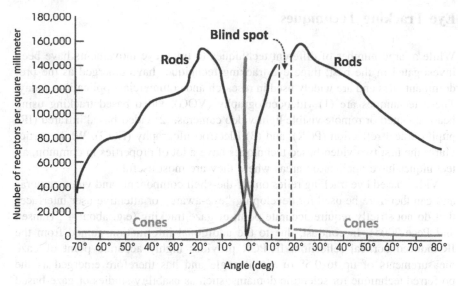

Fig. 3.1 Distribution of rods and cones on the retina (Adapted from Osterberg 1935)

smoothly follow a moving target; this is known as (smooth) pursuit movement. For more information about other types of eye movements and visual perception in general, see, for example, Mulvey (2012).

The size of the high-acuity field of vision, the fovea, subtends at an angle of about one degree from the eye. The diameter of this region corresponds to an area of about two degrees, which is about the size of a thumbnail when viewed with the arm extended (Duchowski and Vertegaal 2000). Everything inside the fovea can be perceived with high acuity but the acuity decreases rapidly towards the periphery of the eye. The cause for this can be seen by examining the physiology of the retina (see Fig. 3.1). The lens focuses the light coming from the pupil on the center of the retina. The fovea is packed with photoreceptive cells but the density of these cells decreases rapidly in the peripheral area. The fovea mainly contains cones, photoreceptive cells that are sensitive to color and provide acuity. In contrast, the peripheral area contains mostly rods, i.e. cells that are sensitive to light, shade and motion. The remaining peripheral vision provides cues about where to look next and also gives information on movement or changes in the scene in front of the viewer. For example, a sudden movement in the periphery can thus quickly attract the viewer's attention (Hillstrom and Yantis 1994).

We only see a small fraction of the visual scene in front of us with high acuity at any point in time. The need to move our eyes toward the target is the basis for eye tracking: it is possible to deduct the gaze vector by observing the "line-of-sight".

Eye Tracking Techniques

While a large number of different techniques to track eye movements have been investigated in the past, three eye tracking techniques have emerged as the predominant ones and are widely used in research and commercial applications today. These techniques are (1) videooculography (VOG), video based tracking using head-mounted or remote visible light video cameras, (2) video-based infrared (IR) pupil-corneal reflection (PCR), and (3) Electrooculography (EOG). While particularly the first two video-based techniques have a lot of properties in common, all techniques have application areas where they are most useful.

Video-based eye tracking relies on off-the-shelf components and video cameras and can therefore be used for developing "eye-aware" or attentive user interfaces that do not strictly require accurate point of gaze tracking (e.g. about 4°, Hansen and Pece 2005). In contrast, due to the additional information gained from the IR-induced corneal reflection, IR-PCR provides highly accurate point of gaze measurements of up to 0.5° of visual angle and has therefore emerged as the preferred technique for scientific domains, such as usability studies or gaze-based interaction, and commercial applications, such as in marketing research. Finally, EOG has been used for decades for ophthalmological studies as it allows for measuring relative movements of the eyes with high temporal accuracy. In addition to different application areas, each of these measurement techniques also has specific technical advantages and disadvantages that we will discuss in the following sections.

Video-Based Tracking

A video-based eye tracking system can be either used in a remote or head-mounted configuration. A typical setup consists of a video camera that records the movements of the eye(s) and a computer that saves and analyses the gaze data. In remote systems, the camera is typically based below the computer screen (Fig. 3.2) while in head-mounted systems, the camera is attached either on a frame of eyeglasses or in a separate "helmet". Head-mounted systems often also include a scene camera for recording the user's point of view, which can then be used to map the user's gaze to the current visual scene.

The frame rate and resolution of the video camera have a significant effect on the accuracy of tracking; a low-cost web camera cannot compete with a high-end camera with high-resolution and high sample rate. The focal length of the lens, the angle, as well as the distance between the eye and the camera have an effect on the working distance and the quality of gaze tracking. With large zooming (large focal length), it is possible to get a close-up view of the eye but it narrows the working angle of the camera and requires the user to sit fairly still (unless the camera follows the user's movements). In head-mounted systems, the camera is placed

Fig. 3.2 The eye tracker's camera is placed under the monitor. Infrared light sources are located on each side of the camera. IR is used to illuminate the eye and its reflection on the cornea provides an additional reference point that improves accuracy when tracked together with the center of the pupil (© 2008, www.cogain. org. Used with permission)

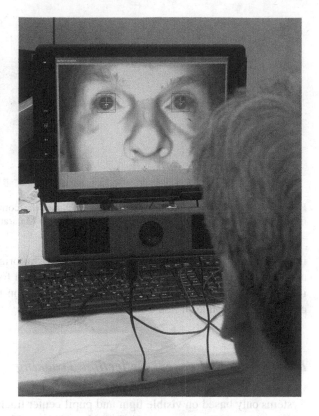

near the eye, which means a bigger image of the eye and thus more pixels for tracking the eye. If a wide angle camera is used, it allows more freedom of movement of the user but also requires a high-resolution camera to maintain enough accuracy for tracking the pupil (Hansen and Majaranta 2012).

Since tracking is based on video images of the eye, it requires an unobstructed view of the eye. There are a number of issues that can affect the quality of tracking, such as varying light conditions, reflections of eyeglasses, droopy eyelids, squinting the eyes while smiling, or even heavy makeup (for more information and guidelines, see Goldberg and Wichansky 2003).

The video images are the basis for estimating the gaze position on the computer screen: the location of the eye(s) and the center of the pupil are detected. Changes in their position are tracked, analyzed and mapped to gaze coordinates. For a detailed survey of video-based techniques for eye and pupil detection and gaze position estimation, see Hansen and Ji (2009). If only the pupil center is used and no other reference points are available, the user must stay absolutely still for an accurate calculation of the gaze vector (the line of sight from the user's eye to the point of view on the screen). Forcing the user to sit still may be uncomfortable, thus various methods for tracking and compensating the head movement have been

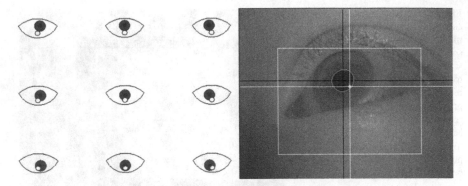

Fig. 3.3 The relationship between the pupil center and the corneal reflection when the user fixates on different locations on the screen (Adapted from Majaranta et al. 2009b)

implemented (e.g. Sugioka et al. 1996; Murphy-Chutorian and Trivedi 2009; Zhu and Ji 2005). Head tracking methods are also required for head-mounted systems, if one wishes to calculate the point of gaze in relation to the user's eye and the environment (Rothkopf and Pelz 2004).

Infrared Pupil-Corneal Reflection Tracking

Systems only based on visible light and pupil center tracking tend to be inaccurate and sensitive to head movement. To address this problem, a reference point, a so called "corneal reflection" or glint, can be added. Such a reference point can be added by using an artificial infrared (IR) light source aimed on- or off-axis at the eye. An on-axis light source will result in a "bright pupil" effect, making it easier for the analysis software to recognize the pupil in the image. The effect is similar to the red-eye effect caused by flash in a photograph. The off-axis light results in "dark pupil" images. Both will help in keeping the eye area well lit but they do not disturb viewing or affect pupil dilation since IR light is invisible to the human eye (Duchowski 2003).

By measuring the corneal reflection(s) from the IR source relative to the center of the pupil, the system can compensate for inaccuracies and also allow for a limited degree of head movement. Gaze direction is then calculated by measuring the changing relationship between the moving pupil center of the eye and the corneal reflection (see Fig. 3.3). As the position of the corneal reflection remains roughly constant during eye movement, the reflection will remain static during rotation of the eye and changes in gaze direction, thus giving a basic eye and head position reference. In addition, it also provides a simple reference point to compare with the moving pupil, and thus enables calculation of the gaze vector (for a more detailed explanation, see Duchowski and Vertegaal 2000).

While IR illumination enables fairly accurate remote tracking of the user it does not work well in changing ambient light, such as in outdoors settings. There is an ongoing research that tries to solve this issue (see e.g. Kinsman and Pelz 2012; Bengoechea et al. 2012). In addition, according to our personal experience, there seems to be a small number of people for whom, robust/accurate eye tracking does not seem to work even in laboratory settings. Electrooculography is not dependent or disturbed by lighting conditions and thus can replace VOG-based tracking in some of these situations and for some applications.

Electrooculography-Based Tracking

The human eye can be modeled as a dipole with its positive pole at the cornea and its negative pole at the retina. Assuming a stable cornea-retinal potential difference, the eye is the origin of a steady electric potential field. The electrical signal that can be measured from this field is called the electrooculogram (EOG). The signal is measured between two pairs of surface electrodes placed in periorbital positions around the eye (see Fig. 3.4) with respect to a reference electrode (typically placed on the forehead). If the eyes move from the center position towards one of these electrodes, the retina approaches this electrode, while the cornea approaches the opposing one. This change in dipole orientation causes a change in the electric potential field, which in turn can be measured to track eye movements. In contrast to video-based eye tracking, recorded eye movements are typically split into one horizontal and one vertical EOG signal component. This split reflects the discretisation given by the electrode setup.

One drawback of EOG compared to video-based tracking is the fact that EOG requires electrodes to be attached to the skin around the eyes. In addition, EOG provides lower spatial POG tracking accuracy and is therefore better suited for tracking relative eye movements. EOG signals are subject to signal noise and artifacts and prone to drifting, particularly if recorded in mobile settings. EOG signals—like other physiological signals—may be corrupted with noise from the residential power line, the measurement circuitry, electrodes, or other interfering physiological sources.

One advantage of EOG compared to video-based eye tracking is that changing lighting conditions have only little impact on EOG signals, a property that is particularly useful for mobile recordings in daily life settings. As light falling into the eyes is not required for the electric potential field to be established; EOG can also be measured in total darkness or when the eyes are closed. It is for this reason that EOG is a well-known measurement technique for recording eye movements during sleep, e.g. to identify REM phases (Smith et al. 1971) or diagnosing sleep disorders (Penzel et al. 2005). The second major advantage of EOG is that the signal processing is computationally light-weight and particularly does not require any complex video and image processing. Consequently, while EOG has traditionally been used in stationary settings (Hori et al. 2006; Borghetti et al. 2007), it can also

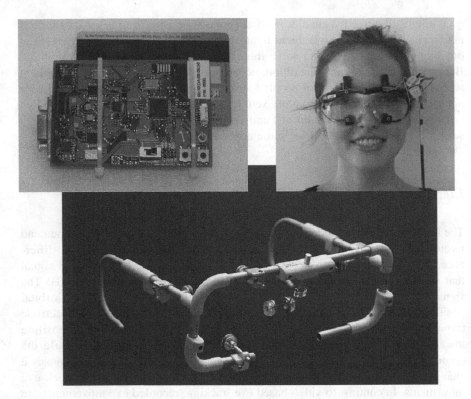

Fig. 3.4 Wearable EOG goggles (Bulling et al. 2008b, 2009b)

be implemented as a low-power and fully embedded on-body system for mobile recordings in daily life settings (Manabe and Fukumoto 2006; Vehkaoja et al. 2005; Bulling et al. 2008b, 2009b). While state-of-the art video-based eye trackers require additional equipment for data recording and storage, such as laptops, and are limited to recording times of a few hours, EOG allows for long-term recordings, allowing capture of people's everyday life (Bulling et al. 2012a, b).

Eye Tracker Calibration and Accuracy

Before a remote video-based eye tracking system can map gaze onto a screen, it must be calibrated to that screen for each user. This is usually done by showing a number of calibration points on the screen and asking the user to consecutively fixate at these points, one at a time. The relationship between the pupil position and the corneal reflections changes as a function of eye gaze direction (see Fig. 3.3). The images of the eye and thus its orientation in space are analyzed by the computer for each calibration point, and each image is associated with corresponding screen coordinates. These main points are used to calculate any other point on-screen via interpolation of the data.

Gaze mapping is more challenging for mobile head-mounted eye trackers as, in contrast to remote eye trackers, the user and thus eye tracker cannot be assumed to be positioned in a fixed location or distance relative to the screen to which the tracker was initially calibrated. The system can be calibrated by asking the user to fixate at certain points in the environment (e.g. indicated by a laser pointer) and the system obtains the eye angle during each calibration point (Schneider et al. 2005). If a scene camera is used, it is possible to overlay the gaze point on top of the scene video for offline analysis. For real-time use, the most common solution to this problem is to place visual markers in the environment, calibrate the eye tracker relative to these markers, and to use computer vision techniques to detect and track them and map gaze accordingly in real time. The robustness of recognizing the markers can be improved by using reflective markers (Essig et al. 2012). Given that visual markers can only be tracked with a certain accuracy, gaze estimates obtained from head-mounted eye trackers are typically less accurate than those from remote systems. In addition, the eye glass frames or the helmet where the camera is attached may occasionally move, causing some drifting.

Calibration is a key factor defining the accuracy of any eye tracker. If the calibration is successful, the accuracy is typically about 0.5° of visual angle. This corresponds to about 15 pixels on a 17″ display with the resolution of 1024 × 768 pixels, viewed from a distance of 70 cm. Even with successful calibration, the practical accuracy may be less due to drifting which will cause an offset between the measured point of gaze and the actual gaze point. Such drifting may be caused by changes in lighting and pupil size. In head mounted systems, it is also possible that the camera has moved along with the frames. Various methods have been implemented to prevent drifting (Hansen et al. 2010) or to cope with it (Stampe and Reingold 1995). If both eyes are tracked, it usually not only improves accuracy in general but also limits drifting. Since calibration takes time and may be seen as an obstacle for using eye tracking in everyday applications, techniques requiring only one calibration point, automatic calibration procedures, and "calibration-free" systems have been developed (see e.g. Nagamatsu et al. 2010).

Even if the eye tracker was perfectly accurate, it may still be impossible to know the exact pixel the user is focused on. This is because everything within the fovea is seen in detail and the user can move attention within this area without voluntarily moving her eyes. Besides, the eyes perform very small, rapid movements, so-called micro saccades, even during fixations to keep the nerve cells in the retina active and to correct slight drifting in focus. Thus, if the cursor of an "eye mouse" were to follow eye movements faithfully, the cursor movement would appear jerky and it would be difficult to concentrate on pointing (Jacob 1993). Therefore, the coordinates reported by the system are often "smoothed" by averaging data from several raw gaze points. This may have an effect on the responsiveness of the system, especially if the sample rate of the camera is low.

Eye-Based Interaction

While gaze may not be as accurate an input device as, for example, a manual mouse, if the target objects are large enough, gaze can be much faster at pointing (Sibert and Jacob 2000; Ware and Mikaelian 1987). Gaze not only shows where our current visual attention is directed at but it also often precedes action, meaning we look at things before acting on them. Thus, there is a lot of potential in using gaze in human-computer interfaces either as an input method or as an information source for proactive interfaces.

Using gaze as an input method can be problematic, since the same modality is used for both perception and control. The system needs to be able to distinguish casual viewing of an object from intentional control, in order to prevent the "Midas touch" problem where all items viewed are selected (Jacob 1991). Gaze is also easily distracted by movement in the peripheral vision, resulting in unwanted glances away from the object of interest. Eye movements are also largely unconscious and automatic. When necessary, however, one can control gaze at will, which makes voluntary eye control possible.

Implementation Issues

We will now discuss issues involved in implementing gaze-control in HCI and give practical hints on how to avoid typical caveats using the different eye tracking techniques. We will then review gaze-based applications and real life examples that demonstrate successful gaze interaction.

Accuracy and Responsiveness

There are several ways to cope with the spatial inaccuracy of the measured point of gaze. Increasing the size of the targets makes them easier to hit by gaze. The drawback of increasing the target size is that fewer objects fit on the screen at any time. This increases the need to organize them hierarchically in menus and sub-menus, which, in turn, slows down interaction. Other methods include for example dynamic zooming and fish-eye lenses (Ashmore et al. 2005; Bates and Istance 2002). It is also possible to combine gaze with other modalities. For example, the user can look at the target item and confirm the desired object by speech (Miniotas et al. 2006), touch input (Stellmach and Dachselt 2012), or head movement (Špakov and Majaranta 2012).

If the eye is used as a replacement for the mouse cursor, poor calibration means the cursor may not be located exactly at the point of the user's focus, but offset by a few pixels. In addition, the constant movement of the eye may make it hard to hit a target with the eye. Eyes not only move during saccades but they also make small movements during a fixation. The jittery movement of the cursor may distract concentration as the user's attention is drawn by the movement in the parafoveal vision. If the user tries to look at the cursor, he may end up chasing it as the cursor is always is a few pixels away from the point they are looking at (Jacob 1995). Experienced users may learn either to ignore the cursor or to take advantage of the visual feedback provided by the cursor in order to compensate for any slight calibration errors by adjusting their gaze point accordingly to bring the cursor onto an object. Nevertheless, it is useful to smooth the cursor movement. A stable cursor is more comfortable to use and it is easier to keep it long enough upon a target for it to be selected. The level of the smoothing should be adjusted to suit the application, because extensive smoothing may slow down the responsiveness of the cursor too much for tasks requiring fast-paced actions (e.g. action games).

A video-based system places the cursor at the point of the user's gaze. However, since the EOG potential is proportional to the angle of the eye in the head, an EOG-based mouse pointer is moved by changing the angle of the eyes in the head. This means the user can move the mouse cursor by moving the eyes, the head, or both. Thus, even if EOG as such may not be as accurate as VOG-based tracking methods, it allows head movements to be used for fine-tuning the position of the cursor.

Midas Touch

Coping with the Midas touch problem is maybe the most prominent challenge of gaze interaction. Various methods have been implemented and tested over the years (Velichkovsky et al. 1997). An easy way to prevent unintentional selections is to combine gaze pointing with an additional modality. This can be a spoken confirmation, a separate manual switch, a blink, a wink, a sip, a puff, a wrinkling, or any muscle activity available to the user (Skovsgaard et al. 2012).

For systems based solely on gaze-control, the most common method for preventing erroneous activations is to introduce a brief delay, a so-called "dwell time", to differentiate viewing and gaze-control. The duration should match the specific requirements of the task and the user. Expert eye typists require only a very short dwell time duration (e.g. 300 ms) while novices may prefer longer dwell time durations (e.g. 1000 ms) that give them more time to think, react and cancel the action (Majaranta 2012). A long continuous dwelling (fixation) can be uncomfortable and tiring to the eyes. On the other hand, the possibility to adjust dwell time supports efficient learning of the gaze-controlled interface and increases user satisfaction (Majaranta et al. 2009a).

Other ways to implement eye-based selection include, for example, specially designed selection areas and gaze gestures. Ohno (1998) divided the menu objects into two areas: command name and selection area (located side by side on each menu item). This enabled the user to glance through the items by reading their labels (command name) and select the desired item by moving the gaze to the selection area. In gesture based systems, the user initiates commands by making a sequence of "eye strokes" (Drewes and Schmidt 2007). Such gaze gestures can either be made by looking at certain areas on or off-the screen (Isokoski 2000; Wobbrock et al. 2008), or by making relative eye strokes without focusing on any specific target. The latter is useful especially in EOG-based systems where the user may execute commands simply by moving eyes up-down or left-right (Bulling et al. 2008a, b). Gestures are also useful in low-cost systems as they do not require accurate calibration (Huckauf and Urbina 2008). Simple gestures up, down, left or right can be used as a joystick, for example, to remotely control a toy car by gaze (Fig. 3.5).

Using gaze-initiated selection, corresponding feedback must be provided by the application. When manually pressing a button, the user makes the selection and physically executes it. In comparison, when using dwell time, the user only initiates the action; the system executes it after a predefined interval. Appropriate feedback plays an essential role in gaze-based interfaces; the user must be given clear indication of the status of the system: is the tracker following the gaze accurately, has the system recognized the target the user is looking at (feedback on focus), and has the system selected the intended object (feedback on selection).

It is also important to note that the user cannot simultaneously control an object and view the effects of the action, unless the effect appears on the object itself. For example, if the user is entering text by gaze, he or she cannot see the text appear in the text input field while simultaneously selecting a letter by "eye pressing" a key on an on-screen keyboard. Majaranta et al. (2006) showed that proper feedback significantly reduces errors and increase interaction speed in gaze-based text entry. For example, a simple animated feedback of the progression of the dwell time helped novices to maintain their gaze on the target for the full duration required for the item to be selected, thus reducing errors caused by premature exits. Successful feedback was also reflected in the gaze behavior and user satisfaction; as the users became more confident they no longer felt the need to repeatedly swap their gaze between the keyboard and the input field.

As discussed above, the calibration offset and the constant cursor movement may distract attention. Thus, it is often useful to give the visual feedback on the target item itself. If the item is highlighted on focus, the system appears as accurate and responsive to the user. It may also be useful to design the gaze-reactive button so that the user will look at the center of it, which will help in preventing errors and maintaining good accuracy. If the calibration is off by a few pixels, a look near the edge of the button may result in an error (e.g. a button adjacent to the target may get selected instead). If the user will always look at the center of the successfully selected button, this may also act as a checkpoint for dynamic re-calibration.

Fig. 3.5 The toy car (described in Fejtová et al. 2009) is controlled by relative eye movements that act like a joystick to move the car forward or backward, or turn it *left* or *right* (© 2006, www. cogain.org. Used with permission)

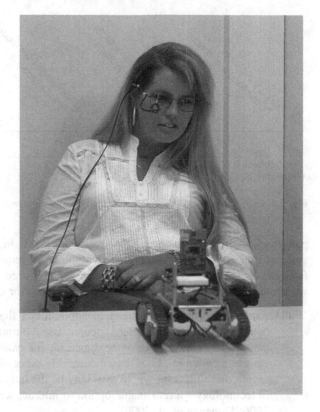

Gaze Interaction Applications

Information from eye movements and gaze direction can be utilized on various levels in a wide variety of applications. Some applications require the user to move her eyes voluntarily while other systems monitor the eye movements subtly in the background and require no special effort from the user.

Fairclough (2011) suggested a four-group classification to describe the different kinds of physiological computing system. The categories start from the overt, intentional systems (such as conventional input devices) and end with the covert, unintentional systems (e.g. ambulatory monitoring). Each individual system can be placed on this continuum and some systems may also be hybrids that contain features from different categories. A similar continuum can also be used to describe different types of gaze-based systems, starting from applications where the intention is the driving force, requiring full, overt, conscious attention from the user (see Fig. 3.6). In the middle, we have attentive applications that somehow react to the user's behavior but do not require any explicit control from the user. An advanced form of this are adaptive applications that learn the user's behavior

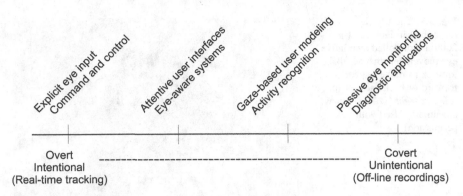

Fig. 3.6 Continuum of eye tracking applications from intentional to unintentional systems

patterns and are able to model the user's behavior. In the other end, we have systems that passively monitor their eye behavior, requiring no conscious input from the user whose behavior is monitored and analyzed. In the following section, we provide examples of representative applications for each category.

(1) *Explicit eye input* is utilized in applications that implement gaze-based command and control. Here, people use voluntary eye movements and consciously control their gaze direction, for example, to communicate or control a computer. Gaze-based control is especially useful for people with severe disabilities for whom eyes may be the only or—due to developments in technology—a reckonable option to interact with the world (Bates et al. 2006; Donegan et al. 2009).

In its simplest form, the eye can be used as a switch. For example, the user may blink once or twice, or use simple vertical or horizontal eye movements as an indication of agreement or disagreement (obtainable even with a low-cost web camera based tracker). The most common way to implement gaze-based control is to use the eye's capability to point at the desired target (requiring a more accurate tracker). Mouse emulation, combined with different techniques and gaze-friendly tools for dragging, double-click, screen magnification etc. make it possible to control practically any graphical interface based on windows, icons, menus, and pointer devices (WIMP). It should be noted, though, that gaze control of WIMP is noticeably slower and more error prone than control by conventional mouse and keyboard (e.g. gaze typing reaches about 20 wpm which is far from the 80 wpm by a touch typist, see Majaranta et al. 2009a). However, with special techniques such as zooming to overcome the inaccuracy problems, gaze becomes comparable with other special access methods such as head pointing where head movement is used to control the cursor movement (Bates and Istance 2002; Hansen et al. 2004; Porta et al. 2010). Other example applications include gaze-based text entry, web browsing, gaze-controlled games, music, etc. (see e.g. (Majaranta and Räihä 2002;

Castellina and Corno 2007; Isokoski et al. 2009; Vickers et al. 2010). For a review of different techniques and applications for gaze-based computer control, see (Skovsgaard et al. 2012).

Some applications, such as eye drawing or steering of a wheelchair with the eyes, are not best suited for a simple point-and-select interface. For example, drawing a smooth curve is not possible with fixations and saccades but would require smooth pursuit type of eye movement. Such continuous smooth movement is not easy for the human eyes but require a target to follow or some other visual guidance (e.g. the after image effect, see Lorenceau 2012). Similarly, in steering tasks or navigation in e.g. virtual worlds require special techniques that take into account the special characteristics of eye input (Bates et al. 2008; Hansen et al. 2008).

Most current assistive gaze-controlled systems utilize video and infrared based eye trackers. However, a lot of research has been conducted on EOG-based systems and some of them are currently in real use by people with disabilities (see EagleEyes, www.eagleeyes.org). Patmore et al. (1998) developed an EOG-based system intended to provide a pointing device for people with physical disabilities. Basic eye movement characteristics detected from EOG signals, such as saccades, fixations, blinks and deliberate movement patterns, have been used for hands-free operation of stationary human-computer (Ding et al. 2005; Kherlopian et al. 2006) and human-robot (Kim et al. 2001; Chen and Newman 2004) command interfaces. As part of a hospital alarm system, EOG-based switches provided immobile patients with a safe and reliable way of signaling an alarm (Venkataramanan et al. 2005).

Bulling et al. (2008b, 2009a) investigated EOG-based interaction with a desktop using eye gestures, sequences of consecutive relative eye movements. Since EOG measures relative eye movements, it is especially useful for mobile settings, e.g. for assistive robots (Wijesoma et al. 2005) and as a control for an electric wheelchair (Barea et al. 2002; Philips et al. 2007). These systems are intended to be used by physically disabled people who have extremely limited peripheral mobility but still retain eye motor coordination. Mizuno et al. (2003) used basic characteristics of eye motion to operate a wearable computer system for medical caregivers.

A current trend in gaze-controlled applications seems to be to move gaze interaction away from the desktop environment, to support environmental control by gaze, mobile applications and gaze-based mobility, and control of physical objects and human-robot interaction (e.g. Corno et al. 2010; Dybdal et al. 2012; Fejtová et al. 2009; Mohammad et al. 2010).

(2) *Attentive user interfaces* can be considered as non-command interfaces (Nielsen 1993) where the user is not expected to change his or her gaze behavior to give explicit commands. Instead, the information of the user's natural eye movements is used subtly in the background. In its simplest form, an attentive interface may implement a "gaze-contingent display" that shows a higher resolution image on the area the user is focusing on

while maintaining a lower resolution in the periphery in order to save bandwidth (Duchowski et al. 2004). Another example is given by Vesterby et al. (2005) who experimented with gaze-guided viewing of interactive movies where the plot of the movie changes according to the viewer's visual interest. The movie contained scenes where the narrative would branch based on the level of visual interest paid by the viewers on the key objects in the movie. The choice did not require any special effort from the viewer as it was based on their viewing behavior. If the user is explicitly required to give commands and if gaze-reactive areas are emphasized by explicit feedback, it might disturb the immersion and the viewer might lose track of the story line.

There is a thin line between attentive interfaces and explicit gaze input. An attentive system may assist the user's conventional manual interactions. For example, information from the eye movements may be used to automatize part of the task. For example, the eyes are used to set the focus (e.g. on viewed window/dialog) while manual input is used to select the focused item (Fono and Vertegaal 2005). Some systems constantly monitor the user's natural gaze behavior and may assist for example by automatically fetching information so that it can be shown immediately as the user moves her gaze to the information window (Jacob 1991; Hyrskykari et al. 2000). If the user knows her gaze is being tracked, she may also learn to adapt her gaze behavior in order to take better benefit of the gaze-aware features of the system (Hyrskykari et al. 2003). For example, a gaze-aware reading assistant provides automatic translations for foreign words and phrases when it detects deviations in reading behavior. The reader may also explicitly trigger the translation by staring at the difficult word (Fig. 3.7).

An attentive system may be gaze-aware or eye-aware. For some applications, simply detecting the presence of the eye(s) may be useful, without knowledge of the gaze direction. Eye-contact detection is useful for example in home appliances which know they are being attended to. For example, an attentive TV knows when it is looked at and could pause the movie if the viewer turns her gaze away. Another example is a multimodal "look-to-talk" application that reacts to spoken commands only when the user is visually attending it (Shell et al. 2004). As the application reacts to the user's natural behavior by explicit commands, it is important to provide enough information of the system state so that the user does not lose control and is able to react to potential problems caused by the inaccuracy of gaze.

It has been argued (e.g. by Jacob 1993), that the eye, as a perceptual organ, is best suited for interaction as an additional input. It is thus unlikely that systems based solely on gaze input would attract wider audiences. However, attentive applications that incorporate eye input into the interface in a natural way, have a lot of potential for mainstream applications that may help able-bodied and disabled users alike. For a review and more information about attentive applications, see Räihä et al. (2011) or Istance and Hyrskykari (2012).

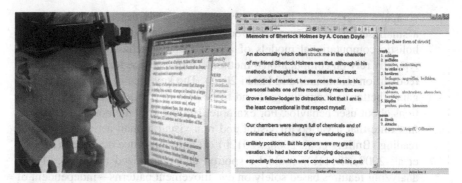

Fig. 3.7 iDict (Hyrskykari et al. 2000) is an attentive reading aid that automatically shows a translation above the word the user gets stuck with. A full dictionary entry for the word is shown on the side windows as soon as the user moves her gaze to it (© 2001, Aulikki Hyrskykari and Päivi Majaranta. Used with permission)

Since gaze often precedes action, an attentive system may try to predict user intentions from the gaze behavior and respond proactively (Kandemir and Kaski 2012). This is possible by monitoring and analyzing the user's behavior over time, which leads us to the next category of the continuum.

(3) *Gaze-based user modeling* provides a way to better understand the user's behavior, cognitive processes, and intentions.

All of the previous gaze-based applications explicitly or implicitly assume that the sole entity of interest is the user's point of gaze on a specific interactive surface or interface. In addition, the vast majority of these applications use gaze as an explicit input. The complementary approach to using the absolute POG is to monitor and analyze the dynamics of visual behavior over time and thus use information on visual behavior implicitly in a computing system from the point of view of the user. The fundamental difference between both approaches can be illustrated by thinking of the former as analyzing "where (in space) somebody is looking" and the latter as analyzing "how somebody is looking". Automated analysis of eye movements has a long history as a tool in experimental psychology to better understand the underlying cognitive processes of visual perception. For example, Markov processes have been used to model fixation sequences of observers looking at objects with the goal of quantifying the similarity of eye movements (Hacisalihzade et al. 1992), to identify salient image features that affected the perception of visual realism (ElHelw et al. 2008), or to interpret eye movements as accurately as human experts but in significantly less time (Salvucci and Anderson 2001). Others demonstrated that different tasks, such as reading, counting, talking, sorting, and walking, could be compared with each other by using eye movement features, such as mean fixation duration or mean saccade amplitude (Canosa 2009).

All of these works analyzed differences of eye movements performed by users while viewing different visual stimuli. A recent trend in human-computer interaction is to move beyond such purely descriptive analyses of a small set of specific eye movement characteristics toward developing holistic computational models of a user's visual behavior. These models typically rely on computational methods from machine learning and pattern recognition (Kandemir and Kaski 2012). The key goal of these efforts is to gain a better understanding of and to be able to perform automatic predictions about user behavior. For example, Bulling et al. demonstrated for the first time that a variety of visual and non-visual human activities, such as reading (Bulling et al. 2008a, 2012b) or common office activities (Bulling et al. 2009c, 2011b), could be spotted and recognized automatically by analyzing features based solely on eye movement patterns—independent of any information on gaze.

As evidenced by research in experimental psychology, visual behavior is closely linked to a number of cognitive processes of visual perception (Rayner 1995). In the first study of its kind, Bulling et al. (2011a, b) demonstrated that they could automatically recognise visual memory recall from eye movements by predicting whether people were looking at familiar or unfamiliar pictures. Using a support vector machine classifier and person-independent classifier training they achieved a top recognition performance of 84.3 %. In another study, Tessendorf et al. (2011) showed that high cognitive load during concentrated work could be recognized from visual behavior with up to 86 % accuracy. Finally, Bednarik et al. (2012) investigated automatic detection of intention from eye movements. However, Greene et al. (2012) were not able to automatically recognize the task that elicited specific visual behaviors using linear classifiers.

(4) *Passive eye monitoring* is useful for diagnostic applications in which the user's visual behavior is only recorded and stored for later offline processing and analysis with no immediate reaction or effect on the user's interaction with the world (Duchowski 2002). While passive eye monitoring has traditionally been conducted in laboratory settings a current trend is to move out from the laboratory and to study people in their natural, everyday settings. For example, Bulling et al. (2013) proposed and implemented passive long-term eye movement monitoring as a means for computing systems to better understand the situation of the user. Their system allowed to automatically detect high-level behavioral cues, such as being socially or physically active, being inside our outside a building or doing concentrated work. This information could, for example, be used for automatic annotation and filtering in life logging applications. More information of passive eye monitoring and its applications can be found in Hammoud (2008).

Conclusion and Future Directions

Eye tracking is no longer a niche technology used by specialized research laboratories or a few select user groups but actively exploited in a wide variety of disciplines and application areas. When choosing an eye tracking system, one should pay attention to the hardware's gaze tracking features as well as the accompanying software and additional accessories. Many eye tracking manufacturers provide different models targeted at different purposes. The systems may use the same basic technical principles of operation, but what makes a certain system suitable for a specific purpose are the applications (software) that utilize the raw eye data, e.g. software for recording and analyzing the gaze path, or assistive software that allow the eye to be used as an substitute for the mouse.

Issues to consider from the technical part that affect the suitability of the system for a specific purpose include: spatial and temporal resolution (accuracy), camera angle, freedom of head movements, tolerance to ambient light, tolerance to eye glasses and contact lenses, possibility to track only one or two eyes.

As shown above, video-based eye tracking, especially if implemented as a remote tracker, provides a fairly comfortable non-invasive (contact-free) option for the users. Systems that combine the video with infrared (i.e. track both the pupil and the IR corneal reflection) also provide reasonable freedom of head movement without sacrificing the accuracy too much. However, those systems, especially IR-PCR, are very sensitive to ambient light and changes in the light levels and only provide limited temporal accuracy and recording time. EOG-based eye trackers are not sensitive to lighting conditions. The downside is that EOG can be considered invasive and may be seen as impractical for everyday use, because it require electrodes to be placed around the eye to measure the skin's electrical potential differences. Since EOG is based on the changes in the electrical potential, it can also track all types of eye movements and blinks; this is an option for those for whom VOG-based calibration fails. EOG also continues tracking eye movements even if the user squints or closes the eyes for example during laughing.

There are also differences in the data produced by each of the trackers. Since an EOG-based system provides information on relative eye movements, it is especially useful in situations where only changes in the gaze direction are required (e.g. gaze gestures, navigation and steering tasks, or research on saccades and smooth pursuit). However, VOG based systems may work better if an exact point of gaze is important (e.g. point-and-select tasks).

For some tasks, a combination of EOG and VOG might provide the best results. Apart from a few exceptions (e.g. Du et al. 2012) their combined use has not been applied much. We believe there might be high potential in using a method that combines the best features of each technology, especially for passive eye monitoring and clinical studies conducted in challenging outdoor environments.

Depending on the context and the target environment, one should also consider issues such as the portability, support for wireless use, battery life and modularity of the tracker. The eye tracking device (camera) can be embedded into the edge of the computer monitor or be shipped as a separate unit which can be attached to any laptop or other device, or it can be head-worn. Some manufacturers also sell eye tracking modules and tailored solutions that can be integrated into the customer's devices.

From the human factors point of view, the system's invasiveness, ease of use, setup time and available customer support are important issues. For a disabled person, an eye control system is a way of communicating and interacting with the world and may be used extensively in varying conditions. Thus, reliability, robustness, safety, and mounting issues must be carefully taken into account, in addition to ease of use and general usability. In addition, one should be able to tailor the system to match each user's abilities, needs and challenges induced by disease (Donegan et al. 2009). With increased availability, reliability and usability of the state-of-the-art trackers, the focus on gaze assistive technology research is slowly moving from technical challenges toward the human point of view, presenting a need to also study user experience (Mele and Federici 2012).

A current trend in both eye tracking research and application development is the move away from the laboratory to more natural mobile settings both indoors and outdoors (Bulling and Gellersen 2010). It is for this reason that there is a high demand for systems that can operate in varying mobile contexts. In addition to improved VOG and EOG based techniques, also novel eye tracking approaches are under investigation. Future eye tracking systems may be based on technology and sensory systems that mimic the biological sensing and eye structure. For example, the so-called "silicon retina" shows high potential for high speed eye tracking that can provide robust measurements also in ambient light conditions (Liu and Delbuck 2010). The pixels in the silicon retina are able to asynchronously respond to relative changes in intensity. This enables fast and robust detection of movement and tracking of object in varying light conditions where traditional video and IR based eye tracking typically fail.

In addition to gaze direction and eye movement patterns, also other eye-related measurements such as the pupil size and even microsaccades can contribute to the interpretation of the user's emotional and cognitive state. Gaze behavior can also be combined with other measurements from the user's face and body, enabling multimodal physiological computing. Gaze-based user modeling may offer a step toward truly intelligent interfaces that are able to facilitate the user in a smart way that complements the user's natural behavior.

Advances in the technology open new areas for eye tracking, widening the scope of gaze-based applications. Current hot topics include all kinds of mobile applications and pervasive systems where the user's visual behavior and attention is tracked and used for eye-based interaction everywhere and at any time, also called pervasive eye tracking and pervasive eye-based human-computer interaction (Bulling et al. 2010, 2012a, b; Zhang et al. 2013; Vidal et al. 2013). Other emerging areas include, for example, automotive industry (drowsiness, attention alarms, safety), attentive navigation and location awareness, information retrieval and enhanced visual search, human-robot interaction, attentive intelligent tutoring systems (e.g. Jokinen and Majaranta 2013; Nakano et al. 2012; Zhang et al. 2012). For people with special needs, mobile eye tracking may give more freedom by wheelchair control, tele-presence and tele-operation of technology (Wästlund et al. 2010; Alapetite et al. 2012).

Eye tracking is becoming an increasingly interesting option even in traditional computing. Major technology companies and the gaming industry are starting to show growing interest in embedding eye tracking in their future products, such as laptops and tablets (Tobii 2011; Fujitsu 2012). Vision based technologies are already widely used in the gaming field, enabling players to use gestures and full body movement to control the games, and eye tracking is envisioned to be part of future gaming (Larsen 2012). The hype on smart glasses (such as the Google Glass) indicates that it is only a matter of time, when the first eye-controlled consumer product will enter the market. Wider use would mean lower costs. Thus, a breakthrough in one field can give a boost also to other areas of eye tracking.

References

Alapetite A, Hansen JP, MacKenzie IS (2012) Demo of gaze controlled flying. In: Proceedings of the 7th Nordic conference on human-computer interaction: making sense through design, NordiCHI'12. ACM, New York, pp 773–774

Ashmore M, Duchowski AT, Shoemaker G (2005) Efficient eye pointing with a fisheye lens. In: Proceedings of graphics interface 2005, GI'05. Canadian Human-Computer Communications Society, Waterloo, Ontario, pp 203–210

Barea F, Boquete L, Mazo M, Lopez E (2002) System for assisted mobility using eye movements based on electrooculography. IEEE Trans Neural Syst Rehabil Eng 10(4):209–218

Bates R, Donegan M, Istance HO et al (2006) Introducing COGAIN—communication by gaze interaction. In: Clarkson J, Langdon P, Robinson P (eds) Designing accessible technology. Springer, London, pp 77–84

Bates R, Istance H (2002) Zooming interfaces!: enhancing the performance of eye controlled pointing devices. In: Proceedings of the 5th international ACM conference on assistive technologies, Assets'02. ACM, New York, pp 119–126

Bates R, Istance HO, Vickers S (2008) Gaze interaction with virtual on-line communities. Designing inclusive futures. Springer, London, pp 149–162

Bednarik R, Vrzakova H, Hradis M (2012) What you want to do next: a novel approach for intent prediction in gaze-based interaction. In: Proceedings of the symposium on eye tracking research and applications, ETRA'12. ACM, New York, pp 83–90

Bengoechea JJ, Villanueva A, Cabeza R (2012) Hybrid eye detection algorithm for outdoor environments. In: Proceedings of the 2012 ACM conference on ubiquitous computing, UbiComp'12. ACM, New York, pp 685–688

Brigham FJ, Zaimi E, Matkins JJ et al (2001) The eyes may have it: reconsidering eye-movement research in human cognition. In: Scruggs TE, Mastropieri MA (eds) Technological applications. Advances in learning and behavioral disabilities, vol 15. Emerald Group Publishing Limited, Bingley, pp 39–59

Borghetti D, Bruni A, Fabbrini M et al (2007) A low-cost interface for control of computer functions by means of eye movements. Comput Biol Med 37(12):1765–1770

Bulling A, Cheng S, Brône G et al (2012a) 2nd international workshop on pervasive eye tracking and mobile eye-based interaction (PETMEI 2012). In: Proceedings of the 2012 ACM conference on ubiquitous computing, UbiComp 2012. ACM, New York, pp 673–676

Bulling A, Ward JA, Gellersen H et al (2008a) Robust recognition of reading activity in transit using wearable electrooculography. In: Proceedings of the 6th international conference on pervasive computing, Pervasive 2008, pp 19–37

Bulling A, Gellersen H (2010) Toward mobile eye-based human-computer interaction. IEEE Pervasive Comput 9(4):8–12

Bulling A, Roggen D, Tröster G (2008b) It's in your eyes—Towards context-awareness and mobile hci using wearable EOG goggles. In: Proceedings of the 10th international conference on ubiquitous computing. ACM, New York, pp 84–93

Bulling A, Roggen D, Tröster G (2009a) Wearable EOG goggles: eye-based interaction in everyday environments. In: Extended abstracts of the 27th ACM conference on human factors in computing systems, CHI'09. ACM, New York, pp 3259–3264

Bulling A, Roggen D, Tröster G (2009b) Wearable EOG goggles: seamless sensing and context-awareness in everyday environments. J Ambient Intell Smart Environ 1(2):157–171

Bulling A, Ward JA, Gellersen H et al (2009c) Eye movement analysis for activity recognition. In: Proceedings of the 11th international conference on ubiquitous computing, UbiComp 2009. ACM, New York, pp 41–50

Bulling A, Roggen D (2011a) Recognition of visual memory recall processes using eye movement analysis. In: Proceedings of the 13th international conference on ubiquitous computing, UbiComp 2011. ACM, New York, pp 455–464

Bulling A, Ward JA, Gellersen H et al (2011b) Eye movement analysis for activity recognition using electrooculography. IEEE Trans Pattern Anal Mach Intell 33(4):741–753

Bulling A, Ward JA, Gellersen H (2012b) Multimodal recognition of reading activity in transit using body-worn sensors. ACM Trans Appl Percept 9(1):2:1–2:21

Bulling A, Weichel C, Gellersen H (2013) EyeContext: recognition of high-level contextual cues from human visual behavior. In: Proceedings of the 31st SIGCHI international conference on human factors in computing systems, CHI 2013. ACM, New York, pp 305–308

Canosa RL (2009) Real-world vision: selective perception and task. ACM Trans Appl Percept 6(2):article 11, 34 pp

Castellina E, Corno F (2007) Accessible web surfing through gaze interaction. In: Proceedings of the 3rd Conference on communication by gaze interaction, COGAIN 2007, Leicester, 3–4 Sept 2007, pp 74–77

Chen Y, Newman WS (2004) A human-robot interface based on electrooculography. In: Proceedings of the international conference on robotics and automation, ICRA 2004, vol 1, pp 243–248

Corno F, Gale A, Majaranta P et al (2010) Eye-based direct interaction for environmental control in heterogeneous smart environments. In: Nakashima H et al (eds) Handbook of ambient intelligence and smart environments. Springer, New York, pp 1117–1138

Ding Q, Tong K, Li G (2005) Development of an EOG (ElectroOculography) based human-computer interface. In: Proceedings of the 27th annual international conference of the engineering in medicine and biology society, EMBS 2005, pp 6829–6831

Donegan M, Morris DJ, Corno F et al (2009) Understanding users and their needs. Univ Access Inf Soc 8(4):259–275

Drewes H, Schmidt A (2007) Interacting with the computer using gaze gestures. In: Proceedings of INTERACT '07. Lecture notes in computer science, vol 4663. Springer, Heidelberg, pp 475-488

Du R, Liu R, Wu T et al (2012) Online vigilance analysis combining video and electrooculography features. In: Proceedings of 19th international conference on neural information processing, ICONIP 2012. Lecture notes in computer science, vol 7667. Springer, Heidelberg, pp 447–454

Duchowski AT (2002) A breadth-first survey of eye-tracking applications. Behav Res Meth 34(4):455–470

Duchowski AT (2003) Eye tracking methodology: theory and practice. Springer, London

Duchowski AT, Cournia NA, Murphy HA (2004) Gaze-contingent displays: a review. CyberPsychol Behav 7(6):621–634

Duchowski AT, Vertegaal R (2000) Eye-based interaction in graphical systems: theory and practice. Course 05, SIGGRAPH 2000. Course notes. ACM, New York. http://eyecu.ces. clemson.edu/sigcourse/. Accessed 23 Feb 2013

Dybdal ML, San Agustin J, Hansen JP (2012) Gaze input for mobile devices by dwell and gestures. In: Proceedings of the symposium on eye tracking research and applications, ETRA '12. ACM, New York, pp 225–228

ElHelw MA, Atkins S, Nicolaou M et al (2008) A gaze-based study for investigating the perception of photorealism in simulated scenes. ACM Trans Appl Percept 5(1):article 3, 20 pp

Ellis S, Cadera R, Misner J et al (1998) Windows to the soul? What eye movements tell us about software usability. In: Proceedings of 7th annual conference of the usability professionals association, Washington, pp 151–178

Essig K, Dornbusch D, Prinzhorn D et al (2012) Automatic analysis of 3D gaze coordinates on scene objects using data from eye-tracking and motion-capture systems. In: Proceedings of the symposium on eye tracking research and applications, ETRA'12. ACM, New York, pp 37–44

Fairclough SH (2011) Physiological computing: interacting with the human nervous system. In: Ouwerkerk M, Westerlink J, Krans M (eds) Sensing emotions in context: the impact of context on behavioural and physiological experience measurements. Springer, Amsterdam, pp 1–22

Fejtová M, Figueiredo L, Novák P et al (2009) Hands-free interaction with a computer and other technologies. Univ Access Inf Soc 8(4):277–295

Fono D, Vertegaal R (2005) EyeWindows: evaluation of eye-controlled zooming windows for focus selection. In: Proceedings of the SIGCHI conference on human factors in computing systems, CHI'05. ACM, New York, pp 151–160

Friedman MB, Kiliany G, Dzmura et al (1982) The eyetracker communication system. Johns Hopkins APL Technical Digest 3(3):250–252

Fujitsu (2012) Fujitsu develops eye tracking technology. Press release 2 Oct 2012. http://www. fujitsu.com/global/news/pr/archives/month/2012/20121002-02.html. Accessed 23 Feb 2013

Goldberg JH, Wichansky AM (2003) Eye tracking in usability evaluation: a practitioner's guide. In: Hyönä J, Radach R, Deubel H (eds) The mind's eye: cognitive and applied aspects of eye movement research. North-Holland, Amsterdam, pp 493–516

Greene MR, Liu TY, Wolfe JM (2012) Reconsidering Yarbus: a failure to predict observers' task from eye movement patterns. Vis Res 62:1–8

Hacisalihzade SS, Stark LW, Allen JS (1992) Visual perception and sequences of eye movement fixations: a stochastic modeling approach. IEEE Trans Syst Man Cybern 22(3):474–481

Hammoud R (ed) (2008) Passive eye monitoring: algorithms, applications and experiments. Series: signals and communication technology. Springer, Berlin

Hansen DW, Ji Q (2009) In the eye of the beholder: a survey of models for eyes and gaze. IEEE Trans Pattern Anal Mach Intell 32(3):478–500

Hansen DW, Majaranta P (2012) Basics of camera-based gaze tracking. In: Majaranta P et al (eds) Gaze interaction and applications of eye tracking: advances in assistive technologies. Medical Information Science Reference, Hershey, pp 21–26

Hansen DW, Pece AEC (2005) Eye tracking in the wild. Comput Vis Image Underst 98(1):155–181

Hansen DW, Skovsgaard HH, Hansen JP et al (2008) Noise tolerant selection by gaze-controlled pan and zoom in 3D. In: Proceedings of the symposium on eye tracking research and applications, ETRA'08. ACM, New York, pp 205–212

Hansen DW, San Agustin J, Villanueva A (2010) Homography normalization for robust gaze estimation in uncalibrated setups. In: Proceedings of the 2010 symposium on eye-tracking research and applications, ETRA'10. ACM, New York, pp 13–20

Hansen JP, Tørning K, Johansen AS et al (2004) Gaze typing compared with input by head and hand. In: Proceedings of the 2004 symposium on eye tracking research and applications, ETRA'04. ACM, New York, pp 131–138

Hillstrom AP, Yantis S (1994) Visual motion and attentional capture. Percept Psychophys 55(4):399–411

Hori J, Sakano K, Miyakawa M, Saitoh Y (2006) Eye movement communication control system based on EOG and voluntary eye blink. In: Proceedings of the 9th international conference on computers helping people with special needs, ICCHP, vol 4061, pp 950–953

Huckauf A, Urbina MH (2008) On object selection in gaze controlled environments. J Eye Mov Res 2(4):1–7

Hyrskykari A, Majaranta P, Aaltonen A et al (2000) Design issues of iDICT: a gaze-assisted translation aid. In: Proceedings of the 2000 symposium on eye tracking research and applications, ETRA 2000. ACM, New York, pp 9–14

Hyrskykari A, Majaranta P, Räihä KJ (2003) Proactive response to eye movements. In: Rauterberg et al (eds) Proceedings of INTERACT 2003, pp 129–136

Isokoski P (2000) Text input methods for eye trackers using off-screen targets. In: Proceedings of the symposium on eye tracking research and applications, ETRA'00. ACM, New York, pp 15–21

Isokoski P, Joos M, Spakov O et al (2009) Gaze controlled games. Univ Access Inf Soc 8(4):323–337

Istance H, Hyrskykari A (2012) Gaze-aware systems and attentive applications. In: Majaranta P et al (eds) Gaze interaction and applications of eye tracking: advances in assistive technologies. IGI Global, Hershey, pp 175–195

Jacob RJK (1991) The use of eye movements in human-computer interaction techniques: what you look at is what you get. ACM Trans Inf Sys 9(3):152–169

Jacob RJK (1993) Eye movement-based human-computer interaction techniques: toward non-command interfaces. In: Hartson HR, Hix D (eds) Advances in human-computer interaction, vol 4. Ablex Publishing Co, Norwood, pp 151–190

Jacob RJK (1995) Eye tracking in advanced interface design. In: Barfield W, Furness TA (eds) Virtual environments and advanced interface design. Oxford University Press, New York, pp 258–288

Jokinen K, Majaranta P (2013) Eye-gaze and facial expressions as feedback signals in educational interactions. In: Barres DG et al (eds) Technologies for inclusive education: beyond traditional integration approaches. IGI Global, Hershey, pp 38–58

Kandemir M, Kaski S (2012) Learning relevance from natural eye movements in pervasive interfaces. In: Proceedings of the 14th ACM international conference on multimodal interaction, ICMI'12. ACM, New York, pp 85–92

Kherlopian AR, Gerrein JP, Yue M et al (2006) Electrooculogram based system for computer control using a multiple feature classification model. In: Proceedings of the 28th annual international conference of the engineering in medicine and biology society, EMBS 2006, pp 1295–1298

Kim Y, Doh N, Youm Y et al (2001) Development of a human-mobile communication system using electrooculogram signals. In: Proceedings of the 2001 IEEE/RSJ international conference on intelligent robots and systems, IROS 2001, vol 4, pp 2160–2165

Kinsman TB, Pelz JB (2012) Location by parts: model generation and feature fusion for mobile eye pupil tracking under challenging lighting. In: Proceedings of the 2012 ACM conference on ubiquitous computing, UbiComp'12. ACM, New York, pp 695–700

Kleinke CL (1986) Gaze and eye contact: a research review. Psychol Bull 100(1):78–100

Land MF, Furneaux S (1997) The knowledge base of the oculomotor system. Philos Trans Biol Sci 352(1358):1231–1239

Larsen EJ (2012) Systems and methods for providing feedback by tracking user gaze and gestures. Sony Computer Entertainment Inc. US Patent application 2012/0257035. http://www.faqs.org/patents/app/20120257035. Accessed 23 Feb 2013

Liu SC, Delbruck T (2010) Neuromorphic sensory systems. Curr Opin Neurobiol 20:1–8

Lorenceau J (2012) Cursive writing with smooth pursuit eye movements. Curr Biol 22(16):1506–1509. doi:10.1016/j.cub.2012.06.026

Majaranta P (2012) Communication and text entry by gaze. In: Majaranta P et al (eds) Gaze interaction and applications of eye tracking: advances in assistive technologies. IGI Global, Hershey, pp 63–77

Majaranta P, Ahola UK, Špakov O (2009a) Fast gaze typing with an adjustable dwell time. In: Proceedings of the 27th international conference on human factors in computing systems, CHI 2009. ACM, New York, pp 357–360

Majaranta P, Bates R, Donegan M (2009b) Eye tracking. In: Stephanidis C. (ed) The universal access handbook, chapter 36. CRC Press, Boca Raton, 20 pp

Majaranta P, MacKenzie IS, Aula A et al (2006) Effects of feedback and dwell time on eye typing speed and accuracy. Univ Access in Inf Soc 5(2):199–208

Majaranta P, Räihä KJ (2002) Twenty years of eye typing: systems and design issues. In: Proceedings of 2002 symposium on eye tracking research and applications, ETRA 2002. ACM, New York, pp 15–22

Manabe H, Fukumoto M (2006) Full-time wearable headphone-type gaze detector. In: Extended abstracts of the SIGCHI conference on human factors in computing systems, CHI 2006. ACM, New York, pp 1073–1078

Mele ML, Federici S (2012) A psychotechnological review on eye-tracking systems: towards user experience. Disabil Rehabil Assist Technol 7(4):261–281

Miniotas D, Špakov O, Tugoy I et al (2006) Speech-augmented eye gaze interaction with small closely spaced targets. In: Proceedings of the 2006 symposium on eye tracking research and applications, ETRA '06. ACM, New York, pp 67–72

Mizuno F, Hayasaka T, Tsubota K et al (2003) Development of hands-free operation interface for wearable computer-hyper hospital at home. In: Proceedings of the 25th annual international conference of the engineering in medicine and biology society, EMBS 2003, vol 4, 17–21 Sept 2003, pp 3740–3743

Mohammad Y, Okada S, Nishida T (2010) Autonomous development of gaze control for natural human-robot interaction. In Proceedings of the 2010 workshop on eye gaze in intelligent human machine interaction (EGIHMI '10). ACM, New York, NY, USA, pp 63–70

Morimoto CH, Mimica MRM (2005) Eye gaze tracking techniques for interactive applications. Comput Vis Image Underst 98(1):4–24

Mulvey F (2012) Eye anatomy, eye movements and vision. In: Majaranta P et al (eds) Gaze interaction and applications of eye tracking: advances in assistive technologies. IGI Global, Hershey, pp 10–20

Murphy-Chutorian E, Trivedi MM (2009) Head pose estimation in computer vision: a survey. IEEE Trans Pattern Anal Mach Intell 31(4):607–626

Nagamatsu N, Sugano R, Iwamoto Y et al (2010) User-calibration-free gaze tracking with estimation of the horizontal angles between the visual and the optical axes of both eyes. In: Proceedings of the 2010 symposium on eye-tracking research and applications, ETRA'10. ACM, New York, pp 251–254

Nakano YI, Jokinen J, Huang HH (2012) 4th workshop on eye gaze in intelligent human machine interaction: eye gaze and multimodality. In: Proceedings of the 14th ACM international conference on multimodal interaction, ICMI'12. ACM, New York, pp 611–612

Nielsen J (1993) Noncommand user interfaces. Commun ACM 36(4):82–99

Ohno T (1998) Features of eye gaze interface for selection tasks. In: Proceedings of the 3rd Asia Pacific computer-human interaction, APCHI'98. IEEE Computer Society, Washington, pp 176–182

Osterberg G (1935) Topography of the layer of rods and cones in the human retina. Acta Ophthalmol Suppl 13(6):1–102

Patmore DW, Knapp RB (1998) Towards an EOG-based eye tracker for computer control. In Proceedings of the 3rd international ACM conference on assistive technologies, ASSETS'98. ACM, New York, pp 197–203

Penzel T, Lo CC, Ivanov PC et al (2005) Analysis of sleep fragmentation and sleep structure in patients with sleep apnea and normal volunteers. In: 27th annual international conference of the engineering in medicine and biology society, IEEE-EMBS 2005, pp 2591–2594

Philips GR, Catellier AA, Barrett SF et al (2007) Electrooculogram wheelchair control. Biomed Sci Instrum 43:164–169

Porta M Ravarelli A, Spagnoli G (2010) ceCursor, a contextual eye cursor for general pointing in windows environments. In: Proceedings of the 2010 symposium on eye-tracking research and applications, ETRA'10. ACM, New York, pp 331–337

Rayner K (1995) Eye movements and cognitive processes in reading, visual search, and scene perception. In: Findlay JM et al (eds) Eye movement research: mechanisms, processes and applications. North Holland, Amsterdam, pp 3–22

Rothkopf CA, Pelz JP (2004) Head movement estimation for wearable eye tracker. In: Proceedings of the 2004 symposium on eye tracking research and applications, ETRA'04. ACM, New York, pp 123–130

Räihä K-J, Hyrskykari A, Majaranta P (2011) Tracking of visual attention and adaptive applications. In: Roda C (ed) Human attention in digital environments. Cambridge University Press, Cambridge, pp 166–185

Salvucci DD, Anderson JR (2001) Automated eye-movement protocol analysis. Human-Comput Interact 16(1):39–86

Schneider E, Dera T, Bard K et al (2005) Eye movement driven head-mounted camera: it looks where the eyes look. In: IEEE international conference on systems, man and cybernetics, vol 3, pp 2437–2442

Shell JS, Vertegaal R, Cheng D et al (2004) ECSGlasses and EyePliances: using attention to open sociable windows of interaction. In: Proceedings of the 2004 symposium on eye tracking research and applications, ETRA'04. ACM, New York, pp 93–100

Sibert LE, Jacob RJK (2000) Evaluation of eye gaze interaction. In: Proceedings of the SIGCHI conference on human factors in computing systems, CHI '00, ACM, pp 281–288

Skovsgaard H, Räihä KJ, Tall M (2012) Computer control by gaze. In: Majaranta P et al. (eds) Gaze interaction and applications of eye tracking: advances in assistive technologies. IGI Global, Hershey, pp 78–102

Smith JR, Cronin MJ, Karacan I (1971) A multichannel hybrid system for rapid eye movement detection (REM detection). Comp Biomed Res 4(3):275–290

Špakov O, Majaranta P (2012) Enhanced gaze interaction using simple head gestures. In: Proceedings of the 14th international conference on ubiquitous computing, UbiComp'12. ACM Press, New York, pp 705–710

Stampe DM, Reingold EM (1995) Selection by looking: a novel computer interface and its application to psychological research. In: Findlay JM, Walker R, Kentridge RW (eds) Eye movement research: mechanisms, processes and applications. Elsevier Science, Amsterdam, pp 467–478

Stellmach S, Dachselt F (2012) Look and touch: gaze-supported target acquisition. In: Proceedings of the 2012 ACM annual conference on human factors in computing systems, CHI'12. ACM, New York, pp 2981–2990

Sugioka A, Ebisawa Y, Ohtani M (1996) Noncontact video-based eye-gaze detection method allowing large head displacements. In: Proceedings of the 18th annual international conference of the IEEE engineering in medicine and biology society. Bridging disciplines for biomedicine, vol 2, pp 526–528

Ten Kate JH, Frietman EEE, Willems W et al (1979) Eye-switch controlled communication aids. In: Proceedings of the 12th international conference on medical and biological engineering, Jerusalem, Israel, August 1979

Tessendorf B, Bulling A, Roggen D et al (2011) Recognition of hearing needs from body and eye movements to improve hearing instruments. In: Proceedings of the 9th international conference on pervasive computing, Pervasive 2011. Lecture notes in computer science, vol 6696. Springer, Heidelberg, pp 314–331

Tobii (2011) Tobii unveils the world's first eyecontrolled laptop. Press release, 1 March 2011. http://www.tobii.com/en/eye-tracking-research/global/news-and-events/press-release-archive/archive-2011/tobii-unveils-the-worlds-first-eye-controlled-laptop. Accessed 23 Feb 2013

Vehkaoja AT, Verho JA, Puurtinen MM et al (2005) Wireless head cap for EOG and facial EMG measurements. In: Proceedings of the 27th annual international conference of the engineering in medicine and biology society, IEEE EMBS 2005, pp 5865–5868

Velichkovsky B, Sprenger A, Unema P (1997) Towards gaze-mediated interaction: collecting solutions of the "Midas touch problem". In: Proceedings of the IFIP TC13 international conference on human-computer interaction, INTERACT'97. Chapman and Hall, London, pp 509–516

Venkataramanan, A Prabhat P, Choudhury SR et al (2005) Biomedical instrumentation based on electrooculogram (EOG) signal processing and application to a hospital alarm system. In: Proceedings of the 3rd international conference on intelligent sensing and information processing, ICISIP 2005, IEEE Conference Publications, pp 535–540

Vesterby T, Voss JC, Hansen JP et al (2005) Gaze-guided viewing of interactive movies. Digit Creativity 16(4):193–204

Vickers S, Istance H, Smalley M (2010) EyeGuitar: making rhythm based music video games accessible using only eye movements. In: Proceedings of the 7th international conference on advances in computer entertainment technology, ACE'10. ACM, New York, pp 36–39

Vidal M, Bulling A, Gellersen H (2013) Pursuits: spontaneous interaction with displays based on smooth pursuit eye movement and moving targets. In: Proceedings of the 2013 ACM international joint conference on pervasive and ubiquitous computing, UbiComp 2013. ACM, New York

Wade NJ, Tatler BW (2005) The moving tablet of the eye: the origins of modern eye movement research. Oxford University Press, Oxford

Ware C, Mikaelian HH (1987) An evaluation of an eye tracker as a device for computer input. In: Proceedings of the SIGCHI/GI conference on human factors in computing systems and graphics interface, CHI and GI'87. ACM, New York, pp 183–188

Wijesoma WS, Wee Ks, Wee OC et al (2005) EOG based control of mobile assistive platforms for the severely disabled. In: Proceedings of the IEEE international conference on robotics and biomimetics, ROBIO 2005, pp 490–494

Wobbrock JO, Rubinstein J, Sawyer MW et al (2008) Longitudinal evaluation of discrete consecutive gaze gestures for text entry. In: Proceedings of the symposium on eye tracking research and applications, ETRA 2008. ACM, New York, pp 11–18

Wästlund W, Sponseller K, Pettersson O (2010) What you see is where you go: testing a gaze-driven power wheelchair for individuals with severe multiple disabilities. In: Proceedings of the 2010 symposium on eye-tracking research and applications, ETRA 2010. ACM, New York, pp 133–136

Zhang Y, Rasku J, Juhola M (2012) Biometric verification of subjects using saccade eye movements. Int J Biometr 4(4):317–337

Zhang Y, Bulling A, Gellersen H (2013) SideWays: a gaze interface for spontaneous interaction with situated displays. In: Proceedings of the 31st SIGCHI international conference on human factors in computing systems, CHI 2013. ACM, New York, pp 851–860

Zhu Z, Ji Q (2005) Eye gaze tracking under natural head movements. In: IEEE computer society conference on computer vision and pattern recognition, CVPR 2005, vol 1, pp 918–923

Chapter 4
Towards BCI-Based Implicit Control in Human–Computer Interaction

Thorsten O. Zander, Jonas Brönstrup, Romy Lorenz
and Laurens R. Krol

Abstract In this chapter a specific aspect of Physiological Computing, that of implicit Human–Computer Interaction, is defined and discussed. Implicit Interaction aims at controlling a computer system by behavioural or psychophysiological aspects of user state, independently of any intentionally communicated command. This introduces a new type of Human–Computer Interaction, which in contrast to most forms of interaction implemented nowadays, does not require the user to explicitly communicate with the machine. Users can focus on understanding the current state of the system and developing strategies for optimally reaching the goal of the given interaction. For example, the system can assess the user state by means of passive Brain-Computer Interfaces, which the user needs not even be aware of. Based on this information and the given context the system can adapt automatically to the current strategies of the user. In a first study, a proof of principle is given, by implementing an Implicit Interaction to guide simple cursor movements in a 2D grid to a target. The results of this study clearly indicate the high potential of Implicit Interaction and introduce a new bandwidth of applications for passive Brain-Computer Interfaces.

T. O. Zander (✉) · J. Brönstrup · R. Lorenz · L. R. Krol
Team PhyPA, Berlin Institute of Technology, MAR 3-2, 10587 Berlin, Germany
e-mail: tzander@gmail.com

J. Brönstrup
e-mail: jonas.broenstrup@gmail.com

R. Lorenz
e-mail: lorenz.romy@googlemail.com

L. R. Krol
e-mail: lrkrol@mailbox.tu-berlin.de

S. H. Fairclough and K. Gilleade (eds.), *Advances in Physiological Computing*,   67
Human–Computer Interaction Series, DOI: 10.1007/978-1-4471-6392-3_4,
© Springer-Verlag London 2014

Introduction

Technology affects almost every aspect of our lives—our jobs, transportation, entertainment, communication and social integration. As advances in technology serve as a catalyst for the steady progress of our society, industrial, scientific and governmental efforts focus on stimulating the development of new hard- and software which become more powerful day by day. As a result, information can be processed, analyzed and distributed by technical systems at a speed, in an amount and with an accuracy which far exceed the capabilities of human beings. Nevertheless, a human user is needed to control most technical systems because computers still lack the capabilities of intelligent thinking. However, a Human-Machine System (HMS) would work most efficiently if many parts of the human information processing system could be delegated to a machine. The user would just be observing and interpreting the current state of the interaction and deciding on strategies to reach the goal of the HMS based on information smartly distilled by the machine. An example for this line of reasoning would be an adaptive, open-ended electronic book. While reading, the reader evaluates the current story as either 'good' or 'bad'. If the book could assess these evaluations, it could 'steer' the story accordingly, in the direction desired by the reader. Regardless of the reader's evaluations being conscious or not—they may simply be automatic, affective reactions—the reader is not composing a story, nor instructing the system how it should continue: The focus is on reading and interpreting the story as it unfolds, while the actual changes to the book happen automatically, potentially even unbeknown to the reader. In a highly automated way, the computer would understand the concepts developed by the user. Humans would give guidance to machines to efficiently solve a task.

Currently, Human–Computer Interaction (HCI) is far from such an ideal system. Firstly, users have to request information manually and they secondly need to give very detailed commands, usually in a cumbersome way. The first problem results from the fact that computers can store and process large amounts of information, and do that very differently from humans. Think about a log file storing network activity over one day. Such information can be processed in a short amount of time by a computer, but is hardly accessible by users. The second problem is 2-fold. Firstly, humans usually think in larger concepts, while a computer is controlled by triggering small actions leading to the realization of such concepts. If you want to change the colour of a two dimensional figure of a cube, you easily could advise a human painter to do this by a simple sentence ("Please, paint the cube blue."), but if communicating this concept to a computer you have to go step by step (defining areas, select specific shades of blue etc). Secondly, input mechanisms like mouse and keyboard are cumbersome and often unnatural means for communicating intentions and instructions. The user has to spend effort on translating commands, such that they can be processed by the machine. All of these problems lead to a high user-workload resulting from tasks in infrastructural areas.

A lot of effort has gone into increasing the usability of technical systems by resolving one aspect of this problem. Current systems smartly represent and aggregate available information such that it is easily accessible for the user when needed and can be perceived quickly and effortlessly. However, the other direction of HCI, that of sending information from the user to the machine, is also highly relevant. Communicating to the computer is still complicated and demanding. It mainly works based on explicitly sending detailed and small-stepped commands formulated by the user, as described in the examples above. Each communication in this direction increases the effort by the user to keep the interaction running. Hence, an increase in the overall efficiency of a given HCI could be achieved by dissolving most of the direct and explicit communication, which is unwieldy due to form, style and complexity from a human perspective. In that way the user could focus on the task of guiding the interaction to its goal.

In such a scenario, the machine would still need to have information about the users concepts, in order to process and provide appropriate information and pre-pare specific tasks in the interaction. But with *Implicit Interaction*, the machine is expected to infer this information automatically. This can only be achieved by extending the user model used by the machine—which is currently restricted to directly formulated commands—by information about the users emotions, inten-tions and situational interpretations. Passive Brain-Computer Interfaces can be a tool for this as they provide information about even covert aspects of the user state in real time. They can be used for implementing a secondary, implicit interaction loop which supports users in their main interaction, leading to an automated adaptation of the system.

The following parts of this chapter focus on the capabilities of passive Brain-Computer Interfaces for establishing implicit Human–Computer Interaction. An example shows that this could lead to a completely new type of interaction which reaches its goals even without the need for any command that is consciously generated. The user only needs to focus on understanding the current state of the interaction and the machine learns to reach the goal by investigating the users cognition and interpretation automatically.

Brain-Computer Interfaces

The Roots and History of BCI

The idea of "reading thoughts" with the electroencephalogram (EEG) was first mentioned by Berger in 1929 (as cited in Birbaumer 2006). He speculated on the possibility of processing human EEG waveforms using sophisticated mathematical analyses. The development of the first EEG-based "Brain-Computer Interface" (BCI) was pioneered in the early 1970s by Vidal (1973, 1977), who also coined the term BCI. Since then BCI has evolved "into one of the fastest-growing areas of scientific research" (Mak and Wolpaw 2009).

A BCI was originally defined as a new, non-muscular communication and control channel for sending messages and commands in real-time to the external world (Wolpaw et al. 2002). By measuring brain activity associated with the user's intent and translating it into control signals for communication systems or external devices, a BCI bypasses the brain's normal output channels of peripheral nerves and muscles. Brain activity can be recorded from electrodes in the skull (invasive BCIs) or outside (non-invasive BCIs). Invasive BCI involves brain signals such as action potentials from nerve cells or nerve fibers, synaptic and extracellular field potentials and electrocorticography (ECoG) (for a review see Birbaumer 2006). A variety of methods may serve as non-invasive BCI. Besides EEG, these methods include magnetoencephalography (MEG, e.g. Lal et al. 2005; Mellinger et al. 2007), functional magnetic resonance imaging (fMRI, e.g. Lee et al. 2009; Weiskopf et al. 2003), and near-infrared spectroscopy (NIRS, e.g. Coyle et al. 2004). Due to its relatively simple and inexpensive equipment and high temporal resolution, BCI research mainly focused on EEG as preferred recording method in recent decades.

From the early beginning in the 1970s, EEG-based BCIs have given rise to the hope of restoring independence to people suffering from diseases that disrupt the neural pathways through which the brain communicates with and controls its external environment. Among these are neurodegenerative and genetic neuromuscular diseases such as amyotrophic lateral sclerosis (ALS), Friedreich's ataxia or muscular dystrophies, multifactorial and polygenic disorders like multiple sclerosis, cerebral palsy or the Guillain-Barré syndrome, as well as severe neuromuscular impairments due to brainstem stroke or brain and spinal cord injuries. For severely paralyzed patients for whom the remaining control (e.g. eye movement) is weak, easily fatigued, or unreliable (Wolpaw et al. 2002) BCI serves as the only remaining channel for communicating with the outside world. The resulting condition is called locked-in state (LIS) if the basic control of at least one muscle is present (Birbaumer 2006). However, for most cases an easier and more efficient communication can be established by exploiting any remaining muscle rather than employing a BCI (e.g. communication via eye blinks or cheek muscles). As neuronal degeneration progresses the patients become completely paralyzed (e.g. late-stage ALS). They lose control over all voluntary muscles including eye movement and respiration and are "locked into their bodies, unable to communicate in any way" (Wolpaw et al. 2002). For completely locked-in state (CLIS) patients, research has shown that basic communication cannot be restored with BCI (Birbaumer 2006; Kübler and Birbaumer 2008). Whether CLIS constitutes a unique BCI-resistant condition or if individuals are able to retain the capacity for BCI use if they begin employing it before becoming completely locked-in, remains an open empirical question (Kübler and Birbaumer 2008). Beyond this initial motivation for BCI research to enable communication, other BCI applications can be used to transmit brain signals to muscles or to external orthotic devices in order to restore movements in paralyzed limbs. Such so-called neuroprostheses generally use functional electrical stimulation (FES) to "elicit action potentials of the efferent nerves, which provoke contractions of the innervated but paralyzed muscles" (Müller-Putz et al. 2006b). Based on this principle, neuroprostheses artificially compensate for the loss of voluntary muscle control. These originally intended BCI applications have in common that they usually require voluntary and directed commands by the user to enable spelling or the control of an external device.

Categorization of BCIs

Alongside these accomplishments, a recent direction within the research field of BCI attempts to broaden the general BCI approach by substituting the user's command with passively conveyed implicit information. Based on this thought, a new categorization of BCI systems was proposed by Zander and colleagues (Zander et al. 2010b), dividing BCI-driven applications into active, reactive and passive BCI systems.

Active BCI: An active BCI derives its outputs from brain activity which is directly and consciously controlled by the user, independent of external events, for controlling an application.

Reactive BCI: A reactive BCI derives its outputs from brain activity arising in reaction to external stimulation which is indirectly modulated by the user to control an application.

Passive BCI: A passive BCI derives its outputs from arbitrary brain activity arising without the purpose of voluntary control, for enriching a human-machine interaction with implicit information on the user state.

Important Applications of BCIs

Active BCI

Early examples of active BCI systems are based on slow cortical potentials (SCP). SCPs are slow voltage changes generated in the cortex that can last from less than half a second up to several seconds (Birbaumer et al. 1990). With frequencies down to 1 Hz they are among the lowest frequency features of the EEG. It could be shown that both healthy users and paralyzed patients can be trained to self-regulate these positive and negative voltage shifts in order to control external devices by means of a BCI (Birbaumer and Cohen 2007). Most commonly SCP-based BCIs are used for cursor control and target selection, such as spelling (Birbaumer et al. 1999, 2003; Hinterberger et al. 2004). Despite acceptable accuracy rates, a SCP-based BCI needs long training time, sometimes up to several months, and provides only slow communication with usually around one letter per minute (Birbaumer 2006).

More popular active BCI systems utilize the sensorimotor rhythm (SMR). SMR comprise "mu and beta rhythms, which are oscillations in the brain activity localized in the mu band (7–13 Hz) (…) and beta band (13–30 Hz)" (Nicolas-Alonso and Gomez-Gil 2012). SMR-based BCIs operate on the principle of movement-related frequency changes in the ongoing EEG activity over sensori-motor areas. Due to decreased synchrony of the underlying neuronal populations during the performance of such movements, the power in the mu-rhythm decreases (Pfurtscheller and Lopes da Silver 1999). This phenomenon is called event-related desynchronization (ERD, Pfurtscheller 1977) and is measured to effect control in SMR-based BCIs. Besides ERD, post-movement beta rebound (event-related synchronization (ERS), Pfurtscheller 1992) can also be employed for classification (Bai et al. 2008). For BCI, the significance of SMR definitely lies in the fact that it is not only attenuated by actual movements, but also by intended (Kübler et al. 2005) or imagined ones (Wolpaw et al. 2000) in paralyzed patients and healthy subjects respectively. For the latter, the term motor imagery (MI)–based BCI has been established in the field of research. SMR-based BCIs have been extensively investigated since the mid-1980s (Wolpaw et al. 2002). Similar to SCP-based BCIs they are most commonly used for cursor control in order to select letters or icons on a screen (Daly and Wolpaw 2008). Besides one-dimensional control, both two-dimensional (Blankertz et al. 2007; Wolpaw 2004 and three-dimensional control (McFarland et al. 2010) can be achieved by employing MI of several limbs, such as right hand, left hand and foot. Furthermore, the multidimensional control of neuroprostheses (Müller-Putz et al. 2005; Tavella et al. 2010) and orthotic devices such as robotic arms (McFarland and Wolpaw 2008; Pfurtscheller et al. 2000) has been accomplished with the support of MI-based BCIs. However, due to its relatively low bit rates and only moderate accuracy rates compared to for example reactive BCIs (Guger et al. 2003, 2009), the real-world application of MI-based systems is extremely limited. Beyond that, a non-negligible portion of users (15–30 %)—so-called BCI illiterates—fail to gain any MI-based BCI control (Blankertz et al. 2010).

Reactive BCI

The vast majority of systems based on reactive BCI employ event-related potentials (ERP). An ERP is the brain response to an external or internal event such as a visual, auditory or tactile stimulus. The most prominent and best-studied ERP is the P3 (also P300) component, a large positivity that is elicited in the central-parietal region of the brain 300–500 ms post-stimulus upon rare events. For BCI purposes an oddball paradigm is usually applied. A rare target event (e.g. the target letter) is presented among frequently appearing nontarget events (e.g. remaining letters of the alphabet). The user's focused attention on the presented target leads to a noticeable increase of the P3 amplitude that can be extracted from the EEG. Based on this principle, the target letter will be selected. The first P3-based speller, the so-called matrix speller, was introduced by Farwell and Donchin (1988). Since then, similar P3 spellers have been extensively investigated and developed (Nijboer et al. 2008; Sellers and Donchin 2006. Another constituent of the ERP, the N2 (also N200), a parieto-occipital negativity typically evoked 180–320 ms following the stimulus presentation, appears also to be closely associated with cognitive processes of perception and selective attention (Patel and Azzam 2005). For this reason Treder and Blankertz (2010) advocate the use of the term ERP-based BCI in order to emphasize the fact that "there is a multitude of ERP components that is affected by attention and can be exploited by classifiers". Most recently, advances have been made towards gaze-independent spellers (Acqualagna and Blankertz 2011; Treder et al. 2011) or spellers adapted to non-visual modalities by using auditory (Furdea et al. 2009; Schreuder et al. 2011) and tactile stimulation (Brouwer and van Erp 2010) (for a review also see Riccio et al. 2012).

Other reactive BCIs are frequency-based by exploiting steady-state evoked potentials (SSEP) that occur in response to a visual, auditory or tactile stimulus that is presented at a steady rate. For instance in a steady-state visually evoked potential (SSVEP)-based BCI several stimuli, each flickering at different frequencies (typically in the range of 3.5–75 Hz, Beverina et al. 2003), are presented to the user (Bin et al. 2009; Gao et al. 2003). By the user's focused attention on one of the steadily flashing stimuli, the brain produces detectable oscillations of the same frequency in the visual cortex. Further examples for BCIs utilizing steady-state somatosensory evoked potentials (SSSEP, Müller-Putz et al. 2006a) or steady-state auditory evoked potentials (SSAEP, Hill and Scholköpf 2012) have been proposed.

Passive BCI

Systems based on passive BCI can provide information about Covert Aspects of the User State (CAUS), i.e. task-induced states which can only be detected with weak reliability using conventional methods such as behavioural measures (Zander et al. 2010b). Restricted forms of passive BCIs have in the past proven to be valuable tools for detecting mental workload (Kohlmorgen et al. 2007), working memory load (Grimes et al. 2008), fatigue (Papadelis et al. 2007), self-induced errors (Blankertz et al. 2002a), deception (Fang et al. 2003), or anticipation (Gangadhar et al. 2009). However, those systems only focused on user-state detection alone and the information gained about CAUS has not been fed back into the system to enrich the human-machine interaction. More recent examples pursuing this notion include detecting and correction of self-induced (Schmidt et al. 2012) or machine-induced errors (Zander et al. 2010b).

Extending the Definition of BCI for Applications Including Users Without Disabilities

In contrast to active or reactive systems, a passive BCI does not interfere with other means of the human-machine interaction. It can be "reliant on either the presence or the absence of an ongoing conventional human–computer interaction, or be independent of it" (**complementarity**, Zander and Kothe 2011, p. 4). Furthermore, "a passive BCI application can make use of arbitrarily many passive BCI detectors in parallel with no conflicts, which is more difficult for active and reactive BCIs due to the user's limited ability of consciously interacting with multiple components simultaneously" (**composability**, Zander and Kothe 2011, p. 4). "Since no conscious effort from the user is needed for the use of passive BCIs (besides preparation), their operational cost is determined by the cost of their false alarms. Passive BCIs producing probabilistic estimates, together with the a priori probability of predicting correctly, could potentially be designed allowing for arbitrary levels of cost-optimal decision making at the application level. In that way, theoretically, systems could be designed which would only gain in efficiency by utilizing a passive BCI and could have zero benefit in the worst case" (**controlled costs**, Zander and Kothe 2011, p. 4).

As the concept of passive BCI offers the key properties of complementarity, composability and controlled cost, its application spectrum is not limited to users with disabilities. Moreover, it adds an additional information channel conveying highly relevant information about the user. Besides information about the user state, data of the environment and the technical system could augment the available information space and thereby add *context awareness* to the system (Zander and Jatzev 2012). These additions can be used to "improve the actual state-of-the-art human-machine interaction by enabling the technical system to adapt to the user without any additional effort taken by the user" (Zander and Kothe 2011, p. 3).

Brain-Computer Interfaces and Physiological Computing

Physiological Computing (PC) aims at the integration of interaction within an HMS through psychophysiological activity. Thereby the technical system shall gain in-sights on the cognitive and emotional state of the user and adapt itself accordingly.

Passive Brain-Computer Interfaces for Implicit Human–Computer Interaction

Explicit and Implicit Interaction

In a given HMS, the user and the technical system communicate with each other to reach a predefined goal, as described in Rötting et al. (2009) implicit. In the more specific context of HCI, this is usually done through an interaction cycle where user and computer exchange information in an *explicit* way. Changes in the state of the machine are explicitly communicated to the user so that this information can feed the next cycle. Similarly, all communication from the user to the machine is based on specific commands which are formulated and directed by the user. Hence, we define explicit control as the intentional directing of commands at the interface of an HMS.

We define overt and covert commands as being dependent on, respectively, overt and covert aspects of the user state. Explicit commands are usually overt, but they do not have to be, as in the case of an active BCI (see section "Active BCI"). Other examples of explicit control are the use of a computer through peripheral controls such as mouse or keyboard, or more recently also speech and gesture recognition.

Implicit Control on the other hand, we define as an automatic state change of a technical system based at least in part on an evaluation of the user's current state, without any actual commands to that effect being intentionally communicated to the system by the user (Fairclough 2009) fundamentals. Although the user may be aware of neither the communication nor the system's state changes, these state changes in general are intended by the user, who uses the system to reach a specific goal. Just like explicit commands, implicitly sent commands can be covert or overt. In interpersonal interaction the verbal context of speech is an example of explicit interaction, as described in Schmidt (2000), Rötting et al. (2009). But often implicit information has to be taken into account so that the intent of the message can be understood more easily, as sometimes the speakers intention can hardly be inferred from the words alone. Intonation, volume, gestures or facial expressions are examples of information which can change the meaning of a message entirely. A sarcastic statement is a good example for a message that can change its meaning depending on implicit information. It can be taken as proof for the importance of the affective context of communication that *Emoticons* (Rivera et al. 1996) effects have become an important part of text-based interaction.

In the following we refer to a given HCI based on implicit commands as *Implicit Interaction*.

Forms of Implicit Interaction

Implicit Interaction is not only relevant for interpersonal interaction. As described in Schmidt (2000) information about the context of a given system can also be used for implicit interaction. In addition, forms of HCI can potentially be improved if the technical system is able to detect cognitive processes such as attention, engagement or workload. Such information could be used to enable a system to adapt to the users state and thereby make HCI more usable, comfortable, intuitive and entertaining (Rötting et al. 2009). Also the affective state of the user such as frustration, confusion, disliking or interest (Picard 1999) carries useful information.

An attempt at a Human–Computer Interface that adapted to behavioural measures of the user, which can be seen as an early realization of the ideas stated in (Schmidt 2000), was "Clippy", the automated assistance in Microsoft Office '97 (Microsoft Corp., Redmond, USA.). Most users found "Clippy" to be highly intrusive, as it was inaccurate in estimating the users intentions, which introduced switching costs (Squire and Parasuraman 2010) and led to frustration (whitworth 2005). The reason for the low accuracy of this automated adaptation is that it is based solely on short-termed information about the user's behaviour, which can be an unreliable source of information (Müller et al. 2008). Incorporating implicit information about the user state, i.e. information about the situational interpretation, could potentially have improved this system, without increasing the users workload, and may hence have led to a better user acceptance.

Assessment of Implicit Information

Even though we can assume that adding implicit information about the cognitive or affective state is important it is unclear how it can be assessed in an efficient way. One promising approach is using psychophysiological measures, as these are suited to convey information about changes in the user state. Galvanic skin response, which measures change in conductance of the skin, is sensitive to changes in cognitive constructs such as workload (Shi et al. 2007) or stress (Lazarus et al. 1963) but also to behavioural patterns such as errors committed by the subject (Hajcak et al. 2003). Similarly, cardiac measures such as heart rate or electrocardiogram (ECG) are responsive to cognitive, physical and environmental influences (Hankins and Wilson 1998; LeBlanc et al. 1976). Yet these methods have clear downsides. The relation of such signals to the users cognitive state is inherently indirect. Bodily processes are usually resulting from cognitive or affective changes, and carry only indirect information about these. As bodily processes are also modulated by other factors, they can indeed be sensitive but are usually not highly specific to an investigated aspect of cognition and affect.

For certain aspects of cognitive and affective state the EEG appears to be a more direct and hence better measure. Often changes in cognitive and affective state are initiated in the human brain. As EEG is reflecting changes in cortical activity, it is capable of assessing direct information about the source of certain state changes. As CAUS (see section "Passive BCI") are only hardly reflected in bodily processes, measuring cortical activity might be the only way of accessing information about these specific changes in cognitive and affective state. An example for this can be found in Zander et al. (2011), where a passive BCI is used to detect the (covert) intention of moving an index finger, before the onset of muscular activity.

As the the autonomic nervous system (ANS) and the human brain are inherently inter-connected, changes in cognition also might be triggered by the ANS, and hence, the EEG is not necessarily the most direct link to cognition. Nevertheless, EEG is a multi-channel bio-signal, that can measure direct, physical manifestations of cognition. In addition, even though the EEG has clear limitations in spatial resolution, it allows for simultaneous assessment of different aspects of human cognition (see composability, section "Extending the Definition of BCI for Applications Including Users Without Disabilities"), as we can identify multiple cortical sources contributing to it. EEG provides a comparably fast temporal resolution; modulations in the EKG for example may be as fast as 2–3 s, while

EEG signals usually respond within hundreds of milliseconds. The evaluation of EEG data in real time for Implicit Interaction is one main application for passive BCI and directly follows its definition (see section "Categorization of BCIs"). Hence, it is a direct and worthwhile mean for assessing information about the user state.

Possibilities for Beneficial Multi-disciplinarily of BCI- and PC-Research

The combination of PC- and BCI-based research can provide mutual benefits. The methodology of BCI research can prove valuable to PC, namely single trial classification of physiological measures and PC can open a new variety of applications for BCI technology.

Passive BCI Methodology for Physiological Computing

Over the past four decades of BCI-research machine learning has become a fundamental part of the field. Initially BCIs consisted of predefined classifiers which the users had to adapt to, as described in section "Active BCI". Machine learning made it possible to shift this training-effort from the user to the machine (Müller et al. 2004).

To allow the technical system to learn the characteristics of a certain signal, exemplary data is collected in a calibration phase. Multiple trials for each experimental condition are recorded. Features are extracted from these data sets which may have temporal, spectral or spatial dimensions. Machine learning then derives a model that emphasizes features that provide maximal discriminability between the conditions. This model is used in the BCI to evaluate new data sets and assign them to one of the cognitive states that are of interest. This time consuming calibration has to be undertaken individually for each subject and usually for each session. In future BCIs this problem might be solved through subject-independent classifiers, also called universal classifiers (Reuderink et al. 2011; Zander 2011; Wolpaw et al. 2002). Such classifiers are predefined (for example through training on a group of subjects) and are capable of accurate single-trial classification of an aspect of the users state independent of the subject. Therefore individual training of the subjects can be omitted. The BCI community has developed and advanced many different approaches to feature extraction and machine learning or adopted approaches and techniques from other fields for neurophysiological analysis. For the definition of predictive models many different approaches from machine learning have been used: from support vector machines (SVM) to linear or quadratic discriminant analysis (LDA and QDA), (Duda et al. 2001) to non-linear kernel SVM (Schöllkopf and Smola 2002) and up to advanced methods building on artificial neural networks (Balderas et al. 2011). Because features usually are gaussian and due to the low complexity (low Vapnik-Chervonenkis dimension) of LDA it is less prone to overfitting (Vapnik and Chervonekis 1971). Another major advantage of LDA over SVM is that it is robust against imbalanced trial numbers between classes, as it is based mainly on an estimation of covariance matrices (Duda et al. 1973).

Implementations of these approaches have been made public through toolboxes and platforms such as BCILAB (Kothe and Makeig 2013), BCI2000 (Schalk et al. 2004) or OpenVIBE (Renard et al. 2010) that allow for easy access to BCI-methodology.

New Applications of BCI Technology in Physiological Computing

For a long time, the main purpose for BCI-research was to provide people with severe physical impairments with a form of communication. This was usually achieved through active or reactive BCIs (see sections "The Roots and History of BCI", "Active BCI" and "Reactive BCI"). With the introduction of passive BCI-applications it was shown that new possibilities arise if the initial methodology is extended (Zander et al. 2010a, b) (see also section "Extending the Definition of BCI for Applications Including Users Without Disabilities").

Since then, the main application of passive BCI technology is automated adaptation of a technical system in an HMS. This can be achieved through the interpretation of the user state (Zander and Kothe 2011), containing interpretations of situational events like errors committed (Blankertz et al. 2002b) or perceived (Ferrez and Millán 2008) or user intentions, like intending to interact with the system (Protzak et al. 2013). Passive BCI technology can also be used to monitor the user state or to give neurofeedback.

Since its initial definition, BCI research mainly focused at one input modality reflecting brain activity. Recently, it opened up for multi-modal approaches, as described in Pfurtscheller et al. (2010). This development allows for an interconnection between the field of PC and BCI, such that the bandwidth of applications for BCI technology is extended significantly. PC already found application in different types of HCI, which can now easily be combined with (passive) BCI technology. The main purpose of PC is to extend the range of possible applications and promote the development of hybrid systems, and hence, its methodology allows for combining different sources of information such as galvanic skin response, cardiac measures or even behavioural measures into combined feature spaces. Such measures make it possible to assess the user's emotions quite accurately, which has proven to be difficult through BCI only. Under the term affective computing (AC) emotions such as anger, happiness, sadness and surprise were classified successfully through a combination of psychophysiological measures (Canento et al. 2011).

Another benefit of combining BCI with physiological input was shown through the combination of eye-tracking with a passive BCI. This provides an elegant approach to overcome a common problem in gaze-based interaction. Usually the affirmative action is executed through dwell times, blink patterns or active BCI (Vilimek and Zander 2009) which are not always easy to control and also are not comfortable to use. This is called the *Midas-touch problem* (Jacob et al. 1993). It was shown that one efficient solution is to assess the users intent to interact with an icon through a passive BCI (Protzak et al. 2013) and to combine it with a dwell time selection. In this study Protzak et al. showed that in a dwell-time based interaction the intention to interact can be detected by a passive BCI. Activity in parietal cortex showed a significant difference during trials where subjects interacted with the system compared to trials where they just looked at items on the screen. A pseudo-online evaluation revealed that it is possible to correctly predict the users intend to interact in single trial with an average accuracy of 81 %. A system that uses eye-tracking and a passive BCI combined is an excellent example for a HMS using PC to establish intuitive HCI.

Influences on the EEG-Signal: Artifacts or Features

In PC, eye-movements or muscular activity are considered to be input modalities used for HCI. Contrarily, in BCI research signals generated from such activity are considered artifacts. Strictly speaking a BCI should process input solely from electrical activity within the central nervous system (CNS, Wolpaw et al. 2002). Factually this requirement can hardly be met. Even under laboratory conditions first degree artifacts, such as eye- or neck-muscle movements, and second degree artifacts, such as changes in the electromagnetic field, will always be part of the recorded EEG-signal (Zander 2011). The magnitude of these signals exceeds that of any cortical signal by an order of magnitude. Where the artifacts are independent of the context investigated in the experiment they are uncritical but merely lead to a lower signal-to-noise-ratio. If artifacts are dependent of conditions investigated, they will contribute strongly to the predictive model of the BCI. Then, the resulting BCI model may be more dependent on artifacts than on cortical activity. Whether artifacts can be used as a reliable control signal that can be included in passive BCI is strongly dependent on the type of interaction investigated. In systems where such artifacts are significantly related to the aspects of user state under investigation, they can be useful additions to or even replacements of cortical signals.

Hence, the question whether artifacts should be used for HCI (as proposed in section "New Applications of BCI Technology in Physiological Computing") based on passive BCI is hard to answer. Our behaviour and our physiology are sensitive to changes in environmental context. Think about changes in your mimicry during social interaction compared to it in privacy. Such changes also affect artifacts produced by such behaviour. Therefore, an interaction including artifacts will also be dependent on the context of the interaction. We assume that basal brain activity representing cognitive or affective processes of interest are more robust to contextual modulation. Nevertheless, this still needs to be proven.

Passive BCI for Implicit Interaction Beyond Secondary Input

The differentiation between explicit and implicit interaction is important for HCI because both forms contain information that is needed for comprehensive interaction. In most applications of passive BCIs, it is intended for secondary input supporting the primary interaction (Schmidt et al. 2012; Zander et al. 2010b; Blankertz et al. 2002a). However, passive BCI technology could ultimately be used as the only input. In such a scenario the user acts as a critic of an external autonomous system and controls it thereby. This would be a completely new type of HCI that renders any explicit input from the user unnecessary since the perception and interpretation of the environment would serve as input.

This form of interaction would be highly intuitive to use since it does not need any instructions (Fairclough 2008). The HCI converges to the goal of the HMS by tracking the process of the user learning about and understanding the current system state. The user does not need to intend to interact with the system, and does not need to translate any mental abstract concepts to small-stepped command sequences, which reduces the workload to a minimum. This also satisfies the demand made in the introduction, for an HMS that runs autonomically and only shifts effort to the user that needs intelligent thinking.

In the following section an example is given of a system which only is guided only by Implicit Interaction based on passive BCI.

Passive BCI for Implicit Interaction: An Example Study

The following study by two of the authors may serve to illustrate the concept of implicit interaction.

Krol, Gramann and Zander (in press) investigated the use of a passive BCI to control the movement of a cursor in two dimensions. The cursor was not controlled directly, but moved autonomously: Implicit interaction with the cursor was realised by adapting its directional preferences, based on the presence or absence of error negativities evoked by the cursor's movements. An error negativity is a "negative deflection in the ongoing (EEG) seen when human participants commit errors" (Holroyd and Coles 2002), and can also be seen after the passive observation of errors being committed (Van Schie et al. 2004).

When, for example, an upwards movement of the cursor was followed by an error negativity, as detected by the passive BCI, the probability of repeating that movement was reduced. In short, rather than actively controlling the direction in which the cursor should go, the subjects were passively observing and interpreting the cursor's initially random movements, and the cursor responded to those interpretations by making its movement increasingly less random.

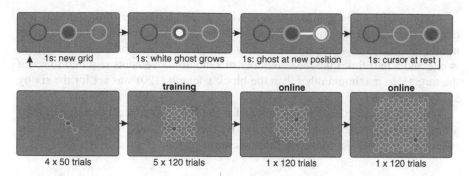

Fig. 4.1 *Above* Stimuli over the course of one (incorrect) trial in the example study, on a one by three grid. *Below* Illustration of the study's blocks and grids. The number of blocks and trials for each grid is indicated. Data from the blocks labelled 'training' were used to train the classifier. The last two blocks, labelled 'online', were BCI-supported

Experimental Design

The cursor as used in the study was a red circle, that could move from one node to any of the adjacent nodes in grids of varying size. These grids consisted of grey open circles, slightly larger than the cursor, connected by grey lines, on a black background. Depending on the cursor's position in the grid, then, there were up to eight possible movements.

An animation allowed the subjects to be able to anticipate the moment of each movement. As illustrated in Fig. 4.1 (top), over the course of one second, a white 'ghost cursor' would grow inside the actual cursor. As soon as this ghost reached the same size as the actual cursor, it would instantaneously jump to the next node, also highlighting the grid line connecting the two nodes in white. The movement remained visible for one second, with the red original cursor still on the initial node, the white ghost cursor on the new node, and a white line connecting them. Following that, the white elements disappeared and the (red) cursor would instantaneously move to and remain at its new position, on the new node, for another second, before the animation would start over for the next movement.

Three different grids were used in the study: One by three nodes, four by four, and six by six. In each grid, a single red node in one of the corners indicated the target. Whenever the cursor reached this target, a new grid was started of the same size. For the one by three grids, each new grid was rotated a random integer multiple of 45 degrees as compared to the previous grid. The four by four and six by six grids did not rotate, but a new target was selected for each new grid, such that no two subsequent grids had a target in the same corner. In all of these grids, the cursor's starting position was one node away from the opposite corner, in a straight line to the target. Each newly started grid was displayed for one second before the first movement was initiated.

Additionally, a new grid was started when a certain number of movements had been made without reaching the target. For the one by three grids, the maximum number of moves was one; for the four by four grids, the maximum was 55, which is one and a half times the mean number of random movements required to reach the target. No maximum other than the block's length (120) was set for the six by six grid.

With the one additional second added for the subjects to orient themselves after a new grid was started, a trial in the one by three grids took four seconds. In the other two grid sizes, a trial took three seconds.

Subjects, Setup, and Procedure

A total of sixteen subjects participated in this study, with an average age of 25.9 years ± 3.4. All had normal or corrected to normal vision.

After preparation and setting up the EEG cap, which took up to 1 h, subjects were seated comfortably in a padded chair in a dimly lit room. In writing, they were instructed to judge every individual movement of the cursor as either 'acceptable' or 'not acceptable' with respect to reaching the goal, and to indicate their verdict by pressing either 'v' or 'b', respectively, on a standard German layout computer keyboard using the same finger of one hand. This task was intended to keep the subjects focused on the cursor's movements. The subjects performed this task during all blocks.

EEG was recorded continuously using 64 Ag/AgCl electrodes mounted according to the extended 10–20 system on an elastic cap (Easy Cap, Falk Minow Services). The signal was sampled at 500 Hz and amplified using a 250 Hz high cutoff filter via Brain Amps (BrainProducts, Munich). All electrodes were referenced to FCz.

The experiment itself took about 1 h. As illustrated in Fig. 4.1 (bottom), subjects were first shown four blocks of 50 trials on a one by three grid, and following that, five blocks of 120 trials on a four by four grid. These latter five blocks were used to train the passive BCI classifier. This classifier was then used in two online blocks: One block of 120 trials on a four by four grid, and one block of 120 trials on a six by six grid.

Feature Extraction and Classification

Two groups of cursor movements were built to train the classifier. One group consisted of those movements that went directly towards the target ('correct' movements), and the other of those whose direction deviated 135 degrees or more from a straight line to the target ('incorrect' movements). Of all 600 trials in the four by four grids, this selection left between 162 and 217 (mean: 185.3) trials per subject for the classifier to be trained on.

Note that the subjects' judgements, indicated using button-presses, were ignored: Only a movement's angle with respect to the target determined its group.

The open-source toolbox BCILAB (Delorme et al. 2010 was used to define and implement the BCI. Features were extracted by the Windowed Means approach (Blankertz et al. 2011), which calculated the average amplitudes of eight sequential time windows of 50 ms each, starting at 300 ms after cursor movement. For this feature extraction, the data was first resampled at 100 Hz, and bandpass filtered from 0.1 to 15 Hz. Classification of these features was done through Linear Discriminant Analysis (Duda et al. 2001), regularised by Shrinkage (Blankertz et al. 2011).

A [5, 5]-times nested cross-validation (Duda et al. 2001) with margins of 5 was used to select the Shrinkage regularisation parameter, and to generate estimates of the model's online reliability, as reported below. A model was trained before the first online block, for each subject individually.

Implicit Control

In the two online blocks, the trained classifier was applied to all cursor movements without any knowledge of the angular difference to the target. Each new grid started with all directions having equal probabilities. If a movement was classified as 'correct', the probability of that movement's direction was increased, as well as, to a lesser extent, the probabilities of its two neighbouring directions. When a movement was classified as 'incorrect', these probabilities were reduced. The cursor did not undo incorrect movements or directly repeat correct movements, but merely altered the relevant probabilities for subsequent trials. Over time, then, this system was hypothesised to gradually "steer" the cursor more and more into the target's direction. This steering would be done on the basis of event-related potentials evoked by the subjects' judgement of the cursor's own, autonomous movements—*not* by any actual *intent* to steer the cursor.

Results

The average classification rate over all sixteen subjects, as estimated using the method described above, was 71 %, with a standard deviation of 7.6 percentage points. This indicates a substantial improvement over chance level, which is 50 % for a binary classifier as used here.

It is important to note that classifiers trained on cursor movements and cursor movements alone, outperformed classifiers that somehow took button presses into account. For example, a classifier trained to distinguish between trials where the subject pressed one or the other button, respectively, had a lower accuracy than a classifier trained to distinguish only between different cursor movements (e.g. deviating $<45°$ vs. $\geq 45°$ from a straight line to the target). This suggests that classification was, at least in part, performed on passive, implicit signals that differed from the subjects' conscious acts.

The performance of the cursor was operationalised as the average number of movements required to reach one target. For the BCI-supported performance, averages were calculated per subject over all 120 online trials of the respective grid size. Trials at the end of a block that did not contribute to reaching a target or hitting the maximum number of trials for that attempt, were discarded. The BCI-supported data was compared to an equal sample size of non-supported (random) performance measures over the same number of trials. A Wilcoxon rank-sum test revealed significant differences between non-supported performance (median = 27.6) and BCI-supported performance (median = 19.9) on both the four by four grid, $W = 171.5$, $z = 3.5$, $p < 0.001$, $r = 0.61$, and on the six by six grid (median = 76, unsupported, vs. 22.6, supported), $W = 123$, $z = 2.7$, $p < 0.01$, $r = 0.53$.

In summary, these results indicate that the classifier was reliably capable of differentiating between movements going towards, and away from the target, without itself knowing where the target was. When this information was used to adapt the cursor's behaviour, a marked improvement was seen in terms of cursor performance. This enabled the subjects to effectively guide the cursor towards the target, even though they were attending to a fundamentally different task.

Discussion and Conclusion

The main result of the theory and the experiment presented in this chapter is that implicit HCI incorporating information about the user state is indeed a realistic concept. The development of and experience with passive BCI provides tools which perfectly fit in this concept. Implicit control theoretically allows for a highly efficient way of interacting with technical systems, as it aims at distributing tasks between the machine and the user along their specific capabilities. In the best case, this distribution is optimal and both machine and human learn from one another during the interaction—their strategies converge efficiently.

The implicit approach might not always be the most effective way to solve a task. In the study presented here it is clear that a user focusing fully on the task and having standard explicit control would reach the target much faster. This is mostly a result of the fact that the scenario is very simple, the optimal strategy to reach the goal is obvious and an intuitive explicit control is easy to establish with eight direction keys. However, a more elaborate passive BCI approach could be applied in scenarios closer to real-world applications. One could envision an example, where a technical system is distributing tasks between a team of experts, i.e. airtraffic controllers in a tower, along their current level of workload or stress. In that scenario mistakes resulting from over- or under loading team members could be reduced. The interpretation of the passive BCI output would then be more complex but it should still be feasible for a computer system. Hence, implicit control might not be the most suitable way of interacting in every given HMS, but it could be for some and it defines a new and more intuitive interaction. This becomes particularly clear when we take into account that most of the systems we currently have available are designed for explicit control. Over several steps such systems could be enhanced by adding implicit control, i.e. for automated error correction during automated adaptation as described in Zander (2011). Future systems, directly designed for implicit control, might then reveal the full potential of this new type of HCI.

From the perspective of BCI research, the main advantage of passive BCI comes into play: Its independence of bitrate Zander (2011). As most BCI approaches, active and reactive, aim at realizing an interface for direct communication and control, but provide only a very limited reliability, they often do not succeed reaching their goal. Additionally, users have to spend a significant amount of effort to keep control and often perceive this as being frustrating Lorenz et al. 2013. With the statistical approach of implicit control based on passive BCI presented here, it is shown that even with a low accuracy of 70 % the system reaches its goal efficiently, and with no additional effort taken by the attentive user.

Nevertheless, from a usability perspective, there are still significant hurdles to be taken. Most realizations of BCIs based on Machine Learning, like the one presented here, need a time-consuming calibration phase. A significant number of prototypes of the features, in current BCI systems typically 40–80 per class, have to be generated to calibrate the BCI model. In currently available BCI frameworks, this has to be repeated before each session, which is time consuming and might be annoying for the user, both depending on the complexity of generating the investigated user state. In addition, the setup of an EEG system is cumbersome and time consuming, as usually several dozens of electrodes need to be gelled to the users head. Several solutions to these problems have been proposed and are currently being investigated. Universal classifiers (Zander 2011) or reduced-training BCIs (Krauledat et al. 2008) could reduce the calibration time to an acceptable level. The time needed for setting up an EEG system can be reduced by using dry electrodes (Zander 2011) and by reducing the number of electrodes by identifying which are the most relevant through applying methods from computational neuroscience. Nevertheless, due to the complex structure of the brain and to volume conduction, a significant number of electrodes will always be needed for a reliable BCI system.

Also, the application of BCIs outside the lab is still mostly uninvestigated. In standard experiments most environmental factors are strictly controlled. As this hardly is possible for real world environments, different approaches have to be investigated. One solution is to model the given HMS completely by incorporating contextual information about user, environment and the technical part. In this approach context-information would counterbalance the lack of control and support the information gain about of the user state (see Zander and Jatzev 2012).

As it is likely that there will be significant advances in solving the above mentioned problems in the near future, BCIs will become more practical and more useable. The theory presented here and the first proof of concept of implicit HCI can be seen as a starting point for a new type of research. It opens up a large variety of applications that need to be investigated in upcoming research endeavors. With passive BCIs a new horizon for HCI is defined, carrying the potential to significantly increase the intuitivity and efficiency of future computer systems.

References

Acqualagna L, Blankertz B (2011) A gaze independent spelling based on rapid serial visual presentation. In: Proceedings IEEE engineering medicine biology society conference, pp 4560–4563

Bai O, Lin P, Vorbach S, Floeter MK, Hattori N, Hallett M (2008) A high performance sensorimotor beta rhythm-based brain-computer interface associated with human natural motor behavior. J Neural Eng 5(1):24–35

Balderas D, Zander TO, Bachl F, Neuper C, Scherer R (2011) Restricted boltzmann machines as useful tool for detecting oscillatory EEG components. In: Proceedings of the 5th international brain-computer interface conference, Graz, pp 68–71

Beverina F, Palmas G, Silvoni S, Piccione F, Giove S (2003) User adaptive BCIs: SSVEP and P300 based interfaces. J Psych Nology 1:331–354

Bin G, Gao X, Yan Z, Hong B, Gao S (2009) An online multi-channel SSVEP-based brain-computer interface using a canonical correlation analysis method. J Neural Eng 6(4):046,002

Birbaumer N (2006) Breaking the silence: brain-computer interfaces (BCI) for communication and motor control. Psychophysiology 43(6):517–532

Birbaumer N, Cohen LG (2007) Brain-computer interfaces: communication and restoration of movement in paralysis. J Physiol 579(3):621–636

Birbaumer N, Elbert T, Canavan AG, Rockstroh B (1990) Slow potentials of the cerebral cortex and behavior. Physiol Rev 70(1):1–41

Birbaumer N, Ghanayim N, Hinterberger T, Iversen I, Kotchoubey B, Kübler A, Perelmouter J, Taub E, Flor H (1999) A spelling device for the paralysed. Nature 398(6725):297–298

Birbaumer N, Hinterberger T, Kübler A, Neumann N (2003) The thought-translation device (TTD): neurobehavioral mechanisms and clinical outcome. IEEE Trans Neural Syst Rehabil Eng 11(2):120–123

Blankertz B, Schäfer C, Dornhege G, Curio G (2002a) Single trial detection of EEG error potentials: a tool for increasing BCI transmission rates. In: Dorronsoro JR (ed) Artificial neural networks—ICANN 2002, vol 2415., Lecture notes in computer science Springer, Berlin, pp 1137–1143

Blankertz B, Schäfer C, Dornhege G, Curio G (2002b) Single trial detection of EEG error potentials: a tool for increasing BCI transmission rates. In: Artificial Neural Networks—ICANN 2002, Springer, pp 1137–1143

Blankertz B, Krauledat M, Dornhege G, Williamson J, Murray-Smith R, Müller KR (2007) A note on brain actuated spelling with the Berlin brain-computer interface. In: Stephanidis C (ed) Universal access in human-computer interaction, Lecture notes in computer science, vol 4557. Springer, pp 759–768

Blankertz B, Sannelli C, Halder S, Hammer E, Kübler A, Müller KR, Curio G, Dickhaus T (2010) Neurophysiological predictor of SMR-based BCI performance. NeuroImage 51(4):1303–1309

Blankertz B, Lemm S, Treder M, Haufe S, Müller KR (2011) Single-trial analysis and classification of ERP components—a tutorial. NeuroImage 56(2):814–825

Brouwer AM, van Erp J (2010) A tactile P300 brain-computer interface. Frontiers in Neuroscience 4(19):1–11

Canento F, Fred A, Silva H, Gamboa H, Lourenço A (2011) Multimodal biosignal sensor data handling for emotion recognition. In: Sensors, 2011 IEEE, pp 647–650

Coyle S, Ward T, Markham C, McDarby G (2004) On the suitability of near-infrared (NIR) systems for next-generation brain-computer interfaces. Physiol Meas 25(4):815–822

Daly JJ, Wolpaw JR (2008) Brain-computer interfaces in neurological rehabilitation. Lancet Neurol 7(11):1032–1043

Delorme A, Kothe C, Vankov A, Bigdely-Shamlo N, Oostenveld R, Zander TO, Makeig S (2010) MATLAB-based tools for BCI research. In: Tan DS, Nijholt A (eds) Brain-computer interfaces, human-computer interaction series, Springer, London, pp 241–259

Duda RO, Hart PE et al (1973) Pattern classification and scene analysis. Wiley, New York

Duda RO, Hart PE, Stork DG (2001) Pattern classification, 2nd edn. Wiley, New York

Fairclough SH (2008) BCI and physiological computing for computer games: differences, similarities and intuitive control. In: Proceedings of CHIGÇÖ08

Fairclough SH (2009) Fundamentals of physiological computing. Interact Comput 21(1):133–145

Fang F, Liu Y, Shen Z (2003) Lie detection with contingent negative variation. Int J Psychophysiol 50(3):247–255

Farwell LA, Donchin E (1988) Talking off the top of your head: toward a mental prosthesis utilizing event-related brain potentials. Electroencephalogr Clin Neurophysiol 70(6):510–523

Ferrez PW, Millán JdR (2008) Simultaneous real-time detection of motor imagery and error-related potentials for improved BCI accuracy. In: Proceedings of the 4th international brain-computer interface workshop and training course, pp 197–202

Furdea A, Halder S, Krusienski D, Bross D, Nijboer F, Birbaumer N, Kübler A (2009) An auditory oddball (P300) spelling system for brain-computer interfaces. Psychophysiology 46(3):617–625

Gangadhar G, Chavarriaga R, Millán JdR (2009) Fast recognition of anticipation-related potentials. IEEE Trans Biomed Eng 56(4):1257–1260

Gao X, Xu D, Cheng M, Gao M (2003) A BCI-based environmental controller for the motion-disabled. IEEE Trans Neural Syst Rehabil Eng 11(2):137–140

Grimes D, Tan DS, Hudson SE, Pradeep S, Rao RP (2008) Feasibility and pragmatics of classifying working memory load with an electroencephalograph. In: Czerwinski M (ed) Proceedings of the twenty-sixth annual SIGCHI conference on Human factors in computing systems. ACM, New York, pp 835–844

Guger C, Edlinger G, Harkam W, Niedermayer I, Pfurtscheller G (2003) How many people are able to operate an EEG-based brain-computer interface (BCI)? IEEE Trans Neural Syst Rehabil Eng 11(2):145–147 (a publication of the IEEE Eng Med Biol Soc)

Guger C, Daban S, Sellers E, Holzner C, Krausz G, Carabalona R, Gramatica F, Edlinger G (2009) How many people are able to control a P300-based brain-computer interface (BCI)? Neurosci Lett 462(1):94–98

Hajcak G, McDonald N, Simons RF (2003) To err is autonomic: error-related brain potentials, ANS activity, and post-error compensatory behavior. Psychophysiology 40(6):895–903

Hankins TC, Wilson GF (1998) A comparison of heart rate, eye activity, EEG and subjective measures of pilot mental workload during flight. Aviat Space Environ Med 69(4):360–367

Hill NJ, Schölkopf B (2012) An online brain-computer interface based on shifting attention to concurrent streams of auditory stimuli. J Neural Eng 9(2):026,011

Hinterberger T, Schmidt S, Neumann N, Mellinger J, Blankertz B, Curio G, Birbaumer N (2004) Brain-computer communication and slow cortical potentials. IEEE Trans Biomed Eng 51(6):1011–1018

Holroyd CB, Coles MGH (2002) The neural basis of human error processing: reinforcement learning, dopamine, and the error-related negativity. Psychol Rev 109(4):679–708

Jacob RJ, Leggett JJ, Myers BA, Pausch R (1993) Interaction styles and input/output devices. Behav Inf Technol 12(2):69–79

Kohlmorgen J, Dornhege G, Braun M, Blankertz B, Müller KR, Curio G, Hagemann K, Bruns A, Schrauf M, Kincses W (2007) Improving human performance in a real operating environment through real-time mental workload detection. In: Dornhege G, Millán JdR, Hinterberger T,

McFarland DJ, Müller KR (eds) Toward brain-computer interfacing, Neural information processing series, MIT Press, Cambridge, pp 409–422

Kothe CA, Makeig S (2013) BCILAB: a platform for brain-computer interface development. J Neural Eng 10(5):056,014

Krauledat M, Tangermann M, Blankertz B, Müller KR (2008) Towards zero training for brain-computer interfacing. PLoS one 3(8):e2967

Kübler A, Birbaumer N (2008) Brain-computer interfaces and communication in paralysis: extinction of goal directed thinking in completely paralysed patients? Clin Neurophysiol 119(11):2658–2666

Kübler A, Nijboer F, Mellinger J, Vaughan TM, Pawelzik H, Schalk G, McFarland DJ, Birbaumer N, Wolpaw JR (2005) Patients with ALS can use sensorimotor rhythms to operate a brain-computer interface. Neurology 64(10):1775–1777

Lal TN, Schröder M, Hill NJ, Preissl H, Hinterberger T, Mellinger J, Bogdan M, Rosenstiel W, Hofmann T, Birbaumer N, Schölkopf B (2005) A brain computer interface with online feedback based on magnetoencephalography. In: ICML '05 Proceedings of the 22nd international conference on machine learning, pp 465–472

Lazarus RS, Speisman JC, Mordkoff AM (1963) The relationship between autonomic indicators of psychological stress: heart rate and skin conductance. Psychosom Med 25(1):19–30

LeBlanc J, Blais B, Barabe B, Cote J (1976) Effects of temperature and wind on facial temperature, heart rate, and sensation. J Appl Physiol 40(2):127–131

Lee JH, Ryu J, Jolesz FA, Cho ZH, Yoo SS (2009) Brain-machine interface via real-time fMRI: preliminary study on thought-controlled robotic arm. Neurosci Lett 450(1):1–6

Lorenz R, Pascual J, Blankertz B, Vidaurre C (2013) Towards a holistic assessment of the user experience with hybrid BCIs. J Neural Eng (submitted)

Mak JN, Wolpaw J (2009) Clinical applications of brain-computer interfaces: current state and future prospects. IEEE Rev Biomed Eng 2:187–199

McFarland DJ, Wolpaw JR (2008) Brain-computer interface operation of robotic and prosthetic devices. Computer 41(10):52–56

McFarland DJ, Sarnacki WA, Wolpaw JR (2010) Electroencephalographic (EEG) control of three-dimensional movement. J Neural Eng 7(3):036,007

Mellinger J, Schalk G, Braun C, Preissl H, Rosenstiel W, Birbaumer N, Kübler A (2007) An MEG-based brain-computer interface (BCI). NeuroImage 36(3):581–593

Müller KR, Krauledat M, Dornhege G, Curio G, Blankertz B (2004) Machine learning techniques for brain-computer interfaces. Biomed Eng 49(1):11–22

Müller KR, Tangermann M, Dornhege G, Krauledat M, Curio G, Blankertz B (2008) Machine learning for real-time single-trial EEG-analysis: from brain-computer interfacing to mental state monitoring. J Neurosci Methods 167(1):82–90

Müller-Putz G, Scherer R, Neuper C, Pfurtscheller G (2006a) Steady-state somatosensory evoked potentials: suitable brain signals for brain-computer interfaces? IEEE Trans Neural Syst Rehabil Eng 14(1):30–37

Müller-Putz GR, Scherer R, Pfurtscheller G, Rupp R (2005) EEG-based neuroprosthesis control: a step towards clinical practice. Neurosci Lett 382(1–2):169–174

Müller-Putz GR, Scherer R, Pfurtscheller G, Rupp R (2006b) Brain-computer interfaces for control of neuroprostheses: from synchronous to asynchronous mode of operation. Biomed Tech 51(2):57–63

Nicolas-Alonso LF, Gomez-Gil J (2012) Brain computer interfaces, a review. Sensors 12(2):1211–1279

Nijboer F, Sellers EW, Mellinger J, Jordan MA, Matuz T, Furdea A, Halder S, Mochty U, Krusienski DJ, Vaughan TM, Wolpaw JR, Birbaumer N, Kübler A (2008) A P300-based brain-computer interface for people with amyotrophic lateral sclerosis. Clin Neurophysiol 119(8):1909–1916

Papadelis C, Chen Z, Kourtidou-Papadeli C, Bamidis PD, Chouvarda I, Bekiaris E, Maglaveras N (2007) Monitoring sleepiness with on-board electrophysiological recordings for preventing sleep-deprived traffic accidents. Clin Neurophysiol 118(9):1906–1922

Patel SH, Azzam PN (2005) Characterization of N200 and P300: selected studies of the event-related potential. Int J Med Sci p 147 2(4):147–154

Pfurtscheller G (1977) Graphical display and statistical evaluation of event-related desynchronization (ERD). Electroencephalogr Clin Neurophysiol 43(5):757–760

Pfurtscheller G (1992) Event-related synchronization (ERS): an electrophysiological correlate of cortical areas at rest. Electroencephalogr Clin Neurophysiol 83(1):62–69

Pfurtscheller G, Lopes da Silva FH (1999) Event-related EEG/MEG synchronization and desynchronization: basic principles. Clin Neurophysiol: Off J Int Fed Clin Neurophysiol 110(11):1842–1857

Pfurtscheller G, Guger C, Müller G, Krausz G, Neuper C (2000) Brain oscillations control hand orthosis in a tetraplegic. Neurosci Lett 292(3):211–214

Pfurtscheller G, Allison BZ, Brunner C, Bauernfeind G, Solis-Escalante T, Scherer R, Zander T, Müller-Putz G, Neuper C, Bierbaumer N (2010) The hybrid BCI. Front Neurosci 4(30):1–11

Picard RW (1999) Affective computing for HCI. In: Human computer interaction, vol 1. pp 829–833

Protzak J, Ihme K, Zander TO (2013) A passive brain-computer interface for supporting gaze-based human-machine interaction. In: Universal access in human-computer interaction. Design methods, tools, and interaction techniques for e inclusion, Springer, pp 662–671

Renard Y, Lotte F, Gibert G, Congedo M, Maby E, Delannoy V, Bertrand O, Lécuyer A (2010) Openvibe: an open-source software platform to design, test, and use brain-computer interfaces in real and virtual environments. Presence: Teleoper Virtual Environ 19(1):35–53

Reuderink B, Farquhar J, Poel M, Nijholt A (2011) A subject-independent brain-computer interface based on smoothed, second-order base lining. In: Engineering in medicine and biology society, EMBC, 2011 annual international conference of the IEEE, pp 4600–4604

Riccio A, Mattia D, Simione L, Olivetti M, Cincotti F (2012) Eye-gaze independent EEG-based brain-computer interfaces for communication. J Neural Eng 9(4):045,001

Rivera K, Cooke NJ, Bauhs JA (1996) The effects of emotional icons on remote communication. In: Conference companion on human factors in computing systems, ACM, pp 99–100

Rötting M, Zander T, Trösterer S, Dzaack J (2009) Implicit interaction in multimodal human-machine systems. In: Industrial engineering and ergonomics, Springer, pp 523–536

Schalk G, McFarland DJ, Hinterberger T, Birbaumer N, Wolpaw JR (2004) BCI2000: a general-purpose brain-computer interface (BCI) system. IEEE Trans Biomed Eng 51(6):1034–1043

Schmidt A (2000) Implicit human computer interaction through context. Pers Technol 4(2–3):191–199

Schmidt NM, Blankertz B, Treder MS (2012) Online detection of error-related potentials boosts the performance of mental typewriters. BMC Neurosci 13(1):19

Schöllkopf B, Smola AJ (2002) Learning with kernels: support vector machines, regularization, optimization, and beyond. The MIT Press, Cambridge

Schreuder M, Rost T, Tangermann M (2011) Listen, you are writing! Speeding up online spelling with a dynamic auditory BCI. Front Neurosci 5

Sellers EW, Donchin E (2006) A P300-based brain-computer interface: initial tests by ALS patients. Clin Neurophysiol 117(3):538–548

Shi Y, Ruiz N, Taib R, Choi E, Chen F (2007) Galvanic skin response (GSR) as an index of cognitive load. In: CHI'07 extended abstracts on human factors in computing systems, ACM, pp 2651–2656

Squire P, Parasuraman R (2010) Effects of automation and task load on task switching during human supervision of multiple semi-autonomous robots in a dynamic environment. Ergonomics 53(8):951–961

Tavella M, Leeb R, Rupp R, Millán JdR (2010) Towards natural non-invasive hand neuroprostheses for daily living. In: Proceedings IEEE engineering in medicine biology society conference, pp 126–129

Treder MS, Blankertz B (2010) (C)overt attention and visual speller design in an ERP-based brain-computer interface. Behav Brain Funct 6(1):28

Treder MS, Schmidt NM, Blankertz B (2011) Gaze-independent brain-computer interfaces based on covert attention and feature attention. J Neural Eng 8(6):066,003

Van Schie HT, Mars RB, Coles MG, Bekkering H (2004) Modulation of activity in medial frontal and motor cortices during error observation. Nat Neurosci 7(5):549–554

Vapnik VN, Chervonenkis AY (1971) On the uniform convergence of relative frequencies of events to their probabilities. Theory Probab Appl 16(2):264–280

Vidal JJ (1973) Toward direct brain-computer communication. Annu Rev Biophys Bioeng 2(1):157–180

Vidal JJ (1977) Real-time detection of brain events in EEG. Proc IEEE 65(5):633–641

Vilimek R, Zander TO (2009) BC (eye): combining eye-gaze input with brain-computer interaction. Universal access in human-computer interaction. Springer, Intelligent and Ubiquitous Interaction Environments, pp 593–602

Weiskopf N, Veit R, Erb M, Mathiak K, Grodd W, Goebel R, Birbaumer N (2003) Physiological self-regulation of regional brain activity using real-time functional magnetic resonance imaging (fMRI): methodology and exemplary data. NeuroImage 19(3):577–586

Whitworth B (2005) Polite computing. Behav Inf Technol 24(5):353–363

Wolpaw JR (2004) Control of a two-dimensional movement signal by a noninvasive brain-computer interface in humans. In: Proceedings of the national academy of sciences 101(51):17,849-17,854

Wolpaw JR, McFarland D, Vaughan T (2000) Brain-computer interface research at the Wadsworth Center. IEEE Trans Rehabil Eng 8(2):222–226

Wolpaw JR, Birbaumer N, McFarland DJ, Pfurtscheller G, Vaughan TM (2002) Brain-computer interfaces for communication and control. Clin Neurophysiol 113(6):767–791

Zander TO (2011) Utilizing brain-computer interfaces for human-machine systems. PhD thesis, Universitätsbibliothek TU, Berlin

Zander TO, Jatzev S (2012) Context-aware brain-computer interfaces: exploring the information space of user, technical system and environment. J Neural Eng 9(1):016,003

Zander TO, Kothe C (2011) Towards passive brain-computer interfaces: applying brain-computer interface technology to human-machine systems in general. J Neural Eng 8(2):025,005

Zander TO, Gaertner M, Kothe C, Vilimek R (2010a) Combining eye gaze input with a brain-computer interface for touchless human-computer interaction. Int J Human Comput Inter 27(1):38–51

Zander TO, Kothe C, Jatzev S, Gaertner M (2010b) Enhancing human-computer interaction with input from active and passive brain-computer interfaces. In: Tan DS, Nijholt A (eds) Brain-computer interfaces: applying our minds to human-computer interaction. Human-Computer Interaction Series, Springer, pp 181–199

Zander TO, Ihme K, Gärtner M, Rötting M (2011) A public data hub for benchmarking common brain-computer interface algorithms. J Neural Eng 8(2):025,021

Chapter 5
Biocybernetic Adaptation as Biofeedback Training Method

Alan T. Pope, Chad L. Stephens and Kiel Gilleade

Abstract A method developed for adapting an automated flight control system to user state has been applied to the process of biofeedback training. This repurposing enables alternative mechanisms for delivering physiological information feedback to the trainee via a method referred to as physiological modulation. These mechanisms employ reinforcement principles to motivate adherence to the biofeedback training regime, to foster interactions among users and to enhance the experience of immersion in video game entertainment. The approach has implications for a broader dissemination of biofeedback training. This chapter will introduce the traditional biofeedback training method and its clinical applications, followed by a discussion of how biocybernetic adaptation can be applied to the biofeedback training method. This will be followed by a description of different methods of realising this self-regulation technology and where the technology may go in the future.

Background

It has not been widely appreciated outside the relatively obscure field of psychophysiology that humans, given sufficiently informative feedback about their own physiological processes, have both the capacity and inherent inclination to

A. T. Pope (✉) · C. L. Stephens
NASA Langley Research Center, Hampton, VA 23681, USA
e-mail: alan.t.pope@nasa.gov

C. L. Stephens
e-mail: chad.l.stephens@nasa.gov

K. Gilleade
School of Natural Sciences and Psychology, Liverpool John Moores University, Liverpool, UK
e-mail: gilleade@gmail.com

S. H. Fairclough and K. Gilleade (eds.), *Advances in Physiological Computing*,
Human–Computer Interaction Series, DOI: 10.1007/978-1-4471-6392-3_5,
© Springer-Verlag London 2014

learn to regulate those processes. This phenomenon has, however, been established conclusively in numerous biofeedback training applications across a range of different biological functions, including the training of brain electrical activity and of autonomic responses (Yucha and Montgomery 2008).

Therapeutic conditioning of autonomic and brainwave signals, now well established, was considered to be fantasy no more than five decades ago. The discovery of the human capacity for physiological self-regulation awaited the inventiveness of pioneers, who, in a bold empowering stroke, displayed physiological signals, previously scrutinized only by the researcher, back to the subjects whose signals they were, with the aim of giving the subjects control of these processes. This innovation began the discovery process that has demonstrated that, given the right information about their bodily processes in the right form, people can exert impressive control over those responses.

Early work by Hefferline et al. (1959) demonstrated that, in a traditional psychological reinforcement paradigm, covert physiological responses could be conditioned by attaching consequences to their production without the trainee's conscious and deliberate effort to control them. Many biofeedback training successes do indeed operate without the necessity for the trainee to be able to articulate the exact nature of the efforts they employ in the learning process, and sometimes without them even trying to consciously control the process.

The earliest of the biofeedback pioneers, Kamiya (1971, pp. ix–xvi), specified the requirements for the biofeedback training technique and these have not changed substantially: (1) the targeted physiological function must be monitored in real-time; (2) information about the function must be presented to the trainee so that the trainee perceives changes in the parameter immediately; and (3) the feedback information should also serve to motivate the trainee to attend to the training task. Many of the information delivery methods presented in this chapter are specifically designed to motivate trainees to apply themselves to the learning task.

The Biofeedback and Biocybernetic Loops

A biofeedback system is an example of a closed-loop feedback system. While environmental and engineering feedback control systems regulate physical variables, biofeedback systems take advantage of knowledge-of-results and immediate reinforcement effects to facilitate learning of voluntary physiological self-regulation.

The terms *biofeedback* loop and *biocybernetic adaptation* loop are often used interchangeably; however, it may be useful to draw some distinctions between them. "Biofeedback loop" may be thought of as a general term referring simply to the return of a biological signal to a point in the system from which it originates, thereby closing a loop. There are multiple possible purposes for closing the biological loop. The human body has its own purposes for its myriad internal loops; the synthetic ones that are created by superimposing an external feedback path can be applied to several ends (Stephens et al. 2012; Mulholland 1977).

"Biocybernetic adaptation" is one particular application of the biofeedback loop; employing the "steering" sense of the term "cybernetic", such systems serve a transitory adaptive purpose that makes use of an assessment of transient state to steer a functional aspect of a system that is external to the physiology from which the state assessment is derived. An early example of biocybernetic adaptation was developed by Pope et al. (1995) for use in an automated flight control system. A pilot's level of task engagement was assessed using continuous brainwave activity, which in turn was used to set the status of the auto-pilot. This can be readily applied to videogames, whereby physiological signals can be used to infer relevant mental states to adapt game difficulty to a more desirable level (Pope and Bogart 1994; Palsson et al. 2002). For example in Fairclough and Gilleade (2012), brainwave activity was used to model the player's level of motivation and workload during a game of Tetris. The game used this to adapt the game difficulty so the player was challenged but not overly so.

Of course, biofeedback training also intends to steer, but with a focus on another point in the loop, i.e., to steer a trainee's physiology to a more or less enduring state or to an improved ability to self-regulate state as a consequence of adapting. For clarity in communication, it can be useful to make explicit whether one is referring to the term "biofeedback" simply in the sense of signal loop configuration versus in combination with the term "training" or "therapy" as a physiological self-regulation training process with enduring effects. The enduring effects of training can be both changed physiological functioning and improved self-regulation skill.

One embodiment of biocybernetic adaptation is a central theme of this chapter: a human-computer interaction system designed such that physiological signals modulate the effect that control of a task by other means, usually manual control, has on performance of the task. Physiological modulation technologies designed for self-regulation training merge the previously described processes of adapting a system on the one hand, and reinforcing a physiological response on the other, by having physiological changes toward a training target cause changes in the functioning of an external system—changes that are intended to be rewarding to the trainee. The information feedback in this biofeedback training configuration is implicit in the functioning of the external system rather than explicit in a physiological signal display.

Efficacy of Clinical Biofeedback Training

Biofeedback training has been demonstrated for over three decades of clinical experience and research to be effective in the treatment of various physiological and psychological problems and can be used to optimize physiological functioning in many ways. Traditionally, biofeedback training consists of placing sensors on the body to measure biological activity, and showing patients on a computer screen (typically in the form of dynamic graphs) what is going on inside their bodies.

When patients are made aware of the moment-to-moment changes in their physiological activity, they can learn over time to control various body functions that are usually outside of conscious control, such as heart rate, muscle tension or blood flow in the skin. In brainwave based biofeedback training, or neurofeedback training, training systems provide real-time information to trainees showing them how well they are producing brainwave patterns that match a criterion pattern. A common format of neurofeedback training focuses on training people to change the functioning of their brain by showing them the strength of different brainwave frequency bands, and encouraging them to systematically make some brainwave frequencies stronger and others weaker. Success at producing the desired changes in brain activity has been reported to improve sustained attention, concentration and academic performance (Lubar 1991; Monastra 2005). In a recent white paper (Pigott et al. 2013), studies were cited that reported more lasting effects with neurofeedback training as compared with traditional behavior therapy and stimulant medication. A recent structural magnetic resonance imaging (MRI) study demonstrated that neurofeedback training to enhance beta1 brainwaves (12–16 Hz), resulting in improvement in attentional performance, can also lead to microstructural changes in white and gray matter (Ghaziri et al. 2013).

Biofeedback training has been used with considerable success in the treatment of various health problems, such as migraine headaches, hypertension, and muscle aches and pains. In a recent review by Yucha and Montgomery (2008), the clinical efficacy of biofeedback training practices for 44 disorders was rated based upon the strength of current research studies. Training practices were rated on a 5 point scale of 'efficacious and specific', 'efficacious,' 'probably efficacious,' 'possibly efficacious,' and 'not empirically supported'. Training programs without peer reviewed work are considered to be "not empirically supported" at the current time. For a training practice to be rated 'possibly efficacious', there must be at least one study demonstrating a statistically significant outcome on a relevant measure with a 'probably efficacious' rating requiring multiple observations of this outcome and replicable results. For a practice to obtain an 'efficacious' rating, randomized comparisons against no-treatment control groups, alternate treatments, and placebos are required, which the biofeedback treatment needs to demonstrate a similar or superior effect. The highest rating for a biofeedback training practice can only be obtained if the treatment is found to be the superior treatment in at least two independent research settings. As can be seen in Table 5.1, which provides an overview of the 44 disorders rankings, there are a number of evidence-based biofeedback practices including treatments for headaches, hypertension, motion sickness, attention deficit disorder and urinary incontinence, however there are many more disorders which do not have a sufficient evidence base to support the use of biofeedback training at the current time.

Certain human physiological states are associated with the optimal performance of certain activities and behaviors. Biofeedback training directed to self-regulating such physiological states seeks to optimize the performance of their associated actions and behaviors, thereby facilitating mastery in action. For example, a self-induced reduction of an elevated heart rate and blood pressure, a rise typically

Table 5.1 Efficacy rating of biofeedback therapies (Yucha and Montgomery 2008)

Rating	Number	Disorders
Not empirically supported	5	Eating disorders, immune function, spinal cord injury, syncope, emerging applications (e.g. stuttering)
Possibly efficacious	18	Asthma, autism, bell's palsy, cerebral palsy, chronic obstructive pulmonary disease, coronary artery disease, cystic fibrosis, depressive disorder, erectile dysfunction, fibromyalgia, hand dystonia, irritable bowel syndrome, post-traumatic stress disorder, repetitive strain injury, respiratory failure, stroke, tinnitus, urinary incontinence in children
Probably efficacious	11	Alcoholism, arthritis, diabetes, fecal disorders in children and adults, constipation, headache (children), insomnia, traumatic brain injury, urinary incontinence in males, vulvodynia
Efficacious	9	Anxiety, arthritis, attention deficit disorder, chronic pain, epilepsy, headache (adult), hypertension, motion sickness, Raynaud's disease, temporomandibular disorder
Efficacious and specific	1	Urinary incontinence in females

associated with anxiety, may be expected to move a person into a state of superior focus with respect to a challenge and its resolution—a state that is better suited for victory over an opponent in real or simulated combat or completion of a real or simulated task (Edmonds and Tenenbaum 2011). Studies have demonstrated the efficacy of biofeedback training for performance enhancement in a variety of pursuits (Gruzelier and Egner 2005).

Origin of the Physiological Modulation Training Method

Although scientific research has shown biofeedback training to be an effective form of medical treatment for several disorders, some aspects of this treatment have made it less widely used than it otherwise could be: biofeedback training tends to be tedious, the treatment requires numerous sessions, it can be difficult to learn in the first place, and it is an expensive treatment (as it typically requires several visits to a specialized clinic). Biofeedback training, as commonly implemented, is not optimally suited for treating disorders and problems, especially outside the clinical setting, as it has typically been utilized in a way which is too technical, cumbersome and unappealing for individuals to apply on their own.

Non-adherence to the training regimen often undermines biofeedback treatment. Physiologically *driven* video games are specifically designed to overcome this drawback, incorporating engaging graphics and animation to promote adherence to training practice through entertainment appeal. Examples of this type of physiologically based game are CalmPrix (Calmpute 1984), and, more recently, Zukor's Grind (2010) and Space Investor (Hilborn et al. 2013). Prior to physiologically driven video games, biofeedback systems delivered training in bland and minimally motivating task formats. State-of-the-art commercial biofeedback training systems often incorporate game-like graphics that are driven directly with a physiological signal. In contrast, another biofeedback training delivery method, physiologically *modulated* videogames, fully integrates biofeedback training into a truly dynamic video game. It differs from conventional biofeedback training in that the feedback and reward are not explicit on a display, but implicit in the influence of the player's physiological signal on the game scenario or the player's intentional inputs.

The concept of physiological modulation (Pope and Bogart 1994; Palsson et al. 2002) evolved from a physiologically adaptive simulator system that was developed in flight deck research at NASA Langley Research Center (LaRC) studying mental engagement in flight tasks. One of the objectives of a closed-loop biocybernetic method was as an assessment procedure to determine the requirements for operator involvement that promote effective operator awareness states (Pope et al. 1995). In this system, EEG signals of pilots controlled the level of automation in a simulator flight deck. In effect, a feedback control process is implemented wherein stable task engagement, reflected in stable short cycle oscillation of an engagement index, is eventually achieved after systematic adjustment of task demand for operator participation. This testing setup was used to determine what level of automation kept pilots engaged optimally according to this particular criterion of mental engagement derived from brain electrical activity. Testing with the system revealed that, given enough practice, pilots may learn how to deliberately control subtask allocation to the level at which they prefer to work by regulating their EEG. The assessment procedure then functions as a training protocol in that the subject is rewarded for producing the EEG pattern that reflects increasing attention level by having the automated system share more of the work. If the flight simulator is replaced with a video game, the system becomes an engaging way to deliver biofeedback training. As Gilleade et al. (2005) note, "…if through practice, the player becomes proficient in controlling their natural physiological responses; the awareness of volitional control makes the game become a biofeedback game once again." However, this process differs from conventional biofeedback training in that the feedback and reward are not explicit on a display, but implicit in the influence of the subject's EEG on the task's mode of operation. With this method, biofeedback training happens in the background as a person plays the games, and therefore does not become onerous or boring. For example, a neurofeedback training game developed by Palsson et al. (2002) used physiological signals representative of attention to modulate the responsiveness of a conventional game controller. The less attentive players are, the less control they have over the game. The aim of the training program is to improve the player's self-regulation of their attention, and thereby increase their level of concentration. This is achieved by implicitly rewarding players with a better game experience, through more responsive controls, when they self-regulate the desired physiological signals. In this way, physiological modulation integrates physiological self-regulation synergistically with the manual mode of control input. Specific physiological changes are thereby reinforced by success at playing the video game without the requirement for explicit feedback.

The distinction between *driven* and *modulated* here is analogous to the distinction between "brain-computer interfaces primarily intended to support the *control* of computer-based systems using neural signals" (Hettinger et al. 2003, p. 10, emphasis added) and those in "which the system modifies the availability and/or presentation of information to the user as well as the *nature and extent of the control* that the user can exert on the system" (Hettinger et al., p. 6, emphasis added). This latter function may be thought of as physiologically based modulation of the control that the operator is deliberately exerting by other means. This distinction between modulation and control characterizes the biocybernetic paradigm employed in adaptive automation work at NASA Langley Research Center and Old Dominion University (Freeman et al. 2000; Pope et al. 1995; Prinzel et al. 2000). This difference parallels the distinction made by Fairclough (Fairclough et al. 2013; Fairclough 2008) between intentional brain-computer interface (BCI) operation and the biocybernetic adaptation paradigm that is based on spontaneous operator functional state.

The video game format motivates trainees to participate in and adhere to the training process. One effective use of the physiologically modulated game concept is to augment current biofeedback training techniques by providing a rewarding environment in which trainees can demonstrate and improve skills learned in conventional training. The modulated video game training technology transforms an arduous training regimen into game playing time. The popular pastime of playing video games, considered a "social evil" by some, becomes an opportunity for developing valuable mental skills. Physiologically modulated video game technology was created in an effort to find a way for biofeedback training to overcome obstacles to its usefulness, so that it can become more widely used, easier to apply for training, and more appealing to the people it can help. Additionally, physiologically modulated game technology has the potential to enhance the video game playing experience itself. Rani et al. (2005) showed that players' skills improve more and they have a more enjoyable experience when the level of a simulation's challenge is adapted to their affective or mental state rather than their performance.

While biofeedback has been found efficacious for certain treatments, whether particular presentation formats are better in terms of improved outcome measures such as training time and patient retention than other traditional formats, is a question that has yet to be answered, being an area still in its infancy (Knox et al. 2011). In a recent study by Mandryk et al. (2013), physiologically modulated games were found to be capable of maintaining patient motivation in children with fetal alcohol spectrum disorder. Using off-the-shelf videogames, this system modulated a texture-based graphical overlay according to player physiology. At the end of a 12 week treatment course, patients indicated they were still motivated by the game to take part in the training program. However as the study did not use a control for patient motivation, e.g., traditional biofeedback training, it is difficult to judge the impact of physiological modulation. At the present time there is limited evidence (Palsson et al. 2001) that games actually improve adherence by comparison to traditional formats; as a new technology it will take some time before there is enough evidence available to answer this question.

Reinforcement Principles in Biofeedback Training Games

The physiologically modulated video game training method teaches video game players to incorporate autonomic or brainwave physiological self-regulation into video game playing without the need for undivided attention to the self-regulation effort. The method operates through a two-step mechanism of instrumental learning and classic conditioning. Through the player's effort and inherent motivation to master the game task, and through repeated associations in accordance with established psychological learning principles, the healthy changes can generalize to other life situations.

In one embodiment of physiological game modulation (Palsson et al. 2002), the training program explicitly sets up brainwave performance criteria, in addition to the usual hand-eye coordination criteria, for success in playing a video game. For producing particular brainwave patterns, the player is explicitly rewarded by improved capability and performance in playing the game. As a consequence, production of these brainwave patterns is reinforced; that is, the patterns are more likely to occur as the game progresses. A study with this technology (Palsson et al. 2001) showed that both the physiologically modulated game and standard neurofeedback treatments improved the functioning of children with attention deficit hyperactivity disorder (ADHD) substantially over and above the benefits of medication. Use of the video game technology provided advantages over standard neurofeedback treatment in terms of enjoyability for the children and positive parent perception, resulting in lower attrition from treatment. Trends on pre-post quantitative EEG change maps indicated that the video game training may have advantages in creating more quantitative EEG effect in the therapeutic direction. DeBeus et al. (2004) used the physiological game modulation method as the experimental treatment and unmodulated video game playing as a control in a crossover study design and demonstrated reduction of ADHD symptoms with the treatment.

The reinforcement principle involved in this process is known as the Premack prepotent principle, which is stated: "A high probability behavior may be used as the reinforcer for a low probability behavior" (Premack 1965). A high probability behavior may be understood as that activity in which an individual will engage in the given situation, if unconstrained (for example, video game playing.) The "low probability behavior" in this case is production of non-ADHD brainwave patterns. Whether the training produces lasting changes in brainwave activity, and/or improvements in the trainee's ability to recruit these changes when needed, are questions for further research. In a recent white paper, Pigott et al. (2013), investigating the cost-effectiveness of neurofeedback interventions in the treatment of ADHD, identified several promising studies which indicated the carry over effect from training was still measurable two years later.

Implementing Reinforcement Principles

In some implementations, the degree of improvement in the ability to succeed in the video game may be programmed to be inversely proportional to the difference between the player's current momentary physiological signal value or pattern and a pre-selected target value or pattern for the physiological signal. In this way, the player is rewarded for diminishing this difference by an improved ability in controlling the game; this may be termed a physiologically modulated advantage. For example in a racing game, the accelerator might be described as a function of target brainwave activity, therefore the nearer the player's brainwaves are to the target state, the faster the racer will go.

Some game consequences may be set up to reward the player for achieving a psychophysiological goal by diminishing an undesirable effect in the game (analogous to negative reinforcement). Other game consequences may reward the player for achieving a psychophysiological goal by producing a desirable effect (analogous to positive reinforcement) such as additional scoring opportunities. That is, some modulation effects may enable superimposed disadvantages in a digital game or simulation to be reduced by physiological modulation, whereas others enable advantages to be effected through physiological modulation.

Target values of physiological functions are desirable values of physiological functions representing a goal required of a user. Target values may be artificially defined or may be defined on the basis of a baselining procedure for an individual competitor. That is, an individual's physiological performance during a game can be referenced to that individual's baseline physiological performance during a baseline period of interaction in the game when no influence based upon physiological signals is being applied to the game. Baseline performance statistics of central tendency (e.g., mean) and of variability (e.g., standard deviation) are computed. A target physiological state occurs and is rewarded if the measured values of physiological functions indicating or defining the physiological state are within a predefined degree of statistical variability from a statistical measure of central tendency from target values. An individual's physiological performance baseline may be recalibrated at selected points during the participant's game-playing career.

Longer Term Adaptation During Training

The ability to self-regulate physiological state emerges and develops over time with exposure to reinforcement contingencies that encourage that ability. Beginning with the introduction of a computer-assisted training system (Pope and Gersten 1977), technology in the field of biofeedback training has commonly taken into account the fact that the physiological self-regulation behavior of the trainee changes as training progresses. These systems have incorporated algorithms that responded to momentary, transient changes in physiological signals in real time, but also to longer time course measurements that reflected a trainee's emerging ability to voluntarily control physiological parameters. The momentary changes are displayed as information and reward feedback for learning of self-regulation skill, while the longer time course measurements are assessed to guide the setting of higher and higher self-regulation performance goals.

In early systems incorporating this adaptation over the long term, feedback gain (sensitivity) was periodically adjusted along with changes made in the within-session training sequence (Pope and Gersten 1977), or the threshold for the next trial was automatically readjusted based on the performance of the client during the previous trial (Applied Psychophysiology Institutes 1988). A current system employs a fuzzy logic system for autothresholding, issuing rewards (improvement in game play and/or auditory feedback) whenever there is movement in the desired direction of the protocol in place, rather than in excess of a static threshold value as in most neurofeedback training systems (Cyberlearning LLC 2004, p. 9).

Calibration is an issue in setting up biofeedback training systems. In therapeutic environments, manual calibration of reward thresholds to an individual's physiology is common. This requires time and can be problematic in maintaining the patient's motivation over multiple sessions. In Lansbergen et al. (2011), a neurofeedback based system designed for ADHD was trialed with automatic reward thresholds in order to effectively compare the treatment against a sham neurofeedback intervention i.e., automatic rewards are easier to mask in randomized trials from all parties involved. While successful, the researchers noted that this method may not be suited for treatment as questions remain whether automatic thresholds can outperform manually adjusted ones.

O'Shea and Sleeman (1973) developed a conceptual framework useful for considering teaching systems that, in addition to being adaptive, are self-improving. A training strategy implies a set of assertions relating strategy characteristics and their effects on training progress. A database of these assertions could be updated on-line and the training system would be self-improving. In effect, the system evaluates the results of mini-experiments with various strategy versions within a session and modifies the strategy accordingly (Pope and Gersten 1977, p. 168).

There are various ways in which a biofeedback reinforcement paradigm can be implemented. In the following section we will describe a range of different physiological modulation formats. In the first part of this section we will focus on the original physiological modulation concept, developed from the flight management system, for the treatment of ADHD and the spin-offs of this technology in arenas such as motion games. In the second part we will describe adaptations of this technology in multiplayer environments and how biofeedback loops can be combined with traditional control loops to create more adaptable training environments. We conclude this chapter with a discussion of future uses of physiological modulation technologies.

Physiological Modulation Game Concepts

Biocybernetic adaptation as applied to biofeedback training through physiological modulation has shown promise in improving treatment outcomes however the technology is still at a nascent stage and it will be some time before an evidence base becomes available to draw conclusions from its application. In the following section we will present a range of different methods of applying physiological modulation to biofeedback training games both for singular and multiplayer environments.

Physiological Modulation of Gameplay

An early embodiment of the physiological modulation concept was implemented in game software in a "space battle" scenario (Pope and Bogart 1994, 1996). In this modulated prototype, a "difficulty adjuster" is programmed to vary according to an electroencephalogram (EEG) band power ratio, termed an "engagement index". Modulation of difficulty in this game takes the form of changes in elements of the game's scenario, e.g., number or evasiveness of targets. In this way, the player is encouraged to maintain high levels of the ratio index in order to successfully master the challenge.

Changes in the scenario elements can be programmed to challenge or assist (Gilleade et al. 2005), according to the player's preference; it may be more rewarding to some players for difficulty or challenge to increase with improved physiological performance, while others would choose a decreasing difficulty contingency. This approach had the disadvantage of requiring extensive reprogramming of a video game, or the complete construction of an entire new video game in order to implement the modulation concept, while another approach (Palsson et al. 2002) enables the use of off-the-shelf games by modulating game controller signals prior to the control input being used by the computer simulation or game software. The result is that the magnitude of the effect of the game or simulation's input device (e.g., joystick, game pad, steering wheel) is modulated by the strength of the physiological signal(s). These two methods differ in that the first modulates aspects of the game scenario itself, whereas the second modulates the effect that the player's inputs have on the game; however, both afford the opportunity to motivate adherence to training. The controller modulation approach is limited in that the best functionality that a player can be provided is normal operation of the controller, i.e., reward is always provided by diminishing an undesirable effect, impaired functionality of the controller, as described above in "Implementing reinforcement principles." The scenario modulation approach has the advantage that the reinforcement contingency may be tailored to the player's reward preference: positive reinforcement by adding challenge for expert players or negative reinforcement by lessening difficulty for novices.

Another physiologically modulated technology that turns off-the-shelf computer games into biofeedback training games is that of Mandryk et al. (2013). This technology uses texture-based graphical overlays that vary in their obfuscation of underlying screen elements based on the sensed physiological state of the player.

Physiological Modulation of Control Input

Physiologically-modulated game controllers respond to physiological signals as well as to manual input; they embody the concept of rewarding specific body signals with success at playing a video game. The initial implementation of this method (Pope and Bogart 1994, 1996) used physiological signals (e.g., electro-encephalogram frequency band strengths) not simply to drive a display directly, or periodically modify a task as in other biofeedback systems, but to continuously modulate parameters (e.g., game character speed and mobility) of a game task in real time while the game task was being performed by other means (e.g., a game controller). The initial input modulation implementation at NASA LaRC used physiological signals to modulate the manual inputs a player makes to the buttons or joysticks of a traditional video game hand controller, for example, the Play-Station 2 controller (Pope and Bogart 1994; Palsson et al. 2002; Weising 2011).

Physiologically Modulated Control With Motion-Sensing Controllers

In recent years, motion has been introduced as an input to commercial video-games. Released in 2006, the default game controller for Nintendo Wii™ was capable of tracking the player's hand motions and translating them into an equivalent game input. This offered an interesting avenue for exploration with the input modulation developed for traditional controllers, requiring an entirely new technical implementation to integrate psychophysiological signals into game play. To the extent that motion-sensing videogame controllers accurately translate a player's movements into realistic game actions, the player is rewarded for imitating a skilled performer's overt motor behavior. Similarly, physiologically-modulated videogame controllers can additionally challenge the player to experience the expert performer's emotional and cognitive state by setting as a target the psychophysiological responses experienced by the expert in the real-world situation. Prototypes of one design (Pope et al. 2012; Neilson et al. 2013; Balconi-Lamica et al. 2012) enhance the challenge of various games by physiologically modulated attenuation (motion-control dampening) and/or disruption (cursor control perturbation).

Intuitive Mapping With Physiologically Modulated Controllers

The Wii™-based prototypes translate exaggerated effects of the physiological concomitants of emotion and cognition into game play. In one game example, an autonomic concomitant of nervousness, heart rate, is translated into modulated disruption of control of a surgical instrument. A simulated nervous unsteadiness, proportional in degree to the heart rate value's departure from a target expert performer's level, is superimposed on the intentional movement of the manually controlled game object. The exaggeration of effect, superimposed on manual control, is an intuitive way of simulating the effect of nervousness on motor behavior that would not otherwise be experienced in the game situation, at least not to the degree that it would be experienced in the real situation. These modulation influences can simulate the amplification of nervousness when performing a task under pressure.

Early biofeedback training displays that delivered information in the form of simple graphs employed intuitive mapping of signal changes to display changes. For example, if peripheral temperature was being monitored and the trainee was told that hand warming was the goal, a line scrolling on a graph could be designed to rise with temperature increase; if the training goal was specified as relaxation, a line could be designed to fall with temperature increase, indicating a "calming down." Similarly, muscle tension feedback for relaxation usually involved a line that fell with electromyographic (EMG) signal decrease. Intuitive mapping also appears in the functional magnetic resonance imaging (fMRI) feedback technology of deCharms et al. (2005), where a pain brain signal is represented by a graphically rendered flame. The simulation of the effects of nervousness by disrupting targeting, as described above, is an example of intuitive mapping in the context of physiologically modulated video games or simulations. Nacke et al. (2011) notes: "Natural mappings may present more intuitive game interfaces, but also limit the flexibility and generality of the sensors for game control. This tension between innovating new uses of physiological controls and sticking with standard mappings will present future challenges for physiological game designers."

Physiologically Modulated Controller Implementations

In one embodiment (Pope et al. 2012; Hodges 2010, Sept. 3), the standard sensor bar of the Wii™ video game system that the Wii™ remote uses to triangulate its position is replaced with an array of infrared light-emitting diodes (LEDs) that are individually controllable. This embodiment turns LEDs in the array on and off in dynamic patterns to produce a disturbance in the player-directed control of the infrared-sensing videogame controller, resulting in a disruption in the stability of the player-controlled object (e.g., a scalpel) on the screen. The degree of the disruption is programmed to be proportional to the difference between the player's current momentary physiological signal value and a pre-selected target value.

In this way, the player is rewarded for diminishing this difference by an improved ability to accurately position the player-controlled object on the screen.

In another Wii^{TM}-based prototype, a stroke in golf, tennis or baseball is physiologically modulated (Hodges 2010, Sept. 3; Pope et al. 2012). The strength of the stroke with the Wii^{TM} remote is attenuated by an amount proportional to the deviation of the physiological signal from a target. The skilled performer state that is targeted in this case can be relaxed frontalis muscle tension if relaxation during performance is the goal, moderate forearm muscle tension if appropriately non-excessive grip force is the goal (Fay 2007; Moyer 2005; Wei et al. 2006) or particular EEG patterns that are associated with successful golf strokes (Crews and Landers 1993; Abrahams 2001) or marksmanship (Dingfelder 2008).

Games and simulations that are appropriate for these manipulations include first person shooter games using crosshairs position disturbance and point of view perturbations, medical simulations that use surgical instrument position pertur-bation based on autonomic measures reflecting anxiety to teach stress management during medical procedures, and sports simulations that adjust the virtual strength of a golf stroke based on electroencephalographic signals reflecting "being in the zone".

The Microsoft® Kinect® is a full-body 3D motion-sensing controller system that does not involve the use of a handheld device. Recent embodiments of the modulation training concept utilize physiological signal inputs to change the response of a user's avatar to inputs from the Kinect® system. Various aspects of a user's avatar response can be modified based on derived signals representing a user's psychophysiological state. For example, the steadiness of an avatar's hand or arm response to a user's movement may be made to vary with a physiological signal.

At NASA LaRC, a prototype third-person role-playing game was created which allows the Emotiv® EPOC® to modulate the effect of the Microsoft® Kinect® output in the game. Creation of a game from scratch allowed for manipulation of the movement controls affected by the player via the Kinect®. Subtle changes, such as force with which a player's avatar can exert with a sword as well as precision of targeting of projectile weaponry were altered according to concor-dance or discordance with psychophysiological states. This approach to modula-tion permits a seamless mapping of the various controls a player exerts in game and the mismatch between goal psychophysiological states.

Whereas this first method of modulation using the Kinect® controller involves programming an entire custom game, a second method has been used to enhance games such as The Elder Scrolls V: Skyrim® (Bethesda Game Studios 2011) and Fallout: New Vegas® (Obsidian Entertainment 2010), both of which are open-world role-playing game and Moonbase Alpha® (Virtual Heroes, Inc. 2010), a simulation of life on a moon base. With this method, the Kinect® translates the player's physical gestures and movements into game commands which control the movement and actions of the player's avatar. Simultaneously, the player's psy-chophysiological state, sensed by the Emotiv® headset, modulates the weapon skill or ability skill of the avatar. Normally in the Skyrim® and New Vegas® games, the player's established skill rank in a certain weapon or ability is a feature that grows over time through practicing that ability, and results in improving the player's competency with that weapon or ability. However, with this modulation method, the level of a player's rank in a specific skill is tied to certain levels of the player's physiological signals; as such, individual skills are manipulated to feedback the player's momentary psychophysiological state through control of character actions. For example, in Skyrim® the player's sword skill would be optimally modulated by maximizing level of excitement sensed by the Emotiv EEG headset, such that increased excitement results in increased sword skill. Other skills in Skyrim® which were modulated include archery (based on frustration), stealth (based on minimizing excitement), and magic (based on maximizing meditation); in New Vegas® weapon aim skill is modulated based on increased excitement. In Moonbase Alpha a player's skill at completing tasks such as repairing/welding damaged life support technology is modulated based on their ability to minimize frustration.

This form of modulation, while affecting the player's competency in a certain skill, does not directly modulate signals from the Kinect® input device, but, rather, changes the response of the player's avatar to a given command (e.g. a physiologically modulated sword skill will affect how many times the player must cause the avatar to swing the sword to defeat an opponent). Such dynamic feedback presents naturalistic challenge to the player to improve their self-regulation skill and potentially enhances immersion through psychophysiologically based modulation.

Physiological Modulation of the Physical Environment

Another embodiment of the physiological modulation concept (Hodges 2009, May 11; Prinzel et al. 2014) is a "physiomechatronic" apparatus that disrupts the physical practice environment of golf putting by physiological modulation. This apparatus modulates, for example, the stability of the surface of a putting practice green and the size of the aperture that the putting green hole presents to a golf ball. The idea here is analogous to the game mechanic previously described in which components of the game scenario itself, as opposed to the player's inputs, are modulated.

The modulation of the task element has the effect of altering the probability of successfully performing a physical action or maneuver essential to completing the task successfully, such as, for example, successfully sinking a putt with a single stroke in a game of golf. In this embodiment, the capture probability—the probability of successfully performing the physical task—is made an inverse function of the extent to which a measured physiological state of the subject performing the task departs from a predefined or selectable physiological state that is consistent with the optimal performance of the task. This technology thus enables the simultaneous practice of the motor skill and the physiological state conducive to successful putting; the technology is likewise applicable to other activities involving skilled movement and physiological self-regulation (Prinzel et al. 2014).

Research in precision control sports helps define the skilled performer state that is the target with this training technology. Crews and Landers identified EEG measures of attentional patterns prior to successful golf putts (Crews and Landers 1993; Abrahams 2001), and more recently, Mahoney identified individual differences in the optimal EEG patterns for trapshooting (Dingfelder 2008).

Interpersonal Biocybernetic Technologies

The physiological modulation concept described thus far may be termed an intrapersonal biocybernetic design; the interpersonal biocybernetic concept is an extension of the intrapersonal design (Pope and Stephens 2012). In the intrapersonal design, a participant's own physiological signals are made to influence or modulate the effect of their manual control of an interface. As explained previously, the intrapersonal design has been implemented by modulating manual videogame controllers and wireless motion videogame controllers.

Extending intrapersonal modulation into the interpersonal domain is intended to catalyze interaction among participants around physiological self-regulation performance challenge. These interpersonal interactions may be mixes of competition and cooperation for simulation training and/or videogame entertainment.

Physiological modulation technologies that operate by altering the functioning of game controllers, i.e., externally to game consoles, may be readily set up to allow players to interact with the game, and compete with each other, on a psychophysiological level, adding a new dimension to play—as well as expanding the skill set required. Competitive interaction with these intrapersonal modulation functionalities may be implemented with the standard multi-player capability of off-the-shelf game systems.

However, a multiplayer format may also be envisioned wherein physiological self-regulation skill contributes to success in ways analogous to traditional game-playing skills, i.e., scoring, power-ups, etc. In the following section we discuss several multiplayer setups.

Physiological Modulation for Multiplayer Environments

Multi-User Modulation Design

Norris (1986, p. 11–12) pointed out that:

> Top athletes [...] make excelling in their chosen type of psychophysiological control of the craniospinal system and striate muscles the major focus of their efforts. Here in the West, we value objectivism, material things, and have turned our attention outward toward controlling the external world. In the East, it has been quite different; the orientation of

science and society values subjectivism and numinal experiences, and they have turned
their attention inward, toward control of the internal world. Therefore, their champion
'acrobats' are those individuals who can assert and demonstrate control over autonomic
and other internal processes. […] in India, they have a sort of autonomic Olympics, where
yogis and adepts come from far and wide to demonstrate their prowess at such things….

In the present day, this sort of event might take place in a multi-player environment such as a videogame tournament.

The design of a psychophysiologically competitive, as well as cooperative,
environment is proposed in "Physiological Interface for a Multi-User Virtual
Environment (MUVE)" (Pope and Palsson 2011a). The aim is to make any multi-
user videogame or multi-user computer-simulated task more engaging and hence
more effective as a device for teaching physiological self-regulation, by incorporating, as a competitive or cooperative interactive feature, each user's ability to
self-regulate aspects of their physiology. This MUVE design is intended as an
enhancement of multiplayer videogames that computes physiological scores
standardized on an individual's baseline responses—to level the playing field, and
compares a selected score with a benchmark target or benchmark normative value.
Depending on the results of the comparison, a game consequence is selected which
may change a user's point score, change some game capability, or modulate the
user's control of the MUVE control input device. Based on the user's performance,
game consequences may also take the form of similar competitive or cooperative
consequences for the user's opponents or teammates.

One component of a user's performance is determined by each user's skill in
using an input device to control the actions of their avatar in various scenarios and
encounters arising within the MUVE, such as the outcome of combat with an
enemy avatar in a videogame embodiment of a MUVE, or the outcome of a
cooperative effort with a teammate avatar in a computer-simulated task embodiment of a MUVE. A second component is determined by each user's skill in self-
regulating their own physiological functioning while controlling their avatar using
an input device. The second component reflects the competition or cooperation
engaged in by each user of the MUVE using measured values of their physiologic
functions.

Collaborative Modulation Design

The entertainment value and social interaction experience of electronic gameplay
may be enhanced by distributing the control and modulation of inputs to electronic
games among two or more players, so that joint game goals are collaboratively
pursued and accomplished by separate players who provide different means of
control and modulation (Pope and Palsson 2011b). For example, one player may
provide physical activity control via game controller(s) (this player may be termed
the physical operator) and another player may influence the game through physiological activity measured via body sensors (this player may be termed the

physiological operator). When applied to neurofeedback training, such collaboration encourages the therapist or parent to provide social support by engaging in a training session as the physical operator, while the trainee practices self-regulation as the physiological operator. In a training simulation context, collaboration would consist of a physiological operator (e.g., the pilot-monitoring) practicing a psychophysiological state associated with sustained attention while the physical operator (e.g., pilot-flying) practices manual operation. This interdependent mode of operation could provide novel material for the communication component of crew resource management (CRM) training (Kanki et al. 2010).

Some physiologically modulated game systems (Palsson et al. 2002; Pope and Bogart 1994; Pope et al. 2012) lend themselves readily to collaborative interaction by enabling different players to assume the physical and physiological operator roles with the same modulated controller. This design modulates some players' game controllers (i.e., game input device operated by physical activity) using the physiological signals of other, collaborating players who are not providing input to the game via a game controller. This function is accomplished by transmitting control signals derived from some players' physiological signals to modulate the control over the game of other players who are using electronic game controllers, in a way that either limits or boosts the game performance influence of the game controllers.

Such an embodiment avoids the problem of movement disruption of physiological sensing by modulating one player's game controller using the physiological signals of another, collaborating player who is physically inactive. This functionality further enables collaborative team play by multiple players with different roles on the team—some providing physiological mastery to facilitate game performance while others simultaneously provide manual or physical skills needed to operate the game. This creates richer and more complex gaming opportunities than present games provide, enabling engaging and rewarding team social interactions among people who have different skill sets and interests or who take turns playing different roles on a team—either providing the physiological self-mastery skill or providing physical performance action skills.

Individuals who are physically challenged may participate in electronic game play by collaborating with a player who is able to manipulate controls that the challenged player cannot, and enables individuals with different skill sets and interests (physiological self-control versus physical performance skills) to join together in rewarding game play.

Unprecedented electronic games can be created that incorporate a classic motif in superhero comics and movies in which differently-abled protagonists collaborate and/or interact, such as Professor X and his cohorts in the X-Men series, and provides opportunities for new kinds of games where the application of "mental powers" of particular individuals (e.g., particular deliberately produced EEG characteristics) can enable or enrich the performance of other individuals playing a game.

Socially Interactive Biofeedback

Biofeedback training techniques for physiological self-regulation are fundamentally grounded upon repetition and the frequency of repetition, techniques for which persons have varying and limiting tolerances, particularly if their practice of self-regulation skill is undertaken in an environment that is not motivating because it fails to engender excitement, enthusiasm, challenge, stimulation, or curiosity. The absence of such motivating feelings can result in nonadherence to biofeedback training—a persistent and pervasive problem that has limited the prevalence and effectiveness of biofeedback training. Recent biofeedback training technology innovations (Neilson et al. 2012, 2013; Pope and Bogart 1994; Palsson et al. 2002; Pope et al. 2012) have solved this problem to a degree, by blending biofeedback training into videogames, thereby making training inherently motivating.

However, biofeedback training programmed into videogames or computer simulations has been limited to single-user videogames or single-user computer simulations, where the user is made aware of only their own monitored physiological functions, and the user's interaction with the videogame or computer simulation is modulated only by the control of their own physiological functions. In effect, the user competes only with themselves, and this may limit commitment to play and participation, with a concomitant decline in biofeedback training-mediated self-regulation of the user's physiological state.

On the other hand, physiologically modulated videogame or computer simulation systems also enable a variety of human-human interactions based upon physiological self-regulation performance. As seen herein, these interpersonal interactions may be mixes of competition and cooperation for simulation training and/or videogame entertainment. Also as explained in this chapter, physiologically modulating games and simulations has the effect of projecting exaggerated effects of the physiological concomitants of emotion and cognition into the interaction. Incorporating social interactivity into physiologically modulated games and simulations further engages users in human-computer interaction (HCI) experiences that have the capacity to train valuable mental skills beyond hand-eye coordination.

The approaches to physiological computing described in this chapter represent a unique blending of conventional computer interface capabilities with contemporary psychophysiological monitoring and biofeedback training techniques. The use of physiologically modulated videogames and simulations involving multiple players using traditional manual control and BCIs as intelligent sensors promises to augment HCI and human-human interaction (HHI) applications (Pope and Stephens 2012). Tapping into the natural social experience that occurs when players compete or collaborate in gaming or simulated environments leverages subtle interpersonal interactions. The addition of the challenge of physiological self-regulation in a social context elevates the motivation to perform in order to enable team success or victory over opponents in simulated environments. Further, implementing this challenge in the ways described herein has the potential to foster dialogue around self-regulation among the participants. These implementations can require dividing attention between one's own self-regulation performance and that of others, a potentially valuable skill for team settings. Modulated game systems can be designed to inherit the benefit of social interplay that occurs between humans. The application of readily available physiological information from BCI technology can be used to enable such a user experience.

Future Applications

Interactions with computers or computer-controlled objects will be the predominant daily activity of both adults and children in the years to come, if not so already. Biofeedback training, with its ability to optimize functioning and to maintain well-being and health will be embedded in these activities. Below we discuss several applications of biofeedback training in the future.

Instrument Functionality Feedback

Both inattention and stress overload play a substantial role in impairing pilot performance and producing flight hazards. Kellar et al. (1993, July) cite studies to support the assertion that "Reasonable evidence exists to conclude that pilots may lose control of their aircraft as a direct result of reactive stress. The condition in which a high state of physiological arousal is accompanied by a narrowing of the focus of attention can be referred to as autonomous mode behavior. ... A number of studies have produced evidence that this type of training [physiological self-regulation training] effectively reduces arousal which affects operational efficiency in student pilots." Biofeedback training can foreseeably help reduce the occurrence of these "hazardous states of awareness" (Pope and Bogart 1992) by teaching pilots to maintain the necessary physiological conditions for good cognitive and psychomotor performance under the circumstances that are most likely to produce inattention or dysfunctional stress. The modulation concept embodied in the videogame biofeedback training technology may be adapted for use in task simulators.

Instrument Functionality Feedback (IFF) Training is a concept for training pilots in maintaining the physiological equilibrium suited for optimal cognitive and motor performance under emergency events in an airplane cockpit (Palsson and Pope 1999). It is a training concept for reducing pilot error during demanding or unexpected events in the cockpit by teaching pilots self-regulation of excessive autonomic nervous system (ANS) reactivity during simulated flight tasks. The training method (a) adapts biofeedback training methodology to train physiological balance during simulated operation of an airplane, and (b) uses graded impairment of control over the flight task to encourage the pilot to gain mastery over their autonomic functions. In Instrument Functionality Feedback Training, pilots are trained to minimize their autonomic deviation from baseline values while operating a flight simulation. This is done by making their skin conductance and hand temperature deviations from baseline impair the functionality of the aircraft controls. Trainees also receive auditory and visual cues about their autonomic deviation, and are instructed to keep these within pre-set limits to retain full control of the aircraft.

Recreation Embedded State Tuning for Optimal Readiness and Effectiveness

Long-duration space missions will include crew recreation periods that will afford physiological self-regulation training opportunities. However, to promote adherence to the regimen, the practice experience that occupies their recreation time must be perceived by the crew as engaging and entertaining throughout repeated reinforcement sessions on long-duration missions. The physiological modulated games and simulations approach provides the opportunity to deliver physiological self-regulation training in an entertaining and motivating fashion. The Recreation Embedded State Tuning for Optimal Readiness and Effectiveness (RESTORE) concept is designed to provide a physiological self-regulation training counter-measure for maintaining and reinforcing cognitive readiness, resilience under psychological stress, and effective mood states in long-duration crews (Pope and Prinzel 2005). RESTORE aims to reduce the risk of future manned exploration missions by enhancing the capability of individual crewmembers to self-regulate cognitive states through recreation-embedded training protocols to effectively deal with the psychological toll of long-duration space flight.

Intrasomatic Biofeedback

The biofeedback training method is an effective health-enhancement technique, which exemplifies the integration of biotechnology and information technology with the reinforcement principles of cognitive science. Adding nanotechnology to this mix will enable researchers to explore the extent to which physiological self-regulation can be made more specific and even molecular, and may lead to an entire new class of effective health-enhancing and health-optimizing technologies (Pope and Palsson 2002).

The exclusive reliance upon sensing of physiological functions from the surface of the body has limited biofeedback training's specificity in targeting the physiological processes that underlie human performance and the physiological dys-regulation implicated in several disorders. Biofeedback technology has yet to incorporate recent advances in biotechnology, including nanoscale biosensors, etc., perhaps because biofeedback training research and practice is dominated by a focus on traditional and proven training protocols rather than on biotechnology.

The integration of nanotechnology with the biofeedback training method opens an entirely new frontier, inviting the pioneers of a new era in psychophysiology to explore the extent to which this physiological self-regulation can be made more precise, perhaps even to the point of reliably modifying specific molecular events. These developments will enable human beings to willfully induce inside their own bodies small and highly specific biological changes with large health-and performance-enhancing consequences.

Projection

When physiological signal(s) are the target of physiological self-regulation or biofeedback training, modulated game play reinforces therapeutic changes in related physiological processes. However, the reinforcing feedback is implicit in the game play and not explicit in the form of direct feedback (bar and line graphs), as in conventional biofeedback training. In this way, contingencies for subtle conditioning of the desirable physiological response(s) are set up.

The added benefit of the physiologically modulated approach is the improvement of self-regulation capabilities that directly impact a player's health in a positive manner. Videogames and simulations can be designed such that success in the virtual world is predicated upon self-regulation skills demonstrative of healthy autonomic function and/or optimal cognitive states. Evoking certain psychophysiological states is a design choice that developers are currently making de facto, but with the result that games and simulations are often devices that produce frustration and foster poor attention abilities. The decision by designers to incorporate physiological modulation can be considered a next step in a more informed and healthy direction for gaming and simulation products. Making this choice allows users to choose technology that is entertaining as well as beneficial to their physical, mental and interpersonal health.

The biofeedback training technologies described in this chapter demonstrate how biofeedback training can be applied to develop a range of emotional and cognitive skills using biofeedback technology embedded in a variety of new contexts, making the opportunities for training ubiquitous. As projected by Palsson and Pope (2002):

> Embedding biofeedback training into people's *primary daily activities,* whether work or play, is a largely untapped and rich opportunity to foster health and growth. It may soon be regarded to be as natural and expected as is the addition of vitamins to popular breakfast cereals. Toymakers of the future might get unfavorable reviews if they offer computer games that only provide "empty entertainment." In the same vein, worker unions may frown upon computer workstations that do not help safeguard the health and well-being of employees through physiological monitoring and protective biofeedback training.

... we predict that biofeedback training will be widely employed in the health and well-being of coming generations. Unlike the biofeedback implementations we know today, almost all of tomorrow's biofeedback training will take place in everyday life in society rather than in clinics or labs.

References

Abrahams J (2001) Putting under stress. Golf magazine. p. 30–32

Applied Psychophysiology Institutes (1988) USE language and PC interface manual. J & J Enterprises, Poulsbo, WA

Balconi-Lamica C, Neilson BN, Stephens CL, Pope AT (2012) Experiment design for study of neuro-biofeedback: mindshift. In: Proceedings of the association for applied psychophysiology and biofeedback 43rd annual meeting, Baltimore, AAPB, p 308

Calmpute (1984) CalmPrix car racing game. Thought Technology Ltd

Crews DJ, Landers DM (1993) Electroencephalographic measures of attentional patterns prior to the golf putt. Med Sci Sports Exerc 25(1):116–126

Cyberlearning LLC (2004) S.M.A.R.T. Box technical manual. S.M.A.R.T. BrainGames

DeBeus R, Ball JD, DeBeus ME, Harrington R (2004) Attention training with ADHD children: preliminary findings in a double-blind placebo-controlled study. J Neurotherapy 8:145–148

deCharms R, Maeda F, Glover G, Ludlow D, Pauly J, Soneji D, Gabrieli J, Mackey S (2005) Control over brain activation and pain learned by using real-time functional MRI. Proc Natl Acad Sci 102:18626–18631

Dingfelder SF (2008) Elite athletes are using EEG feedback to hone their mental states: but does it work? APA Monitor on Psychology, 39(7):58

Edmonds WA, Tenenbaum G (eds) (2011) Case studies in applied psychophysiology: neurofeedback and biofeedback treatments for advances in human performance. Wiley, West Sussex

Fairclough SH (2008) BCI and physiological computing: differences, similarities & intuitive control. Workshop on BCI and computer games, CHI (08), Florence. http://www.physiologicalcomputing.net/?p=1928

Fairclough SH, Gilleade K (2012) Construction of the biocybernetic loop: a case study. In: ACM international conference on multimodal interaction, New York, pp 571–578

Fairclough SH, Gilleade K, Ewing KC, Roberts J (2013) Capturing user engagement via psychophysiology: measures and mechanisms for biocybernetic adaptation. Int J Auton Adapt Commun Syst 6(1):63–79

Fay C (2007) How to grip a baseball bat. eHow. http://www.ehow.com/how_10084_grip-baseball-bat.html. Accessed 12 Nov 2013

Freeman F, Mikulka P, Scerbo M, Prinzel L, Clouatre K (2000) Evaluation of a psychophysiologically controlled adaptive automation system, using performance on a tracking task. Appl Psychophysiol Biofeedback 25:103–115

Ghaziri J, Tuckolka A, Larue V, Blanchette-Sylvestre M, Reyburn G, Gilbert G, Levesque J, Beauregard M (2013) Neurofeedback training induces changes in white and gray matter. Clin EEG Neurosci 44(4):265–272

Gilleade K, Dix A, Allanson J (2005) Affective videogames and modes of affective gaming: assist me, challenge me, emote me. In: Digital games research association (DiGRA) conference, Vancouver, pp 16–20

Gruzelier J, Egner T (2005) Critical validation studies of neurofeedback. Child and Adolesc Psychiatr Clin North Am 14:83–104

Hefferline RF, Keenan B, Harford RA (1959) Escape and avoidance conditioning in human subjects without their observation of the response. Science 130:1338–1339

Hettinger L, Branco P, Encarnacao LM, Bonato P (2003) Neuroadaptive technologies: applying neuroergonomics to the design of advanced interfaces. Theor Issues Ergon Sci 4:220–237

Hilborn O, Cederholm H, Eriksson J, Lindley C (2013) A biofeedback game for training arousal regulation during a stressful task: the space investor. In: Kurosu M (ed) Human-computer interaction, HCII 2013, Part V. Springer, Berlin, pp 403–410

Hodges J (2009) For langley inventors, it's mind over golf. NASA Langley Researcher News

Hodges J (2010) 'Mindshift' biofeedback gaming technology. NASA Langley Researcher News

Kamiya, J. (1971) Biofeedback and self-control: an Aldine reader on the regulation of bodily processes and consciousness. Aldine-Atherton, Chicago

Kanki BG, Helmreich RL, Anca J (eds) (2010) Crew resource management, 2nd edn. Elsevier, San Diego

Kellar MA, Folen RA, Cowings PA, Toscano WB, Hisert GL (1993) Autogenic feedback training improves pilot performance during emergency flight conditions. Flight safety digest. Flight safety foundation

Knox M, Lentini J, Cummings TS (2011) Game-based biofeedback for paediatric anxiety and depression. Mental Health Fam Med 8:195

Lansbergen MM, Dongen-Boomsma M, Buitelaar JK, Slaats-Willemse D (2011) ADHD and EEG-neurofeedback: a double-blind randomized placebo-controlled feasibility study. J Neural Transm 118:275–284

Lubar JF (1991) Discourse on the development of EEG diagnostics and biofeedback for attention-deficit/hyperactivity disorders. Biofeedback Self-Regul 16(3):201–225

Mandryk RL, Dielschneider S, Kalyn MR, Betram CP, Gaetz M, Doucette A, Taylor BA, Orr AP, Keiver K (2013) Games as neurofeedback training for kids with FASD. In: International conference on interaction design and children. ACM, pp 165–172

Monastra VJ (2005) Electroencephalographic biofeedback (neurotherapy) as a treatment for attention deficit hyperactivity disorder: rationale and empirical foundation. Child Adolesc Psychiatr Clin North Am 14:55–82

Moyer P (2005) Golfers' "Yips" may be caused by a focal dystonia. http://www.medscape.com/viewarticle/503271. Accessed 12 Nov 2013

Mulholland T (1977) Biofeedback as scientific method. In: Schwartz G, Beatty J (eds) Biofeedback: theory and research. Academic Press, New York, pp 9–28

Nacke LE, Kalyn M, Lough C, Mandryk RL (2011) Biofeedback game design: using direct and indirect physiological control to enhance game interaction. In: CHI Conference, Vancouver, ACM, pp 103–112

Neilson BN, Stephens CL, Pope AT (2012) Psychophysiological and performance effects of commercial brain-computer interface technology. In: Proceedings of the association for applied psychophysiology and biofeedback 43rd annual meeting, Baltimore, AAPB, p 309

Neilson BN, Stephens CL, Pope AT (2013) Physiological self-regulation training using two new technologies: commercial off-the-shelf brain-computer interface devices and NASA LaRC MindShift technology. Poster presented at the association for applied psychophysiology and biofeedback 44th annual meeting, Portland

Norris P (1986) Biofeedback, voluntary control, and human potential. Biofeedback Self-Regul 11(1):1–20

O'Shea T, Sleeman DH (1973) A design for an adaptive self improving teaching system. In: Rose J (ed) Advances in cybernetics and systems, vol 3. Gordon & Breach, London

Palsson O, Pope AT (1999) Stress counterresponse training of pilots via instrumental functionality feedback. In: Proceedings of the association for applied psychophysiology and biofeedback 30th annual meeting, Vancouver, AAPB

Palsson OS, Harris R, Pope AT (2002) Method and apparatus for encouraging physiological self-regulation through modulation of an operator's control input to a video game or training simulator. Washington, DC, USA Patent 6450820

Palsson OS, Pope AT (2002) Morphing beyond recognition: the future of biofeedback technologies. Biofeedback 30(1):14–18

Palsson OS, Pope AT, Ball JD, Turner MJ, Nevin S, DeBeus R (2001) Neurofeedback videogame ADHD technology: results of the first concept study. In: Proceedings of the association for applied psychophysiology and biofeedback. http://www.hp-add.com/articles/AAPB%20 Videogame%20NASA%20Study%20Slides.pdf

Pigott HE, Bodenhamer-Davis E, Davis RE, Harbin H (2013) The evidence-base for neurofeedback as a reimbursable healthcare service to treat attention deficit/hyperactivity disorder

Pope A, Bogart E, Bartolome D (1995) Biocybernetic system validates index of operator engagement in automated task. Biol Psychol 40:187–195

Pope AT, Bogart E (1992) Identification of hazardous awareness states in monitoring environments. SAE 1992 Trans J Aerosp 101:449–457 (Section 1)

Pope AT, Bogart E (1994) Method of encouraging attention by correlating video game difficulty with attention level. Washington, DC, Patent 5377100

Pope AT, Bogart E (1996) Extended attention span training system: video game neurotherapy for attention deficit disorder. Child Study J 26:39–50

Pope AT, Gersten CD (1977) Computer automation of biofeedback training. Behav Res Methods Instrum 9:164–168

Pope AT, Palsson OS (2002) Converging technologies for physiological self-regulation. In: Roco MC, Bainbridge WS (eds) Converging technologies for improving human performance: nanotechnology, biotechnology, information technology and cognitive science, NSF/DOC-sponsored report. National Science Foundation, Arlington, pp 231–239

Pope AT, Palsson OS (2011a) Physiological user interface for a multi-user virtual environment. Washington, DC, USA Patent 8062129

Pope AT, Palsson OS (2011b) Team electronic gameplay combining different means of control. Washington, DC, USA Patent Application 20110300523

Pope AT, Prinzel L (2005) Recreation embedded state tuning for optimal readiness and effectiveness. In: 11th international conference on human-computer interaction, MIRA Digital Publishing, Las Vegas

Pope AT, Stephens CL (2012) Interpersonal biocybernetics: connecting through social psychophysiology. In: ACM international conference on multimodal interaction, Santa Monica, pp 123–190

Pope AT, Stephens CL, Blanson NM (2012) Method and system for physiologically modulating videogames or simulations which use motion-sensing input devices. Washington, DC, USA Patent Application 20120004034

Premack D (1965) Reinforcement theory. In: Jones MR (ed) Nebraska symposium on motivation. University of Nebraska Press, Lincoln

Prinzel L, Freeman F, Scerbo M, Mikulka P, Pope A (2000) A closed-loop system for examining psychophysiological measures for adaptive task allocation. Int J Aviat Psychol 10:393–410

Prinzel L, Pope AT, Palsson OS, Turner MJ (2014) Method and apparatus for performance optimization through physical perturbation of task elements. Washington, DC, USA Patent Application 8628333

Rani P, Sarkar N, Liu C (2005) Maintaining optimal challenge in computer games through real-time physiological feedback. In: Proceedings 11th international conference on human computer interaction. Las Vegas, NV, 184–192

Stephens CL, Scerbo MW, Pope AT (2012) Adaptive automation for mitigation of hazardous states of awareness. In: Matthews G, Desmond PA, Neubauer C, Hancock PA (eds) The handbook of operator fatigue. Ashgate, Farnham, pp 415–440

Wei SH, Chiang JY, Shiang TY, Chang HY (2006) Comparison of shock transmission and forearm electromyography between experienced and recreational tennis players during backhand strokes. Clin J Sport Med 16(2):129–135

Weising (2011) Biometric interface for a handheld device. Washington, DC, USA Patent Application 20110260830

Yucha C, Montgomery D (2008) Evidence-based practice in biofeedback and neurofeedback. Association for Applied Psychophysiology and Biofeedback, Wheat Ridge, CO

Zukor's Grind (2010) Zukor interactive. http://zukor.com/interactive/grind.html

Chapter 6
Using fNIRS to Measure Mental Workload in the Real World

Evan M. Peck, Daniel Afergan, Beste F. Yuksel, Francine Lalooses
and Robert J. K. Jacob

Abstract In the past decade, functional near-infrared spectroscopy (fNIRS) has seen increasing use as a non-invasive brain sensing technology. Using optical signals to approximate blood-oxygenation levels in localized regions of the brain, the appeal of the fNIRS signal is that it is relatively robust to movement artifacts and comparable to fMRI measures. We provide an overview of research that builds towards the use of fNIRS to monitor user workload in real world environments, and eventually to act as input to biocybernetic systems. While there are still challenges for the use of fNIRS in real world environments, its unique characteristics make it an appealing alternative for monitoring the cognitive processes of a user.

Introduction

As brain sensing technology has become more unobtrusive, portable, and inexpensive, it has become a more viable technology for evaluating everyday work environments. The ability to access physiological parameters that correlate with

E. M. Peck (✉) · D. Afergan · B. F. Yuksel · F. Lalooses · R. J. K. Jacob
Tufts University, Medford, USA
e-mail: evan.peck@tufts.edu

D. Afergan
e-mail: afergan@cs.tufts.edu

B. F. Yuksel
e-mail: beste.yuksel@tufts.edu

F. Lalooses
e-mail: francine.lalooses@tufts.edu

R. J. K. Jacob
e-mail: jacob@cs.tufts.edu

S. H. Fairclough and K. Gilleade (eds.), *Advances in Physiological Computing*,
Human–Computer Interaction Series, DOI: 10.1007/978-1-4471-6392-3_6,
© Springer-Verlag London 2014

brain activity is an appealing option for researchers who are trying to capture cognitive state at its primary source. Monitoring cognitive states such as workload, attention, or emotion provide valuable information that aids in the evaluation of interfaces design, task design, or individual cognitive abilities.

In particular, researchers have sought to capture working memory because it has been labelled as the information bottleneck in the brain, and is necessary for reasoning, anticipation, and planning (Baddeley 1992). However, working memory is also limited by both duration and capacity (Miller 1956). When multiple elements compete for space, there is a loss of information and often a decrease in performance. Thus, preventing users from overloading their working memory, by understanding when and how it is overloaded, is a critical component of supporting analytical thought.

We pursue the use of brain sensing to capture these processes not only because it may lend insight into periods of overload, but because overload can be difficult to observe through other means—increasing load on working memory does not always result in a decrease in performance (Hockey 1997). Performance may be maintained with an increased reliance on extra resources and with extra subjective effort, behavioral, and physiological costs.

In addition, observing load on working memory often hints at the overall mental workload of the user. Wickens (2002) demonstrates how closely the two are connected and how the distinctions are not always so clear with his four-dimensional multiple resources model. Wickens' theory dictates that two tasks that both need the same level of a dimension will yield more conflict than two non-overlapping tasks. Thus, multiple working memory tasks that require the same modalities are likely to yield an overload on that resource. If we can observe working memory (or mental workload) in real-time, then we may be able to improve the user's environment to better support these processes, improving interaction and increasing performance.

To capture measures of mental workload in the brain, most research has focused on the use of electroencephalography (EEG) to monitor the electrical activity of the brain. However, there has also been increasing interest in functional near-infrared spectroscopy (fNIRS) as an alternative brain sensing technique. This is largely due to the fact that fNIRS measures a unique set of physiological parameters (oxygenated and deoxygenated hemoglobin) in a relatively unobtrusive manner. Thus, fNIRS has seen increased use for scenarios where it is necessary to capture cognitive state without applying too many physical restrictions on the user.

In this chapter, we give an overview of why fNIRS is well-suited to observe a user's working memory, specifically, the central executive (Repovš and Baddeley 2006). In particular, we focus on fNIRS work that is geared towards the field of human-computer interaction and ecologically valid evaluations.

To accomplish this goal, we build from a technical description of fNIRS to the use of fNIRS in real world scenarios. First, we describe fNIRS as a brain sensing technology, highlighting its advantages and disadvantages in comparison to other brain sensing techniques. Next, we describe Repovš and Baddeley's (2006) multi-component model of working memory and then dive into the existing neuroscience literature, exploring why the prefrontal cortex is an ideal place to observe increases in working memory. Then, beginning with highly controlled psychology tasks, we highlight experiments that use fNIRS to investigate working memory load in the prefrontal cortex. Finally, we look at the potential of using fNIRS as real-time input to adaptive brain-computer interfaces. We find this last section to be most exciting, as using the brain as input to a computer expands the interaction bandwidth between a user and the computer in unique and powerful ways.

There are still serious challenges for the use of fNIRS, which we will also discuss in this chapter, but it also provides researchers with a unique set of properties that can compliment other physiological signals. We hope to highlight the potential of fNIRS in this chapter, as well as outline its future development.

Introduction to fNIRS

How Does it Work, What Does it Measure?

Functional near infrared spectroscopy (fNIRS) is an optical brain sensing technique developed in the 1990 s that is portable, resistant to movement artifacts (Solovey et al. 2009), and observes similar physiological parameters to functional magnetic resonance imaging (fMRI) (Chance et. al 1998). These characteristics have made it an attractive alternative for researchers seeking to observe the brain in natural working environments.

fNIRS uses near-infrared light to measure concentration and oxygenation of the blood in the tissue at depths of 1–3 cm (Villringer and Chance 1997). Light is sent into the forehead in the near infrared range (650–900 nm), where it is diffusely reflected by the scalp, skull, and brain cortex. At this wavelength, oxygenated and deoxygenated hemoglobin are the primary absorbers of light. A very small percentage of the light sent into the head returns from the cortex to the detector on the fNIRS probe. By measuring the light returned to the detector, researchers are able to calculate the amount of oxygen in the blood, as well as the amount of blood in the tissue.

Biologically, when a region of the brain is active, there is an increase of blood flow to that region (D'Esposito et al. 1999). This increase of blood flow is typically coupled with decreased levels of deoxygenated hemoglobin and increased levels of oxygenated hemoglobin. Thus, fNIRS can be used to measure activity in localized areas of the brain.

To make this calculation, raw data can be transformed into deoxygenated hemoglobin concentrations using the modified Beer-Lambert Law [5]:

$$\Delta A = \varepsilon \times \Delta c \times d \times B \qquad (6.1)$$

where ΔA is the change in attenuation of light, ε is the molar absorption coefficient of the absorbing molecules, Δc is the change in the concentration of the absorbing molecules, d is the optical pathlength (i.e., the distance the light travels), and B is the differential pathlength factor. The attenuation of light is measured by how much light is absorbed by oxygenated and deoxygenated hemoglobin (which are the main absorbers of near infrared light at these wavelengths). As the attenuation of light is related to the levels of hemoglobin, given ΔA, we can derive the changes in the levels of oxygenated and deoxygenated hemoglobin (Chance et al. 1998).

For the sake of focus, we will primarily discuss fNIRS probes that are placed on the forehead, measuring brain activity in the anterior prefrontal cortex. This placement offers a significant advantage for researchers: fNIRS measurements can be made without the interference of hair follicles, which can absorb light and disrupt the signal. As a result, probes that monitor activity in the prefrontal cortex are often more unobtrusive, and therefore, more interesting for researchers searching for ecologically sound measurements.

Other Techniques: EEG and fMRI

In the past, various brain sensing technologies have been proposed to observe a user's response to activities in a lab setting. Electroencephalography (EEG) and functional magnetic resonance imaging (fMRI) are two of the most prevalent and both have been successful at measurement and classification of brain activities. fMRI requires a person to lie motionless inside a large, loud chamber in which small movements (those larger than 3 mm) often result in discarded data (i.e. Cahill et al. 2004; Davis et al. 2004). fMRI scanners are also expensive to purchase and maintain, requiring technical staff and purpose-built rooms or buildings.

EEG has recently seen commercial success because it is portable, less invasive, and relatively inexpensive. While EEG has a high temporal resolution, it also has a low spatial resolution, which makes it difficult to pinpoint the origin of neural activity. Although EEG is easier to set up and use than fMRI, many configurations require applying gel into a person's hair to create a conductive contact with the skin. Finally, movement artifacts can be problematic with the use of EEG. Without proper filtering methods, minor movements, such as facial muscles can disrupt incoming data. Despite these limitations, EEG has gained popularity because of its quick temporal response (1 ms), the strong existing body of EEG research, and the availability of well-supported commercial setups.

fNIRS Advantages

While fNIRS preserves some of the core features that make EEG a popular brain sensing technology, most notably its ease of use and portability, fNIRS also has a few unique properties that are worth considering. For example, fNIRS has a short setup time and is generally resistant to movement artifacts. Mouse-clicking, typing, eye movement, and blinking in normal computing environments are acceptable during the use of fNIRS (Solovey et al. 2009). Minor head movement, respiration, and heartbeats can be filtered using known signal processing techniques. Only major head and forehead movement (which could be induced by frowning) are disruptive to the signal.

fNIRS also has a spatial resolution on the order of 0.5–1 cm, and readings have been validated against fMRI (Strangman et al. 2002). Furthermore, fNIRS provides access to hemodynamic and metabolic parameters that are not accessible with EEG (which is sensitive to electrical signals and not to blood flow or tissue oxygenation) and fMRI (which is only sensitive to deoxygenated hemoglobin and not oxygenated hemoglobin).

fNIRS Considerations

It's important to note that there are both caveats and considerations to the use of fNIRS as well. Once a region of the brain becomes active, the biological response to support this increase in activity takes several seconds to reach the cortex (Gore 2003). As a result, changes in blood oxygenation that reflect user state cannot be detected immediately using fNIRS.

The impact of this limitation is two-fold. First, we are more likely to measure signal differences in short-term and long-term cognitive states rather than instantaneous one-time events. Second, because the slow biological response impacts how quickly we can identify or classify user state, it also impacts the design of adaptation mechanisms in biocybernetic systems that respond to fNIRS user state. In a later section, we will discuss some design considerations that can help circumvent this issue.

Because light from fNIRS reaches depths of 1–3 cm, activity in deeper areas of the brain is not directly accessible. Additionally, hair can obstruct light, so sources and detectors must be maneuvered to maintain contact with the skin. Although there are several variants of full-head fNIRS devices (Franceschini et al. 2006), most are noticeably less comfortable than probes designed exclusively for the forehead. As a result, many fNIRS researchers currently investigate activity in the prefrontal cortex (PFC).

Working Memory and the Prefrontal Cortex

Working memory has been defined as the "temporary storage and manipulation of the information necessary for such complex tasks such as language comprehension, learning and reasoning" (Baddeley 1992). It is a complex topic that can be explored at different levels (Repovš and Bresjanac 2006), such as neuroanatomical structure, computational cognitive processes, or the more abstract level of modelling its functional capacities. For the purposes of presenting working memory in the context of using fNIRS, we explain working memory in terms of Repovš and Baddeley's (2006) multi-component model. We then motivate the placement of fNIRS on the forehead by reviewing a sample of the existing literature that has linked the PFC to working memory. In this respect, fMRI studies are particularly illuminating, as they access similar physiological parameters as fNIRS and their results have the potential of being directly replicated.

Working Memory

The model proposed by Repovš and Baddeley (2006) for working memory is made up of multiple components: a central executive, a visuospatial sketchpad, a phonological loop, and an episodic buffer. The phonological loop contains verbal information in the form of a short-term acoustic store and an articulatory rehearsal process. The visuospatial sketchpad is comprised of visual and spatial subsystems with independent storage, maintenance and manipulation processes. The central executive seems to have several different functions which are involved in the manipulation of information within the memory stores. The latest addition to the model, the episodic buffer, holds and integrates information from other working memory components and from long-term memory into scenes or episodes. For an in-depth description and discussion of the multi-component model of working memory please see Repovš and Baddeley (2006).

We propose that the increase in mental workload that the fNIRS measures in the PFC is actually related to an increase in working memory, and more specifically, in the central executive. We present evidence of this by discussing studies linking working memory to the prefrontal cortex.

Prefrontal Cortex

It is largely undisputed that the prefrontal cortex is important for higher-order cognitive functions including working memory (Ramnani and Owen 2004). The dorsolateral prefrontal cortex has been associated with working memory and with high-level organization of the contents of working memory. Bor et al. (2003) presented subjects with a spatial working memory task with structured and unstructured sequences. The structured sequences were easier to remember, however, functional magnetic resonance imaging (fMRI) results showed increased activation in the lateral frontal cortex with structured sequences. The results show that even when working memory demand decreases, the frontal cortex is still active in the organization of the contents of working memory (Bor et al. 2003). Similarly, Bor et al. (2004) showed similar results with verbal working memory using structured and unstructured digit sequences. Both of these studies suggest that the lateral frontal cortex structures high-level information into organized groups which can decrease the load on working memory.

The ventrolateral prefrontal-cortex is also associated with working memory and is thought to be linked to the retrieval of a few pieces of information. For example, Jonides et al. (1993) gave participants a memory task by presenting three stimuli concurrently for 200 ms. They then asked participants whether a probe circle displayed 3 s later occupied one of the same locations. Using positron emission tomography (PET), Jonides et al. (1993) found increased activation in the mid-ventrolateral prefrontal cortex in contrast to a simple perception condition. Dove et al. (2001) tested the effects of when participants explicitly intended to remember or retrieve information. Participants looking at pictures of abstract art were instructed either to just look or to explicitly remember similar stimuli for later. The latter condition created increased activation in the mid-ventrolateral cortex (measured with fMRI) (Dove et al. 2001, see also Owen et al. 2005). These findings suggest that the intention to remember may be the cause of the activation in the ventrolateral cortex.

One area of the prefrontal cortex that is not so widely understood but is also associated with working memory is the anterior prefrontal cortex (see Ramnani and Owen 2004 for a review). This constitutes Brodmann area (BA) 10 and is very well developed in humans in comparison to other primates. Some of the neuro-imaging evidence points towards functionalities such as processing of internal states and evaluating ones own thoughts and feelings (Christoff and Gabrieli 2000); memory retrieval, retrieval verification and source memory (Tulving 1983; Rugg 1998); prospective memory such as "at time x, do y" (Burgess et al. 2001); cognitive branching or the ability to hold goals while carrying out secondary goals (Koechlin et al. 2000); and relational knowledge (Kroger et al. 2002; Christoff et al. 2001).

A theory put forward by Ramnani and Owen (2004) is that the anterior pre-frontal cortex is activated when a problem requires more than one cognitive process. Hence, the cognitive operations need to be coordinated in the pursuit of a more general goal. Their hypothesis is broadly consistent with much of the previous functional neuroimaging literature described above, and with the theory of the central executive of Repovš and Baddeley's (2006) model.

Detecting Working Memory with fNIRS

To build towards measuring workload in real world scenarios, we start by using fNIRS to identify it in heavily controlled environments. In particular, we begin by describing the n-back task, a classical workload task in the psychology literature, and review neuroscience work that suggests that fNIRS is capable of detecting activation in the prefrontal cortex.

The N-Back Task

Gevins and Cutillo (1993) created the "n-back" task, a working memory task that has been widely used and quoted in the literature to investigate cognitive working memory processes. The n-back consists of a user being presented with sequentially presented stimuli and answering positively whenever the current stimulus matches the stimulus occurring n positions back in the sequence. The integer n is given to the user at the start and is usually 1, 2 or 3.

The n-back task is demanding and requires on-line storage, monitoring and manipulation of information. The participant must hold information in their working memory whilst incorporating new information and comparing it with the older stimuli. There are different variations of the n-back stimuli: these can be presented verbally (letters and words) or non-verbally (images such as shapes or faces. Another variation is whether the identity of the stimulus has to be remembered or the location of the stimulus (Owen et al. 2005). Below, we show an image of a visuospatial n-back task, labeling the 'yes' responses for both a 1-back and 3-back condition.

The n-back has been shown to produce activation in working memory related cortical regions (Braver et al. 1997; Cohen et al. 1997). Owen et al. (2005) carried out a meta-analysis on 24 functional neuroimaging studies carried out in Talairach space that used the n-back paradigm on healthy subjects. They found that six cortical regions were consistently activated across all studies including the bilateral rostral prefrontal cortex (BA10), the bilateral dorsolateral prefrontal cortex (BA9,46) and the bilateral mid-ventrolateral prefrontal cortex (BA45,47). There were some differences depending on the variation of the n-back task. N-backs that were verbal identity tasks created more activation in the left ventrolateral prefrontal cortex than the non-verbal identity tasks (Owen et al. 2005). Non-verbal location tasks created more activation in the right dorsolateral prefrontal cortex than non-verbal identity tasks. These results suggest that there is functional specialization of working memory systems and that activation of the prefrontal cortex can be identified with n-back tasks to quite a specific degree of accuracy.

N-Back and fNIRS

To validate the use of fNIRS to detect workload in a visual interface HCI task, Peck et al. (2013b) recorded signals in the prefrontal cortex of 16 participants as they interacted with a visuospatial n-back task. In this version of the n-back task, participants were shown a series of slides that have distinct visual patterns and asked whether the pattern in the current slide matched the pattern viewed n slides ago. By increasing the value of n, participants were forced to hold n patterns in their visuospatial short-term memory. Thus, as n increased, the load on their visual short-term memory increased.

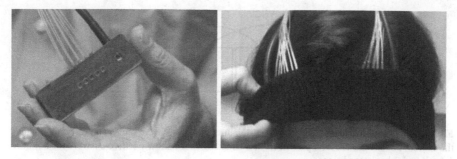

Fig. 6.1 *Left* We display one example of an fNIRS probe with four light sources and one detector. *Right* A researcher uses a headband to secutre two probes to a user's forehead

Fig. 6.2 A participant interacts with a computer while wearing fNIRS probes

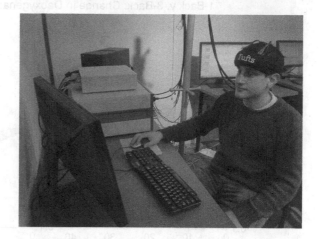

Participants were given eight trials of 1-back and 3-back conditions (representing low and high workload), with each condition consisting of 20 slides. Trials lasted for 40.7 s and were separated by 12-s rest periods. fNIRS sensors, as shown in Figs. 6.1 and 6.2 were applied to the forehead (prefrontal cortex) and changes in deoxy-Hb were compared in the 1-back and 3-back conditions (Figs. 6.3, 6.4).

In agreement with fMRI studies, Peck found more significant decreases in deoxy-Hb during 3-back trials than with 1-back trials. Figure 6.4 shows the mean change in deoxygenated hemoglobin across all trials and all participants of the 1-back and 3-back task. Additionally, participants reported the 3-back to be more mentally demanding than the 1-back and performance degraded as participants interacted with the 3-back in comparison to the 1-back. These results agree with other behavioral studies of the n-back task and validate the use of fNIRS to record changes in visuospatial working-memory in the prefrontal cortex.

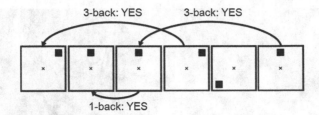

Fig. 6.3 In the visuospatial n-back task, participants view a series of slides and respond whether the current pattern matches the pattern from n slides ago. We show positive answers for both the 1-back and 3-back conditions

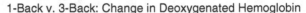

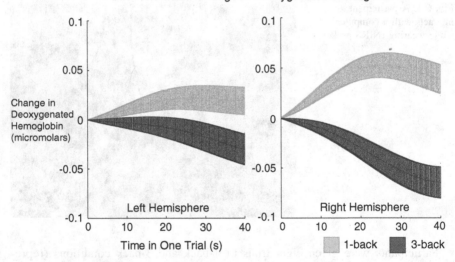

Fig. 6.4 The mean change in fNIRS signal (from a rest state) across all 16 participants in the baseline task since the beginning of the task. The *center line* is the mean for each condition, while the width indicates the standard error. We see a clear separation between the 1-back and 3-back conditions for participants. The more demanding 3-back condition mirrors signals from the graph design that participants believed was more mentally demanding

Detecting Workload in Real World Tasks

So far, we have discussed the potential of fNIRS to detect workload in heavily controlled environments. But can these psychology experiments be generalized to real world environments? As we discussed earlier, fNIRS has the unique advantage of being relatively robust to movement artifacts in a comparison to other brain sensing devices. In this section, we explore techniques that researchers have used to investigate workload in scenarios that are increasingly closer to everyday tasks.

As we review their work, we gradually move from offline statistical analysis of physiological signals, to real-time automated classification of user state.

Analyzing Changes in Oxy-Hb and Deoxy-Hb

One method for using fNIRS to detect changes in workload is statistical analysis of changes in oxy-Hb and deoxy-Hb. Recall that as brain activity increases, we generally observe increases in oxy-Hb and decreases in deoxy-Hb. By analyzing the changes in these parameters during a user's interaction with a complex task, we can hypothesize the level of activity (and the workload) in the user's prefrontal cortex. Here, we share three examples of studies that have performed offline analysis of changes in oxy-Hb or deoxy-Hb to investigate workload levels.

Ayaz et al. (2012) used this approach to detect the level of workload for participants piloting unmanned air vehicles (UAVs). In this task, participants were asked to sit at workstations and direct simulated air traffic, trying to prevent accidents. The number of UAVs was varied (6, 12, 18) between trials and the mean change in oxy-Hb was calculated over the course of each trial.

As users were forced to keep track of more UAVs, fNIRS detected increased levels of oxy-Hb in the PFC. Ayaz found these changes to be comparable to those observed during interacton with the n-back task—a well-characterized psychological task for increasing working (or short-term) memory load. Increased levels of oxy-Hb also correlated with self-reported NASA-TLX workload measures, further validating the detection of signals that point to workload.

In another translation of fNIRS measures to real world environments, activity was recorded as participants were engaged as part of a human-robot team (Solovey et al. 2011). In this task, participants engaged in a multi-tasking assignment that could not be accomplished by the human nor the robot alone. The study investigated three classifications of multi-tasking—delay, dual-task, and branching. While *branching* required participants to maintain the context of a primary task while exploring a secondary task, users did not have to maintain this context in the *dual-task* condition, and they completely ignored the secondary task in the *delay* condition. Analyzing the mean combined hemoglobin (deoxy-Hb + oxy-Hb) for each participant, the branching condition was found to have higher levels of combined hemoglobin than either the dual-task or the delay conditions. In a second experiment that compared changed in deoxy-Hb in random interruptions with interruptions that could be predicted by the user, Solovey found that random interruptions provoked sharper decreases in deoxy-Hb.

Finally, Peck et al. (2013b) used fNIRS to detect working memory differences in a task that derives exclusively from the visual design of information. To explore the potential of fNIRS in evaluating information visualization, a complex visual task was constructed by mapping a well-studied visual judgment task (Cleveland and McGill 1984) with the n-back task. In Cleveland's original study of visual variables, participants made percentage estimates of elements within either bar

Fig. 6.5 An example of the memory-intensive graphical comparison task used by Peck et al. (2013b). Instead of making percentage comparisons of graph elements on the same chart, participants compared an element in the current chart with an element from the previously seen chart

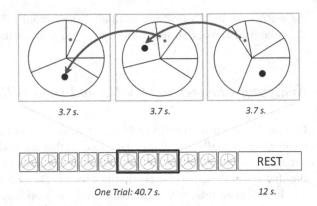

graphs or pie charts. Their results demonstrated that people can more accurately compare information in bar graphs than in pie charts.

In order to modify this simple visual comparison task to mimic more complex, memory-intensive tasks, participants in Peck's experiment compared a graph element in the current graph (bar graphs or pie charts) with a graph element from the *previous* graph (Fig. 6.5). This manipulation required participants to maintain graph elements in their short-term memory, and fNIRS measurements were intended to capture how each graph design (bar graphs or pie charts) supported this mental process. Rather than test on easy and difficult conditions for each graph type, participants engaged with a single 1-back task for each graph to see whether the visual encoding of information would result in low or high workload (Fig. 6.5).

In addition to recording brain activity with fNIRS, participants completed the NASA Task Load Index (NASA-TLX) after interaction. Results showed that levels of deoxy-Hb differed during interaction with bar graphs and pie charts. However, these differences were not categorical. Instead, they correlated with the visualization technique that participants *believed* was more mentally demanding. Similar to the observations made in other workload-intensive tasks, higher mental demand correlated with larger decreases in deoxy-Hb.

These experiments demonstrate that fNIRS can detect workload in a wide variety of tasks that is not limited to a specific type of stimuli or category of working memory.

Automatic Detection of Workload

If fNIRS is to become a viable tool for analyzing mental state during interaction with an interface, it would be ideal for the analysis of fNIRS signals to move from a manual to an automated process. In this section, we discuss work that has employed the use of predictive models to objectively (and automatically) classify user state.

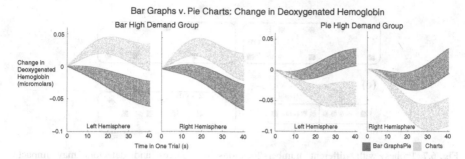

Fig. 6.6 In a study comparing bar graphs (*blue*) and pie charts (*green*), Peck found that a group of participants that subjectively rated bar graphs as more mentally demanding than pie charts (*left*) exhibited reversed fNIRS signals from those who rated pie charts as more mentally demanding than bar graphs (*right*). The plots represent the mean change in deoxygenated hemoglobin (from a rest state) across all trials of each condition. The width of the line represents the standard error at each time point

Classifying Known User State

When the user's intended state is known, some researchers have used predictive models as a statistical method to show that multiple user states is separable. However, the true potential of these models is in the automation of classifying fNIRS signals. This allows evaluators to avoid non-automated analysis—a potentially time-consuming task if fNIRS is to be used as a tool in real user studies. In these circumstances, researchers check the accuracy of their model by using cross-validation techniques.

For example, Luu and Chau (2008) used predictive models to distinguish between fNIRS signals during periods of low and high preference. In their experiment, participants viewed pictures of soft-drinks that they either highly-preferred or did not like at all. After identifying sensors that highly correlated with user preference, they were able to predict the preferred drink with over 80 % accuracy.

Similarly, Moghimi et al. (2012) used fNIRS to measure participants' emotional responses to music, attempting to capture both valence (positive or negative feelings) and arousal. They used linear discriminant analysis (LDA) to build a classifier and found that they could distinguish positive and negative valence with an average accuracy of 71.94 %. They also found they could distinguish between high arousal music and brown noise (low arousal) with an average accuracy of 71.93 %.

Finally, Girouard et al. (2009) measured users as they played a game of Pac-man, interacting with game modes that were both very easy and very difficult. They used a k-nearest neighbor (kNN) algorithm to classify game difficulty levels. While Girouard found that they could distinguish between periods of play and non-play with accuracy levels above 90 %, distinguishing between easy and hard difficulty levels yielded classifications just over 60 %.

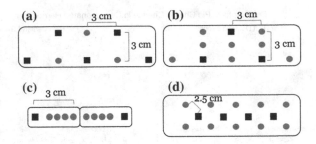

Fig. 6.7 Probes with different numbers/locations of sources and detectors may impact classification accuracy of user state. We show four probe configurations used in studies described in section "Detecting Workload in Real World Tasks". *Red circles* are light sources and *black squares* are detectors. In each case, probes would be centered on the participant's forehead **a** Moghimi et al. (2012), **b** Luu and Chau (2008), **c** Girouard et al. (2009), Hirshfield et al. (2011), Solovey et al. (2011), and Solovey et al. (2012), **d** Ayaz et al. (2012)

As Fig. 6.7 suggests, the discrepancies in classification accuracy in each study may partially stem from the various configurations of fNIRS probes; the first two studies used configurations with significantly more source-detector pairs. This provides two distinct advantages. First, increasing the number of information channels decreases the potential for one noisy channel to adversely impact a model. Second, these configurations provide better coverage of the prefrontal cortex. For example, Moghimi et al. (2012) showed that using information from a source-detector pair on the anatomical midline of the prefrontal cortex yielded the best overall accuracy in their model for capturing emotion. This is information that a smaller probe with a more linear configuration (such as the one used by Girouard) may have difficulty accessing unless it is placed in precisely the right location. However, accuracy is also heavily dependent on analysis methods, and thus far, we have skipped exactly *how* fNIRS is used as input to these models.

Selecting fNIRS Features

When predictive models are created, we need to determine which features of the signal are fed into the models. Choosing too many features with too few training examples may result in the "curse of dimensionality" and low classification rates. Choosing too few features, or incorrect features of the signal, may lead to a set of features that is not truly descriptive of the signal, also resulting in low classification accuracy. Currently, there is no standardized approach to feature extraction. We give four examples from current fNIRS literature:

- Solovey et al. (2012) used the signal value from each time point and each channel over the entire trial as individual features to a support vector machine (SVM).
- Luu et al. (2008) used the average signal value, estimated from a specific channel over a specific time interval within a trial (for example, 15–45 s).

- Hirshfield et al. (2011) extracted the max signal value, min signal value, mean signal value, slope, time to peak, and full width at half maximum.
- Moghimi et al. (2012) used the mean and slope of the signal during each trial. They also used the coefficient of variation, mean difference between signal and noise, and a handful of laterality features.

As these examples suggest, there is yet to be a prevailing consensus about which features of the fNIRS signal potentially result in the highest levels of accuracy. However, there are at least two dominant approaches to feature selection used in current fNIRS literature.

The first is to manually select a set of features based on an expert's knowledge or personal experience. For example, based on the changes of deoxy-Hb in response to load on working memory that we observed in Fig. 6.4, the mean change in deoxy-Hb would appear to be a good indicator of low/high load on working memory. In a finger-tapping task, Cui et al. (2010) show that including both oxy- and deoxy-Hb information to a predictive model improves accuracy. They also found that increasing the number of information channels improves accuracy. Broadly speaking, because the mean change in oxy-Hb is often used in the statistical comparison of fNIRS signals, it stands to reason that this feature is a good starting point for input to a model.

Using this method, context is important. Cui et al. (2010) note that the features they chose were "necessarily dependent" on the classification technique (in their case, support vector machines), and may be dependent on the task. One interesting distinction is that each of the previous examples is event-related—they observe how the fNIRS signals respond following a discrete moment in time. However, to serve as input to biocybernetic systems, it is often desirable for evaluators to view a moment-by-moment picture of workload, introducing new challenges. For example, task starting times, end times, and length may be undefined.

Given these challenges, an alternative approach is to select a large feature space. Then, using the participant's data, automatically determine which features yield the most information for each individual (for example, Luu et al. 2008). While this method often results in higher cross-validation classification rates, there is a danger that we may be building a model that succeeds on a particular dataset rather than one that represents a more general user state. We must take care not to overfit the model to the user's data, making it less flexible and robust for real world environments. In the next section, we describe how research is attempting to construct more generalized models of user state for real-time monitoring.

Classifying Periods of Unknown User State

Unfortunately, in normal user evaluation, researchers often do not know in advance whether a period of interaction *should be* low or high workload, or even when a period of low or high workload may begin. To help solve this problem,

Hirshfield et al. (2009) proposed a methodology for using machine-learning techniques to classify user state in these scenarios.

1. Choose cognitive benchmark tasks from the psychology literature that are known to induce specific user states. For example, if we are investigating the level of verbal working memory that a visual environment might induce, we might run a participant on a demanding 0-back and 3-back task, representing low and high levels of verbal working memory.
2. Next, we build a machine learning classifier to identify and store a cognitive footprint of the fNIRS signal during each level of the benchmark task. We make the assumption that we have stored an accurate representation of verbal working memory for this particular user.
3. Finally, the participant performs a set of tasks in a more complex environment. We run the fNIRS data from those tasks on the classifier we built in the previous steps. The idea is that we are comparing the fNIRS data from this complex environment to the patterns we identified in the cognitive benchmark tasks. Our machine learning classifier returns whether the signal most closely matches low, medium, or high verbal working memory.

Hirshfield used this methodology to explore the working memory demand in a driving task in which the steering controls were reversed (Hirsfield et al. 2011). In comparison to more natural steering controls, the model classified incoming fNIRS data during the reversed control condition as requiring high working-memory. In the same way, Hirshfield used the Stroop test to detect response inhibition during interaction with an interfaces. We use this general structure as a foundation to move towards adaptive brain-computer interfaces.

Using fNIRS in Biocybernetic Interfaces

One of the primary reasons we focus on algorithms that automatically classify the fNIRS signal is that they enable fNIRS to be used as input to intelligent, adaptive systems. Because fNIRS is lightweight and does not place any unreasonable restrictions on the user, it can feasibly be used to augment many operator stations. In a real-time adaptive system, fNIRS data may be used as an additional implicit or explicit input, relaying information about the user to the computer without any further work for the user.

However, while fNIRS devices typically have a sharp temporal resolution, as we have discussed, the biological signal is sluggish. As a result, there are limitations to the systems that can be constructed. In this section, we discuss adaptive systems that use fNIRS as input, the limitations of such systems, and also identify domains where these systems may thrive.

Fig. 6.8 3D View from the robots' perspective in Solovey's multi-tasking navigation environment. Automation was turned on or off based on the user's workload

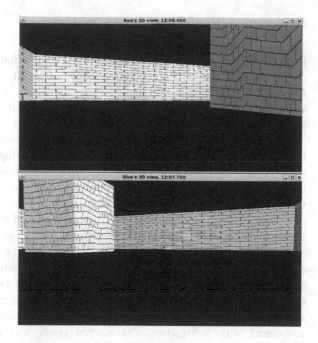

Calibration and Training

Similar to the training method previously described (Hirshfield et al. 2009), in order to create a successful biocybernetic system, users must first perform a task with a known cognitive effect in order for the system to calibrate to the characteristics of brain patterns of each individual. However, the model must be very cautious since users are often in a different mental state during offline calibration and online feedback (Vidaurre et al. 2010).

Ideally, we strive to minimize training time and maximize classification accuracy. Unfortunately, these two objectives typically compete with each other. Many machine learning algorithms are traditionally designed with the assumption that there are hundreds or thousands of training examples. But in an experimental setting, training the user for hours on end is unreasonable. As a result, researchers typically train users for as long as the ordinary time constraints of a user study allows. However, as more research is done in this field, we may find universal patterns that allow us to circumvent the training period. For example, using fNIRS, Herff et al. (2012) found neural responses to speaking modes to be consistent enough to construct a general classifier of accuracy of 71 %. We suspect that similar general models may be constructed for classification of other user states.

Brainput: A Real-Time fNIRS System

In this section, we give a concrete example of previous work that uses passive fNIRS input to an intelligent system. Solovey et al. (2012) created a system, *Brainput*, which was able to adapt a scenario where an interactive human-robot system changed its state of autonomy based on whether it detected a particular state of multitasking (Fig. 6.8).

To train the system to detect these states, they used a well-validated multi-tasking exercise that had previously been explored using fMRI. Participants were shown either lower-case or upper-case letters of the word 'tablet'. Depending on the case of the letter, participants were instructed to perform different actions, thereby resembling a multi-tasking environment. In a previous study (which we described earlier), Solovey et al. (2011) showed that this task could be used to identify multi-tasking scenarios with fNIRS.

In the testing task, users were instructed to direct two robots through a virtual environment to search for areas with strong transmission strengths, and were told to not let the robots go idle or collide with walls or objects in the environment (Fig. 6.8). fNIRS signals from the participants' prefrontal cortex were collected and classified as one of two user states that described the multi-tasking load associated with navigation. The second robot was autonomously controlled whenever the system detected a state of branching, where the user must hold in mind goals while exploring and processing secondary goals (Solovey et al. 2012). The changes occurred in real-time, allowing the system to dynamically respond to the user's individual, situational needs.

Solovey found that more participants completed the task with fewer collisions in this adaptive condition. However, to demonstrate that adaptation mechanism was indeed reacting to correctly classified fNIRS data, Solovey also introduced a maladaptive condition. This condition caused the system to intentionally perform the *opposite* response that should aid the user. In this maladaptive state, users did worse than in a nonadaptive condition, and had a lower overall average transmission strength than either other condition. This experiment provides a successful example of using fNIRS as input to a real-time system that intelligently adapts to the user.

Potential Domains for Adaptive Interfaces

This method has the capability to be used for many other adaptive interfaces, especially operator stations where users may be in charge of complex tasks, such as driving or controlling aerial vehicles. In driving simulators, oxygenated hemoglobin levels for users increased when they were not using cruise control (Tsunashima and Yanagisawa 2009). In addition, prefrontal activation increased when users were preparing to turn, and there were increases in oxygenation levels during a driving task when users were prompted with directions instead of knowing when to turn (Liu et al. 2012). This opens the door for driving applications that may alleviate the user's workload by delivering relevant information (such as directions) in different modes or at different times depending on the user's state.

Turning to another application area, Bunce et al. (2011) found that oxygenated hemoglobin levels increased in an unmanned aerial vehicle (UAV) commander task when the number of UAVs to identify increase. They also found that practice decreased the overall oxygenation change, with experts maintaining higher performance despite lower prefrontal activation. However, at difficult levels, novice performance and oxygenation fell, indicating that they gave up on the task, while experts showed a strong increase (Bunce et al. 2011). This suggests that neural activation can be used to determine a user's expertise in real-time, as well as when the user disengages from a task. The same trend of decreased activation for experts was found using fNIRS on ground operators performing UAVs approach and landing tasks (Izzetoglu et al. 2011). Using fNIRS to detect expertise during interaction may translate from operators to more general educational scenarios, and an adaptive system could potentially calibrate it's instructional aid based on the sensed expertise level of the user.

These measures can be applied to other domains as well. fMRI studies have shown that blood oxygen signals in the prefrontal cortex develop during economic choices where users must make gambling evaluations and expected value decisions (Minati et al. 2012) and when determining decision value for different categories of goods for purchase (Grabenhorst and Rolls 2011). Using these activation patterns, Peck et al. (2013a) demonstrated the use of fNIRS as input to information-filtering systems, constructing a movie recommendation engine that gradually personalized movies to the user based on predicted preference values.

These examples illustrate a small subset of application areas for interfaces that adapt according to physiological input. From gaming to education, there are numerous opportunities to cater the computing environment to each individual's cognitive state.

Challenges of Application

It's important to note that building these systems is not without significant challenge. A real-time adaptive system must filter raw data and determine state as quickly as possible in order to respond before the user's state changes and the adaptation becomes obsolete. Preferably, the system should be flexible and robust in that it is able to detect the user's workload in a variety of environments and tasks.

Aside from the difficulties in classification, the relatively sluggish fNIRS signal limits the appropriate adaptive responses of an interface. For example, using fNIRS to directly control a mouse cursor would likely prove to be frustrating for a user, as their actions would be delayed by 5–7 s. In general, we suggest the use of slow, gentle modifications to the system which the user does not (or hardly) perceive. For example, Solovey's (2012) Brainput system increased performance by adjusting the level of automation. Peck et al. (2013a) recommendation system changed *which* information was emphasized to the user. In both cases, individual changes were imperceptible to the user. These studies suggest that manipulating background processes may present an opportunity for designers to positively impact the user without disruptive adaptation mechanisms. Additionally, these changes minimize the impact of misclassification. Given the current challenges in achieving high classification rates, it is important that incorrect guesses do not result in disrupting the user's workflow or mental model of the system.

Finally, while a primary benefit of measuring activity in the prefrontal cortex stems from its involvement in many high-level user states, the general participation of the PFC in cognition is also a challenge. A variety of user states, from economic judgments to emotion to working memory load, have been correlated with the PFC. As we move the use of fNIRS into increasingly complex environments, it will be important to understand how the interaction of these states impacts changes in oxy-Hb and deoxy-Hb, as it may become difficult to identify them individually.

The Future of fNIRS

Although the work that we have discussed suggests a positive trajectory in using fNIRS to monitor user state, we have also been candid with some of the present challenges in using fNIRS in real world environments. Despite these challenges, recent advances hint that fNIRS will soon become even more lightweight and comfortable.

Moving towards an untethered system, a wireless setup of fNIRS has been implemented by a team at Drexel University (Yurtsever et al. 2003). Other research has seen the development of brush optrodes—sensors that are able to navigate through hair and comfortable measure numerous areas of the brain (Wildey et al. 2010). Finally, there has been preliminary work in no-contact fNIRS sensors, or remote sensing of the brain (Sase et al. 2012). Although these are early proof-of-concept studies, they suggest that someday, optical brain sensing may not require probes of any kind. While the equipment in our laboratory is expensive, the basic technology can eventually be implemented at greatly reduced costs since it consists fundamentally of simply a light source and an optical detector. Given these recent advances, we expect that fNIRS will continue to be considered a viable technology for brain sensing in the coming decades.

Conclusion

In this chapter, we reviewed work that has used functional near-infrared spectroscopy to observe changes in user workload during interaction with a computer interface. We began by describing basic, highly-controlled experiments in which fNIRS recorded changes in workload in classical psychology tasks (the n-back). From there, we moved towards tasks that more closely mirror tasks that users face in everyday life. However, the analysis was performed manually and offline, creating a burden on evaluators that is not ideal for industrial user-studies. Finally, we shared work that uses predictive models to automatically identifies the user's state, requiring little intervention from the evaluator.

Turning an eye towards the future, we painted a picture in which these classifications of user state could be used as passive input to real-time adaptive interfaces. We believe that these interfaces have the potential to specially calibrate the user's computing environment to their individual skills and abilities.

Overall, use of fNIRS is not without its challenges. Signal classification is difficult, and systems must push for increased accuracy in increasingly noisy environments. However, fNIRS provides a unique source of input that can be seen as complimentary to other physiological sensors. We believe that the information that we can gain from fNIRS brain sensing can contribute to evaluation in real world environments, as well as personalization in real-time environments.

References

Ayaz H, Shewokis PA, Bunce S, Izzetoglu K, Willems B, Onaral B (2012) Optical brain monitoring for operator training and mental workload assessment. NeuroImage 59(1):36–47

Baddeley AD (1992) Working memory. Science 255(5044):556–559

Bor D, Cumming N, Scott CEL, Owen AM (2004) Prefrontal cortical involvement in verbal encoding strategies. Eur J Neurosci 19:3365–3370

Bor D, Duncan J, Wiseman RJ, Owen AM (2003) Encoding strategies dissociate prefrontal activity from working memory demand. Neuron 37:361–367

Braver TS, Cohen JD, Nystrom LE, Jonides J, Smith EE, Noll DC (1997) A parametric study of prefrontal cortex involvement in human working memory. Neuroimage 5:49–62

Bunce SC, Izzetoglu K, Ayaz H, Shewokis P, Izzetoglu M, Pourrezaei K, Onaral B (2011) Implementation of fNIRS for monitoring levels of expertise and mental workload. In: Foundations of Augmented Cognition. Directing the Future of Adaptive Systems. Springer, Berlin, pp 13–22

Burgess PW, Quayle A, Frith CD (2001) Brain regions involved in prospective memory as determined by positron emission tomography. Neuropsychologia 39:545–555

Cahill L, Uncapher M, Kilpatrick L, Alkire MT, Turner J (2004) Sex-related hemispheric lateralization of amygdala function in emotionally influenced memory: an fMRI investigation. Learn Mem 11(3):261–266

Chance B, Anday E, Nioka S, Zhou S, Hong L, Worden K, Li C et al (1998) A novel method for fast imaging of brain function, non-invasively, with light. Opt Express 2(10):41123

Christoff K, Gabrieli JDE (2000) The frontopolar cortex and human cognition: evidence for a rostrocaudal hierarchical organisation within the human prefrontal cortex. Psychobiology 28:168–186

Christoff K, Prabhakaran V, Dorfman J, Zhao Z, Kroger JK, Holyoak KJ, Gabrieli JD (2001) Rostrolateral prefrontal cortex involvement in relational integration during reasoning. Neuroimage 14(5):1136–1149

Cleveland WS, McGill R (1984) Graphical Perception: Theory, experimentation, and the application to the development of graphical methods. J Am Stat Assoc 387:531–554

Cohen JD, Perlstein WM, Braver TS, Nystrom LE, Noll DC, Jonides J, Smith EE (1997) Temporal dynamics of brain activation during a working memory task. Nature 386:604–608

Cui X, Bray S, Reiss A (2010) Speeded near infrared spectroscopy (NIRS) response detection. PLoS One 5(11):e15474

Davis MH, Meunier F, Marslen-Wilson WD (2004) Neural responses to morphological, syntactic, and semantic properties of single words: an fMRI study. Brain Lang 89(3):439–449

D'Esposito M, Zarahn E, Aguirre G (1999) Event-related functional MRI: implications for cognitive psychology. Psychol Bull 125(1):155–164

Dove A, Rowe JB, Brett M, Owen AM (2001) Neural correlates of passive and active encoding and retrieval: a 3T fMRI study. Neuroimage 13(Suppl):660

Franceschini MA, Joseph DK, Huppert TJ, Diamond SG, Boas DA (2006) Diffuse optical imaging of the whole head. J Biomed Opt 11(5):054007

Gevins AS, Cutillo BC (1993) Neuroelectric evidence for distributed processing in human working memory. Electroencephalogr Clin Neurophysiol 87:128–143

Girouard A, Solovey E, Hirshfield L, Chauncey K, Sassaroli A, Fantini S, Jacob RJK (2009) Distinguishing difficulty levels with non-invasive brain activity measurements. Interact 2009:440–452

Gore JC (2003) Principles and practice of functional MRI of the human brain. J Clin Investig 112(1):4–9

Grabenhorst F, Rolls ET (2011) Value, pleasure and choice in the ventral prefrontal cortex. Trends Cogn Sci 15(2):5667

Herff C, Heger D, Putze F, Guan C, Schultz T (2012) Cross-subject classification of speaking modes using fNIRS. ICONIP 2012:417–424

Hirshfield LM, Solovey ET, Girouard A, Kebinger J, Jacob RJK, Sassaroli A, Fantini S (2009) Brain measurement for usability testing and adaptive interfaces: an example of uncovering syntactic workload with functional near infrared spectroscopy. In: CHI 2009

Hirshfield LM, Gulotta R, Hirshfield S, Hincks S, Russell M, Ward R, Williams T, Jacob RJK (2011) This is your brain on interfaces: enhancing usability testing with functional near-infrared spectroscopy. In: CHI 2011

Hockey GRJ (1997) Compensatory control in the regulation of human performance under stress and high workload: a cognitive-energetical framework. Biol Psychol 45:73–93

Izzetoglu K, Ayaz H, Menda J (2011) Applications of functional near infrared imaging: case study on UAV ground controller. In: Schmorrow DD, Fidopiastis CM (eds) Foundations of augmented cognition. Springer, New York, pp 608–617

Jonides J, Smith EE, Koeppe RA, Awh E, Minoshima S, Mintun MA (1993) Spatial working memory in humans as revealed by PET. Nature 363:623–625

Koechlin E, Corrado G, Pietrini P, Grafman J (2000) Dissociating the role of the medial and lateral anterior prefrontal cortex in human planning. Proc Nat Acad Sci. 97(13):7651–7656

Kroger JK, Sabb FW, Fales CL, Bookheimer SY, Cohen MS, Holyoak KJ (2002) Recruitment of anterior dorsolateral prefrontal cortex in human reasoning: a parametric study of relational complexity. Cereb Cortex 12:477–485

Liu T, Saito H, Oi M (2012) Distinctive activation patterns under intrinsically versus extrinsically driven cognitive loads in prefrontal cortex: a near-infrared spectroscopy study using a driving video game. Neuroscience letters, 506(2):220–224

Luu S, Chau T (2008) Decoding subjective preference from single-trial near-infrared spectroscopy signals. J Neural Eng 6:058001

Miller G (1956) The magical number seven, plus or minus two: some limits on our capacity for processing information. Psychol Rev 63(2):8197

Minati L, Grisoli M, Franceschetti S, Epifani F, Granvillano A, Medford N, Harrison N et al (2012) Neural signatures of economic parameters during decision-making: a functional MRI (FMRI), electroencephalography (EEG) and autonomic monitoring study. Brain Topogr 25(1):73–96

Moghimi S, Kushki A, Power S, Guerguerian AM, Chau T (2012) Automatic detection of a prefrontal cortical response to emotionally rated music using multi-channel near-infrared spectroscopy. J Neural Eng 9(2):026022

Owen AM, McMillan KM, Laird AR, Bullmore E (2005) N-back working memory paradigm: a meta-analysis of normative functional neuroimaging studies. Hum Brain Mapp 25(1):46–59

Peck EM, Afergan D, Jacob RJK (2013a) Investigation of fNIRS brain sensing as input to information filtering systems. In: Augmented human 2013

Peck EM, Yuksel BF, Ottley A, Jacob RJK, Chang R (2013b) Using fNIRS brain sensing to evaluate information visualization interfaces. In: CHI 2013

Ramnani N, Owen AM (2004) Anterior prefrontal cortex: insights into function from anatomy and neuroimaging. Nat Rev Neurosci 5:184–194

Repovš G, Baddeley A (2006) The multi-component model of working memory: explorations in experimental cognitive psychology. Neuroscience 139:5–21

Repovš G, Bresjanac M (2006) Cognitive neuroscience of working memory: a prologue. Neuroscience 139:1–3

Rugg MD, Fletcher PC, Allan K, Frith CD, Frackowiak RS, Dolan RJ (1998) Neural correlates of memory retrieval during recognition memory and cued recall. Neuroimage 8:262–273

Sase I, Takatsuki A, Seki J, Yanagida T, Seiyama A (2012) Noncontact backscatter-mode near-infrared time-resolved imaging system: preliminary study for functional brain mapping. J Biomed Opt 11(5):054006

Solovey ET, Girouard A, Chauncey K, Hirshfield LM, Sassaroli A, Zheng F, Fantini S, Jacob RJK (2009) Using fNIRS brain sensing in realistic HCI settings: experiments and guidelines. In: UIST 2009

Solovey ET, Lalooses F, Chauncey K, Weaver D, Scheutz M, Sassaroli A, Fantini S, Jacob RJK (2011) Sensing cognitive multitasking for a brain-based adaptive user interface. In: CHI 2011

Solovey ET, Schermerhorn P, Scheutz M, Sassaroli A, Fantini S, Jacob RJK (2012) Brainput: enhancing interactive systems with streaming fNIRS brain input. In: CHI 2012

Strangman G, Culver JP, Thompson JH, Boas DA (2002) A quantitative comparison of simultaneous BOLD fMRI and NIRS recordings during functional brain activation. NeuroImage 17(2):719731

Tsunashima H, Yanagisawa K (2009) Measurement of brain function of car driver using functional near-infrared spectroscopy (fNIRS). Comput Intell Neurosci 2009:164958

Tulving E (1983) Elements of episodic memory. Clarendon, Oxford

Wickens CD (2002) Multiple resources and performance prediction. Theor Issues Ergon Sci 3:159–177

Wildey C, MacFarlane D, Khan B, Tian F, Liu H, Alexandrakis G (2010) Improved fNIRS using a novel brush optrode. In: Laser science

Vidaurre C, Sannelli C, Muller K-R, Blankertz B (2010) Machine-learning-based coadaptive calibration for brain-computer interfaces. Neural Comput 816:791816

Villringer A, Chance B (1997) Non-invasive optical spectroscopy and imaging of human brain function. Trends Neurosci 20(10):43542

Yurtsever G, Ayaz H, Kepics F, Onaral B (2003) Wireless, continuous wave near infrared spectroscopy system for monitoring brain activity. In: Bioengineering conference, pp 53–53

Chapter 7
Psychophysiological Feedback for Adaptive Human–Robot Interaction (HRI)

Esubalew Bekele and Nilanjan Sarkar

Abstract Recent advances in robotics and sensing have given rise to a diverse set of robots and their applications. In recent years robots have increasingly applied in the service industry, search and rescue operations and therapeutic applications. The introduction of robots to interact with humans resulted in a dedicated field called human–robot interaction (HRI). Social HRI is of particular importance as it is the main focus of this chapter. This chapter presents an affect-inspired approach for social HRI. Physiological processing together with machine learning was employed to model affective states for an adaptive social HRI and its application in social interaction in the context of autism therapy was investigated.

Introduction

Traditionally robots equipped with minimal set of sensing and computing abilities were used in industrial settings for specific repetitive tasks (Thrun 2004). However, recent advances in the field have given rise to a diverse set of robots. In recent years robots have increasingly become commonplace in the service industry (Bien and Lee 2007; Severinson-Eklundh et al. 2003), search and rescue operations (Murphy 2004; Nourbakhsh et al. 2005) and therapeutic applications (Kwakkel et al. 2008; Diehl et al. 2012; Scassellati et al. 2012). The introduction of robots to interact with humans resulted in a dedicated field called human–robot interaction (HRI) (Goodrich and Schultz 2007). Social HRI is of particular importance as it is the main focus of this chapter. Social interaction includes social, emotional, and cognitive interactions with a robot. These include learning, imitation, social communication and emotion recognition (Fong et al. 2003).

E. Bekele (✉) · N. Sarkar
Vanderbilt University, 518 Olin hall, 2400 Highland Ave, Nashville, TN 37212, USA
e-mail: bekele@vanderbilt.edu

S. H. Fairclough and K. Gilleade (eds.), *Advances in Physiological Computing*, Human–Computer Interaction Series, DOI: 10.1007/978-1-4471-6392-3_7, © Springer-Verlag London 2014

A vast majority of robots as applied to social interaction have been mostly teleoperated with simplistic and limited behaviors. However, sustained and meaningful social interaction for a more 'natural' human–robot interaction that resembles human–human interaction requires a closed-loop adaptive interaction via a variety of modalities (Agrawal et al. 2008; Fong et al. 2003). Sensors that are used to enable the robot to achieve such intelligence close to natural interactions include audiovisual and physiological signals (Croft 2003). Recent studies employed laser range finders (Feil-Seifer and Mataric 2005), visual processing (Feil-Seifer and Mataric 2011) and adaptation using physiological signals (Agrawal et al. 2008; Liu et al. 2008a) for closed-loop social interactions. In this work we specifically focus on closed-loop interaction between a robot and human based on implicit psychophysiological cues in real-time communication. The rest of the chapter is organized as follows: section "Related Work" reviews the state-of-the-art in psychophysiology sensing and its application to HRI. Section "A Novel HRI System with Psychophysiological Feedback" focuses on our work on HRI with psychophysiology-based emotion understanding whereas section "Extension of the Psychophysiological Feedback Based HRI to Children with Autism" discusses our work on HRI as applied to autism therapy. Section "Discussion, Conclusion and Ongoing Work" highlights our ongoing work on social HRI and psychophysiology as applied to autism intervention. Section "Current Ongoing Psychophysiology Work" summarizes the chapter by discussing the overall impact of endowing robots with emotion recognition ability using wearable psychophysiology computing.

Related Work

Psychophysiology and Intent Recognition

Understanding intent and implicit emotional cues of a human user by a robot is crucial for meaningful and natural interaction since human interactions are characterized by not only explicit but also implicit communications. In particular the implicit emotional cues (e.g. facial expressions, gestures, intonation, and peripheral physiological changes) are presumably expressions of the underlying emotional states (Picard 1997).

Generally, psychophysiology focuses on higher cognitive processes and their integration with central and peripheral processes (Cacioppo et al. 2007). There is good evidence that the physiological activity associated with the affective state can be differentiated and systematically organized (Rani et al. 2004, 2006; Liu et al. 2008b; Welch et al. 2009). The transition from one affective state to another, for instance, from relaxed to anxiety state is accompanied by dynamic shifts in indicators of Autonomic Nervous System (ANS) activity. But, it should be noted that ANS is a general purpose physiological system in which all responses are not exclusively due to emotions. Other aspects of body physiology such as respiration and digestion may also contribute to the ANS response. Moreover, it is not easy to distinguish individual emotions from a particular ANS response since such a response could be due to compound effect of a range of emotions. These factors make emotion recognition from physiological signals a challenging task. The most common measures of ANS responses are electrodermal response via galvanic skin response or conductance (GSR) and peripheral skin temperature (SKT), and cardiovascular response via electrocardiograph (ECG), impedance cardiograph (ICG), phonocardiograph/heart sound (PCG/HS) and pulse plethysmograph (PPG). Whole body responses via muscles can be measured using electromyography (EMG). Although various modalities such as auditory and visual have been used to understand emotions (Pantic et al. 2007; Tao and Tan 2005; D'Mello and Graesser 2010), peripheral psychophysiological signals are used to directly record various responses of the peripheral nervous system (PNS) and understanding of emotional cues. Peripheral physiological signals have been applied to medicine, entertainment (Kim and André 2008), and human–computer interaction (HCI) (Picard 1999), intelligent tutoring systems (Hussain et al. 2011), therapy for autism spectrum disorders (Liu et al. 2008a), cognitive loads (Calvo and D'Mello 2010; Koenig et al. 2011) and their use and application domain is expanding recently (Fairclough 2009).

Physiological responses can be analyzed to infer the underlying emotional or affective states of a human user. Affective state recognition is performed extracting useful features from the raw physiological signals and applying some machine learning algorithms to learn and recognize the states given a certain set of feature vectors. Various machine learning techniques (Calvo and D'Mello 2010; Rani et al. 2006) and representations (Agrawal et al. 2008; Liu et al. 2008a; Hussain et al. 2012) have been proposed for underlying affective state detection from peripheral physiological signals (Wagner et al. 2005). Although a vast body of literature investigated emotion recognition using peripheral psychophysiological signals and their application in an individual specific approach does exist, developing a user independent physiological emotional states recognition system is a challenge yet to be explored (Jerritta et al. 2011).

Adaptive HRI and Psychophysiology

Although, peripheral physiological signals are used widely for other applications, their application to robots in the context of detection of underlying emotional states is limited (Agrawal et al. 2008). A few studies have investigated the use of physiological signals for HRI in tasks ranging from robot safety to ASD therapy. Using GSR, ECG, and EMG and a fuzzy inference engine (Kulić and Croft 2007a) showed physiological states estimated for anxiety, calm, and surprise could be used for monitoring of human reaction for a safe HRI by modifying the robot trajectory in real-time. The same set of physiological signals and inference engine was used in intent estimation (Croft 2003) and anxiety detection (Kulic and Croft 2005) for human–robot interaction in the context of safety for industrial robots. Instead of looking at instantaneous physiological signal changes, a hidden Markov model (HMM) detector based on sequence of physiological changes was proposed by Kulic and Croft (2007b) for an industrial robot and human interaction. ECG, RSP, GSR, PPG and EMG were employed to measure emotional states of human participants in response to search and rescue robots (Bethel et al. 2007; Bethel et al. 2009). Tapus and Mataric (2008) used GSR and SKT as part of a socially rehabilitative robot that assists and encourages human users in social interaction based on personality and preferences.

We have incorporated psychophysiological sensing as the main modality for adaptive HRI for a closed loop interaction in our previous work (Sarkar 2002). An earlier version of the system used ECG together with fuzzy inference model to detect stress online and adapt robot behavior (Rani et al. 2002). An improved version incorporated PPG, GSR and EMG at masseter and corrugator supercilii muscles in addition to ECG and combined them using a fuzzy inference model to deduce anxiety indices (Rani et al. 2004). Another improvement added impedance cardiograph (ICG), phonocardiograph (PCG), SKT, and EMG for three facial and shoulder muscles and employed a regression tree to determine the person's affective state of anxiety (Rani and Sarkar 2005; Liu et al. 2006). Comparative studies were performed to evaluate a range of machine learning algorithms to emotion recognition of three emotions, i.e., liking, engagement, and anxiety was performed (Rani et al. 2006; Liu et al. 2005). Lessons learned from human robot interaction of typical population and feature extraction and machine learning methods developed were later applied to therapy of individuals with ASD (Liu et al. 2007, 2008a; Conn et al. 2010).

A Novel HRI System with Psychophysiological Feedback

We discuss a new HRI framework where a robot monitors and adapts its behavior based on both performance and affective states of the participants. We designed such a HRI framework to emulate typical human-to-human interaction where people monitor each other's action as well as affective cues (e.g., facial expressions, gestures etc.) during interaction. While it is relatively easier for people to use their vision to infer affective cues, it is quite difficult for a robot to infer such cues in real-time through computer vision because several issues such as individual differences in affective facial expressions, peculiar or odd facial expressions and similarity among some facial expressions indicating different emotions may complicate such affect recognition. In this work, we used physiological sensing to infer affective cues. Although individual variations are still present, although in a relatively smaller scale than facial expressions, and the combined effect of various emotions could make the recognition process challenging, it has been shown to be effective in recognizing certain class of emotions (Rani et al. 2006).

Physiological Signals

Although much existing research on affective modeling categorizes affective states into "basic emotions", there is no consensus on a set of basic emotions among the researchers (Cowie et al. 2001). This fact implies that pragmatic choices are required to select target affective states for a given application (Cowie et al. 2001). Notably, evidence shows that several affective states could co-occur at different arousal levels (Vansteelandt et al. 2005) and different individuals could express the same emotion with different characteristic response patterns under the same contexts (i.e., phenomenon of person stereotypy) (Lacey and Lacey 1958). This calls for an individual-specific approach to accommodate the differences encountered in emotional expression. The overall system contains two phases, i.e., the physiological modeling phase to develop an affect recognizer, and the online closed-loop HRI phase, which employs the affect recognizers developed in the first phase for an online adaptive HRI.

The physiological signals that we examined to develop an affect-recognizer were: ECG, ICG, PCG, PPG, GSR, SKT, and EMG (from Corrugator Supercilii, Zygomaticus, and upper Trapezius muscles). These choices were motivated by the existing literature. Cardiovascular and electromyogram (EMG) activities have been used to capture positive and negative affective valence states (Cacioppo et al. 2007; Papillo and Shapiro 1990). Blood pulse volume amplitude and sympathetic activity have been shown to be associated with task engagement (Iani et al. 2004). The relationships between both electrodermal and cardiovascular activities with anxiety were investigated in (Pecchinenda 1996) and (Dawson et al. 2007).

Multiple features (Table 7.1) were derived for each physiological measure. These features are described in Rani et al. (2006) and are described in Table 7.1. Features of cardiovascular activity that were analyzed were: inter-beat interval (IBI), relative pulse volume, pulse transit time (PTT), and pre ejection period (PEP). We also extracted three power spectral features from the cardiovascular signals, i.e., Para, Sym and VLF powers. "Sym" is the power associated with the sympathetic ANS activity of the heart (0.04–0.15 Hz.). "Para" is the power associated with the parasympathetic ANS activity of the heart (0.15–0.4 Hz.) and measures the influence of the vagus nerve in modulating the sinoatrial node and is associated with parasympathetic nervous system activity. "VLF" is the power associated with the Very Low Frequency band (<0.04 Hz.).

PPG measures changes in the volume of blood in the fingertip associated with the pulse cycle, and it provides an index of the relative constriction versus dilation of the blood vessels in the periphery. In addition to the features that are directly extracted from PPG such as inter beat interval (IBI), PTT was derived from a combination of ECG and PPG. PTT is the time it takes for the pulse pressure wave to travel from the heart to the periphery, and it is estimated by computing the time between systole at the heart (as indicated by the R-wave of the ECG) and the peak of the pulse wave reaching the peripheral site where PPG is being measured. Bioelectrical impedance analysis (BIA) measures the impedance or opposition to

Table 7.1 Physiological signals and features

Physiological signals	Features derived	Label used	Units of measurement
Cardiac activity	Sympathetic power (from ECG)	Sym	Unit/square second
	Parasympathetic power (from ECG)	Para	Unit/square second
	Very low frequency power (from ECG)	VLF	Unit/square second
	Ratio of powers	Sym para Para VLF Sym VLF	No unit
	Mean IBI	IBI ECG mean	Milliseconds
	Std. of IBI	IBI ECG std	Standard deviation
	Mean amplitude of the peak values of the PPG signal (Photoplethysmogram)	PPG peak mean	Micro volts
	Standard deviation (std.) of the peak values of the PPG signal	PPG peak std	Standard deviation
	Mean pulse transit time	PTT mean	Milliseconds
Heart sound (Ecocardiography)	Mean of the 3rd, 4th, and 5th level coefficients of the Daubechies wavelet transform of hear sound signal	Mean d3 Mean d4 Mean d5	No unit
	Standard deviation of the 3rd, 4th, and 5th level coefficients of the Daubechies wavelet transform of hear sound signal	Std d3 Std d4 Std d5	No unit
Bioimpedance	Mean pre-ejection period	PEP mean	Milliseconds
	Mean IBI	IBI ICG mean	Milliseconds
Electrodermal activity	Mean tonic activity level	Tonic mean	Micro Siemens
	Slope of tonic activity	Tonic slope	Micro Siemens/second
	Mean amplitude of skin conductance response (phasic activity)	Phasic mean	Micro Siemens
	Maximum amplitude of the skin conductance response (phasic activity)	Phasic max	Micro Siemens
	Rate of phasic activity	Phasic rate	Response peaks/second

(continued)

Table 7.1 (continued)

Physiological signals	Features derived	Label used	Units of measurement
Electromyographic activity	Mean of corrugator supercilii activity	Cor mean	Micro volts/second
	Std. of corrugator supercilii activity	Cor std	Standard deviation
	Slope of corrugator supercilii activity	Cor slope	Micro volts/second
	Mean interbeat interval of blink activity	IBI blink mean	Milliseconds
	Std. of interbeat interval of blink activity	IBI blink std	Standard deviation
	Mean amplitude of blink activity	Amp blink mean	Microvolts
	Std. of blink activity	Blink std	Standard deviation
	Mean of zygomaticus major activity	Zyg mean	Micro volts
	Std. of zygomaticus major activity	Zyg std	Standard deviation
	Slope of zygomaticus major activity	Zyg slope	Micro volts/second
	Mean of upper trapezius activity	Trap mean	Micro volts
	Std. of upper trapezius activity	Trap std	Standard deviation
	Slope of upper trapezius activity	Trap slope	Micro volts/second
	Mean and median frequency of corrugator, zygomaticus, and trapezius	Zfreq median	Hertz
		Cfreq median	
		Tfreq mean	
Skin Temperature	Mean temperature	Temp mean	Degree centigrade
	Std. of temperature	Temp std	Standard deviation
	Slope of temperature	Temp slope	Degree centigrade/second

the flow of an electric current through the body fluids contained mainly in the lean and fat tissue of the thoracic cavity. Changes in thoracic bio impedance has been used to measure cardiac output (Kubicek et al. 1966). A common variable in recent psychophysiology research, PEP—derived from impedance cardiogram (ICG) and ECG, measures the latency between the onset of electromechanical systole, and the onset of left-ventricular ejection. PEP is most heavily influenced by sympathetic innervations of the heart. In addition to the PEP, the thoracic impedance signal has been used to extract the mean inter beat interval of the signal itself as a representative feature. Heart sound (echocardiography) signal measures sounds generated during each heartbeat. These sounds are produced by blood turbulence primarily due to the closing of the valves within the heart. The features extracted from the heart sound signal consisted of the mean and standard deviation of the 3rd, 4th, and 5th level coefficients of the Daubechies wavelet transform as direct features representing the heart sound signal. Similarly, for electrodermal activity we extracted various features from the tonic and phasic response of the GSR as shown in Table 7.1. Tonic skin conductance refers to the ongoing or the baseline level of skin conductance in the absence of any particular discrete environmental events such as stress. Phasic skin conductance refers to the event related changes that occur, caused by a momentary increase in skin conductance (resembling a peak). Several features have also been extracted from three EMG signals. The EMG signal from Corrugator Supercilii muscle (eyebrow) captures a person's frowns and detects the tension in that region. It is also a valuable source of blink information and helps us determine the blink rate. The EMG signal from the Zygomaticus Major muscle captures the muscle movements while smiling. Upper Trapezius muscle activity measures the tension in the shoulders, one of the most common sites in the body for developing stress.

Phase I: Physiological Modeling for Affect Recognition

In this work, we trained a set of classifiers to categorize features derived from the physiological signals into affective states using supervised training methods. An experiment was designed to collect physiological training data for affect recognition to build models. Participants in this experiment were presented with two computer tasks—an anagram word problem solving task and a pong game that elicited various affective states. The anagram task was similar to a word scramble game where the participant was required to complete a word with correct spelling by rearranging the scrambled letters. The pong game was a computer simulated version of the traditional pong game, with the participant controlling the paddle movement using mouse and key strokes. Both tasks were shown to be capable of producing the target affective states by manipulating their difficulty level. Each task consisted of three levels of difficulties and there were three trials in each difficulty level. Various parameters of the games were manipulated to elicit the desired target affective states. For example, for the pong task, ball speed, paddle speed and size, sluggish or over responsive keyboard and random paddle direction were used as parameters to elicit frustration, anxiety and enjoyment. For the anagram task, the length of the words and the number of misplaced words were used as parameters to change the level of difficulties. The levels of difficulties for these tasks were established by a pilot study conducted separately prior to phase one of this study. Six teenagers participated in the pilot study. The affective states elicited by the Pong game include engagement, anxiety, anger, and frustration. These psychological states play an important role in human–machine interaction (HMI). A detailed discussion on the link between these states and HMI can be found in Rani and Sarkar (2005). The affective states were mainly chosen from the domain of negative affective states since they can be more closely related to performance and mental health of humans while interacting with the machines. A total of 15 people participated in this experiment. Each participant took part in six sessions (three 1 h sessions of solving anagrams and three 1 h sessions of playing pong) of the two tasks with each session of about an hour spanning over a month period. Each session was divided into a series of epochs bounded by assessments. Each epoch was 3 min long for anagram and 2–4 min for Pong depending on the difficulty. During the assessment, participants reported their perceived subjective emotional states in relation to the established psychological states using a 10 point Likert scale. These questions assessed the level of engagement, anxiety, anger, frustration and challenge perceived by the participant after each epoch. Self-reports were used as reference points to link the objective physiological data to participants' subjective affective state.

At the beginning of each session, baseline physiological signals were recorded in order to offset day-to-day and individual-variability. The training datasets were formed by merging each epoch's physiological data with the self-report (serving as labels) as shown in Fig 7.1. At the end of this study, we developed models for each participant that would predict a probable affective state (e.g., anxiety) based on their self-labeled physiological markers.

We used 9 channels of physiological signals and about 53 features extracted out of them as shown in Table 7.1. Data points in the training dataset were labeled using self-report by the participants (Fig. 7.1) and the feature sets were included for training if they were correlated with the target affective states (i.e., Anxiety, Engagement, Frustration and Anger) above a certain absolute correlation threshold. Any feature (derived from physiological signals) with an absolute correlation greater than or equal to 0.3 with a given affective state was considered significant and was selected as input to the classifiers. The self-reports were normalized to [0,1] and then converted into a series of banded regions where 0–0.33 was low, 0.34–0.67 was medium, and 0.68–1.0 was high for each of the target states. In order to overcome person-stereotypy we adopted an individual-specific framework where we developed a model for each individual (e.g., we determine the physiological pattern of anxiety for each participant). In this first phase, we targeted various affective states to comparatively evaluate various machine learning techniques. In phase two, described in next section, we chose anxiety only as a target state in a robotic basketball game task.

Fig. 7.1 Formation of
training dataset for input to
classifiers

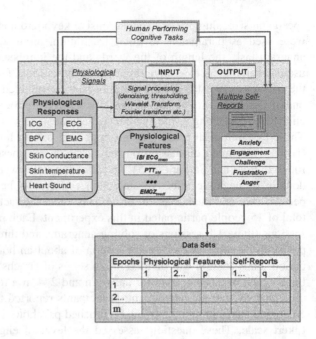

Four machine learning techniques—K Nearest Neighbor (KNN), Regression
Tree (RT), Bayesian Networks (BNT), and Support Vector Machines (SVM) were
used to perform affect-recognition from the data sets that were formed as shown in
Fig. 7.1.

The goal of this study was to determine the performance of the four learning
techniques in predicting the arousal level of unseen instances, given a set of
physiological features each labeled with a particular level of arousal of a given
affective state for training. The overall classification average accuracies over all
the affective states considered were found to be SVM (85.8 %), RT (83.5 %),
KNN (75.1 %), and BNT (74.0 %). Using more informative features based on
absolute correlation improved the classification accuracies of KNN and BNT by
4 %. RT was efficient in both space and time overall. Based on time-space efficiency, comparably higher classification accuracy and effective use of more
informative features, we chose RT for the next phase II robotic basketball
interaction.

Phase II: Closed-Loop RBB HRI

In this section, we describe the various aspects of the human–robot interaction
experiment that was designed to evaluate the effect of the implicit affective
communication using the affective models developed in phase I using anxiety

Fig. 7.2 The robotic basketball (Nerf ball) used in RBB task

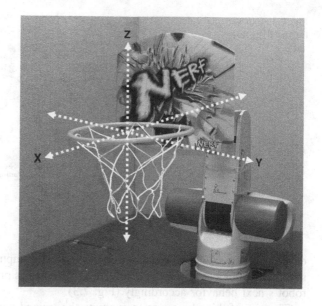

levels as affective states. A closed-loop HRI task, "RBB," was designed to evaluate the effect of implicit affective communication via anxiety (RT models). We named this task as "robot-based basketball (RBB) task". In the RBB task, an undersized basketball hoop was attached to the end-effector of a robotic manipulator, which could move the hoop in different directions (as shown in Fig. 7.1) with different speeds. The difficulty of the game was manipulated by changing the direction and the speed of the hoop using the robot controller. There were three directions of motion with the corresponding Cartesian coordinate axes (X, Y, and Z) and three speeds of motion (100 cm/s, 50 cm/s, and 25 cm/s), which are empirically determined using previous pilot studies. The three speeds and the three directions were combined to produce nine unique configurations. Each participant played each of these configurations in piloting this system to rate the difficulty of each configuration level. Each epoch was 1.5 min long and at the end of each epoch, participants reported the difficulty of the game as they perceived it in a 10 point Likert scale. The nine configurations were then clustered into three levels of difficulty, i.e., Levels I, II, and III.

The real-time implementation of the RBB system is shown in Fig. 7.2. The setup included a 5-degree-of-freedom robot manipulator (CRS Catalyst-5 System) with a small basketball hoop attached to its end-effector. Two sets of IR transmitter and receiver pairs were attached to the hoop to detect small, soft foam balls going through the hoop. The setup also included biological feedback equipment (Biopac system) that collected the participant's physiological signals and the digital output from the IR sensors. The Biopac system was connected to a PC (C1) that (1) acquired physiological signals from the Biopac system and extracted physiological features online; (2) predicted the probable anxiety, level using the affective model

Fig. 7.3 Experimental setup
for the RBB task

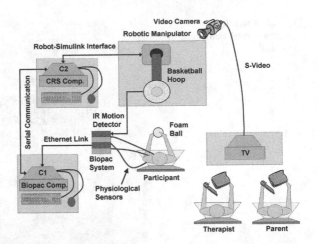

developed (3) acquired IR data through the analog input channels of the Biopac system; (4) ran a program that learns the participant's preference and chooses the robot's next behavior accordingly (Fig. 7.3).

The aim of this phase was to evaluate the trained anxiety model and to effectively adapt the difficulty level of the RBB task using this model. For instance, if a participant's anxiety level was detected as high in previous medium level of difficulty task, the level will be lowered to one level to calm the participant down. In the online phase of interaction, the game difficulty was varied as a function of anxiety to allow each player play at a lower level of anxiety and to study the effect of reducing the anxiety level in improving the participant's performance.

Participants

A total of 14 individuals (8 females, and 6 males) volunteered to participate in the experiments. Out of these, nine of them had also participated in the Phase I experiments. We built the affect-recognizers for the other 5 participants separately as described in phase I above except their first four session of RBB task were used to train their individual classifiers with each session consisting of 10 epochs to collect training data. Their age ranged from 18 to 54 years of age. They were from diverse professional and ethnic backgrounds. Ideally, we would have liked to have all the participants from Phase I study participate in the Phase II experiments. However, some of the participants were not available during the Phase II study.

Experimental Design

In the task design of robot-based basketball, adequate measures were taken to avoid physical effort from overwhelming the psychophysiological response. Test trials were conducted to check if the models built using training data from anagram solving task and a Pong playing task could be used to interpret and classify data from the basketball game. As discussed in the results section below, it was found that the anxiety-based RBB task improved performance and the classifiers trained for anxiety from data collected using pong and anagram tasks generalized for the RBB tasks. Similar conclusions were reached by Leon et al. (2007), where it was shown that physiological data collected from individuals with variable affect intensity or experiencing variable physical exertion could be successfully used to classify positive and negative affective states.

Each of these 14 participants (with 9 of them participated in phase I modeling tasks) took part in two robot basketball sessions (BB1 and BB2). In BB1 the robot changed the difficulty (Level I, II, and III difficulty levels as discussed in above) of the game based on performance without any regard to the anxiety level of the participant. In BB2, the game difficulty was changed based on the anxiety level of the participant without regard to the performance. Each basketball session was approximately 35 min long and consisted of 10 epochs of 1.5 min each. The remaining time was spent in setting-up, attaching sensors, self-reporting and taking breaks.

Three levels of difficulty were designed—Levels I (easy), II (moderately difficult) and III (very difficult)—based on the pilot study discussed above. Furthermore, three levels of performance, i.e. poor, good and excellent, were identified. The performance levels were determined by a threshold number of baskets per epoch where this threshold was set as 10 % more than the average performance of the participants in the pilot study which determined the difficulty levels. Performance in each epoch was computed using the change of the participant's score in that epoch from the threshold set for that level of difficulty as percentage of the threshold. Overall performance in a session was defined as average performance across all epochs in that session. Another metric to measure overall rating of the participant from self–report was satisfaction index (SI). The SI was computed as the combined sum of challenge (C), enjoyment (E), and performance appraisal (P) as reported by the participant, i.e., $SI = C + E + P$.

Three levels of anxiety were defined—low, medium and high as described in phase I using the quantization of the labels that were used to train the anxiety models. Figure 7.4 shows the state flow models that were utilized to switch difficulty based on performance (P) and anxiety (A), in BB1 and BB2, respectively. The switching logic to higher level of difficulty was based on higher performance and lower anxiety level in each of the performance-based and anxiety-based sessions, respectively. As shown in Fig. 7.4, in the performance-based session (Fig. 7.4 top), excellent performance resulted in increase in the level of difficulty (except when the player was already at the highest level), good performance caused the level to remain constant at the current level, and poor performance resulted in decrease in difficulty level (except when the player was already at the lowest level). Similarly, it can be seen that in the anxiety-based session (Fig. 7.4 bottom), low anxiety resulted in increase in the level of difficulty (except when the player was already at the highest level), medium anxiety caused the level to remain

Fig. 7.4 State flow diagram
for performance-based (*top*)
and anxiety-based (*bottom*)
task adaptation

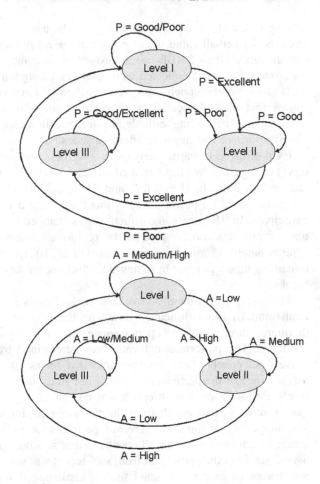

constant at the current level, and high anxiety resulted in decrease in difficulty
level (except when the player was already at the lowest level).

In order to prevent habituation at least 10 days of time interval between any two
BB sessions was enforced. The sessions (performance-based and anxiety-based),
were randomized to avoid any bias due to the order of sessions.

As described above, 5 of the 14 participants did not participate in phase I. Each
new participant took part in a total of four basketball sessions including two
sessions to collect training data and two sessions of BB1 and BB2. Each session
was composed of 10 individual epochs of varying difficulty followed by an interval
of self-reporting. The procedure was similar to the previous anagram and pong
sessions of the remaining 9 participants in phase I. The participants' physiological
data was linked with their self-report and these datasets were utilized to build
individual specific affect-prediction models.

Results

The classification accuracies for the machine learning algorithms considered were presented at the end of section phase I above. Based on these results, anxiety level detection using RT was chosen for phase II classification as discussed above for its lower space complexity while at the same time achieving a classification performance closer to that of SVM. This section discusses the self-report results and the performance improvement results comparing the performance-based (BB1) session vs. anxiety-based session (BB2) of phase II. As described above, the goal of the RBB system as used in phase II was (1) to test the developed models in phase I in real time HRI (2) and to use the self-report and participant's performance to show that using an affect-sensitive (anxiety-based, in this case) system resulted in higher satisfaction and lower anxiety level in HRI as compared to performance only system.

Self-Reported Results

We wanted to assess how the participants themselves felt about the tasks during the performance-based and anxiety-based sessions. We ask the participants to rate their anxiety and satisfaction during these sessions. Figure 7.5 shows the average anxiety of the participants as reported by them (perceived anxiety) during the two sessions. The white bars indicate the anxiety level during the performance-based sessions and the black bars show the anxiety level during the anxiety-based sessions. It can be seen that out of 14 participants, 11 reported decrease in perceived anxiety, 1 reported an increase (P13) and 2 reported no change in anxiety (P9 and P14) during the anxiety-based session as compared to the performance-based session. This was a significant result as the anxiety-based sessions utilized the information regarding the probable anxiety level of the participant to continuously adapt the task difficulty to keep the participant in a lower anxiety state. The majority of the participants felt that they were less anxious when playing the anxiety-based game. Using Chi-square test, it was observed that the null hypothesis (no change in anxiety) could be rejected at 99.99 % confidence interval.

Moreover, physiology based quantitative measure of anxiety matched with 70 % accuracy with that of the subjective rating of anxiety made by the participants. An index called Satisfaction Index (SI) was defined by adding the values of challenge (C), enjoyment (E) and performance appraisal (P) reported by the participants at the end of each session. Figure 7.6 shows the values of the SI during the two sessions for each participant. It can be observed that 10 out of 14 participants reported an increase in the SI during the anxiety-based session. Four participants reported a decrease in SI (P8, P10, P12, and P13). It should be noted that out of the nine participants who showed better performance in anxiety-based session as opposed to performance-based session, eight participants also reported higher satisfaction index in the anxiety-based session. On the other hand, out of the

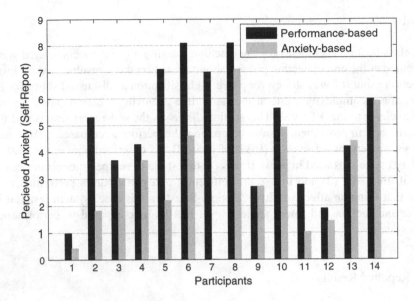

Fig. 7.5 Subjective anxiety as reported by participants

four participants who showed better performance in the performance-based session, three of them reported higher satisfaction in the performance-based session.

It was observed that the null hypothesis that there was no change in satisfaction index between performance-based and anxiety-based sessions could be rejected at 99 % confidence interval Chi-square test.

Performance Results

The performance of a session was computed by the average of performances of each epoch in the session. Figure 7.7 shows the difference in performance between the performance-based and affect-based sessions. It was observed that out of fourteen participants, nine showed better performance during the affect-based session, while four had degradation in performance (P1, P8, P10, and P13) and one did not show any improvement (P14) during the anxiety-based session. It was found that the null hypothesis that there was no change in performance between performance—based and anxiety-based sessions could be rejected at the 99.99 % confidence level.

Figure 7.7 shows, in general, the affect sensitive system was able to reduce anxiety while at the same time resulting in similar performance and satisfaction index to that of the performance-based system. This indicates that incorporating affective cues in human machine interactions could enhance the quality of interaction.

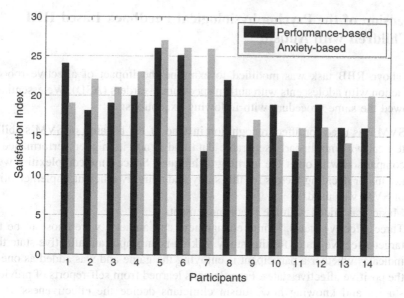

Fig. 7.6 Satisfaction index for all the participants

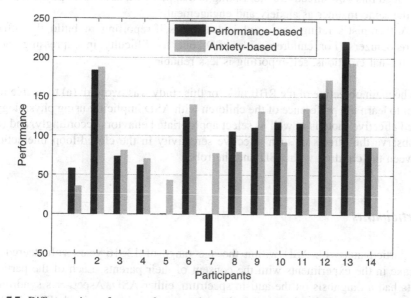

Fig. 7.7 Difference in performance between the performance-based and affect-based sessions

Extension of the Psychophysiological Feedback Based HRI to Children with Autism

The above RBB task was modified to examine the impact of affective robotic interaction with adolescents with autism spectrum disorders (ASD). We essentially followed the same procedure with following exceptions:

(1) SVM was used for affect recognition instead of RT because of SVM's ability to deal with nonlinearly separable data and hence its higher performance in comparison with other the learning techniques. Space-time complexities were not major deciding factors for this study and a highly efficient implementation of SVM was used.
(2) Music was added with the robot movement.
(3) Three affective states, liking, engagement and anxiety, were chose to be the target affective states for this study. Liking is an important affective state that indicates whether a participant is enjoying the game and was added as one of the positive affective states. From lessons learned from self-reports of previous studies and knowing how autism clinicians decide the effectiveness of an intervention task by assessing whether an individual "likes" an activity we added this new affective state. Liking is mapped with associated physiology in the same manner as anxiety and engagement.
(4) A therapist's rating was used instead of self-reporting to build the affect recognizers. For children with ASD, due to difficulty in expressing their internal emotions, self-reporting is less reliable.

The main objective of the RBB task for this study was twofold: (a) to enable the robot to learn the preference of the children with ASD implicitly using physiology-based affective models as well as select appropriate behaviors accordingly, and (b) to observe the effects of such affective sensitivity in the closed-loop interaction between the children with ASD and the robot.

Participants

Six participants with ASD within the age range of 13–16 years volunteered to partake in the experiments with the consent of their parents. Each of the participants had a diagnosis on the autism spectrum, either ASD, Asperger's syndrome (AS), or pervasive developmental disorder not otherwise specified (PDD-NOS), according to their medical records. Each child with ASD was given the Peabody Picture Vocabulary Test III (PPVT-III) (Dunn et al. 1997) to screen cognitive function. Inclusion in our study was characterized as obtaining a standard score of 80 or above on the PPVT-III measure. This test screens participants with cognitive impairments which can hinder completing the study successfully.

Task Design

There were two phases for this study similar to the study described above. A training data collection (phase I) and an actual adaptive robot basketball (phase II) tasks.

Phase I

In a phase I study, similar to the phase I of the study described in the previous section, we used the Anagram and Pong tasks to build individual affect recognizers using SVM. The use of different tasks in the training phase than the actual recognition phase was targeted at reducing the habituation effect, result in more task independent affect recognition and increased generalization. Various parameters of the games were manipulated to elicit the required affective responses. For example, these parameters included ball speed and size, paddle speed and size, sluggish or over-responsive keyboard, random keyboard response, and the level of the computer opponent player in the pong game. Low speeds and large sizes of the ball and paddle made games less engaging after a while; whereas ball and paddle movements at high speeds along with smaller sizes of the two made the game engaging. Very high speeds caused anxiety at times. Playing against a moderate-level computer player usually generated liking. The anagram solving task has also been used in the above study to explore the relationships between physiological indices and anxiety. A long series of trivially easy anagrams caused less engagement while an optimal mix of moderately solvable and difficult anagrams cases increased liking and engagement. Extremely difficult anagrams and adding time deadlines generated anxiety. The difficulty of the anagram task was manipulated through the length of the word and the number of misplaced letters in the word. The task configurations were established through pilot work. Each task sequence was subdivided into a series of discrete trials/epochs that were bounded by the subjective affective state assessments. These assessments were collected using a battery of five questions regarding the three target affective states and the perceived difficulty and performance rated on an 8-point Likert scale where 1 indicated the lowest level and 8 indicated the maximum level. Each participant took part in six sessions—three 1-h sessions of solving anagrams and three 1-h sessions of playing pong on six different days with each epoch being 3 min long for anagram and 4 min for pong game. The rest of the process of labeling the data set for each epoch with the therapist assessment and training the SVM to recognize the target affective states, i.e. liking, engagement, and anxiety is similar to phase I described in section "A Novel HRI System with Psychophysiological Feedback". The SVM-based affect recognition models produced relatively higher average accuracies of 85.0 % for liking, 79.5 % for anxiety, and 84.3 % for engagement.

Table 7.2 Robot behaviors

Behavior ID	Motion direction	Speed	Level	Background music
1	X	Slow	Low	Serene
2	Y	Medium	Medium	Lively
3	Z	Fast	Difficult	Irregular

Phase II

Three robot behaviors were designed, as shown in Table 7.2. For example, in Behavior 1, the robot moved toward and away from the participant (i.e., in the X-direction) at a slow speed with soft background music, and the shooting requirement for successful baskets was relatively low. The parameter configurations were determined based on a pilot study to attain varied impacts on affective experience for different behaviors. From this pilot study, the averaged performance of participants for a given behavior was compiled and analyzed. The threshold of shooting requirement (TSR) was defined as 10 % lower than the average performance. At the end of each epoch, the participant's performance was rated as excellent (baskets ≥ 1.2TSR), above average (0.8TSR $\leq$ baskets < 1.2TSR), or below average (baskets < 0.8TSR). Behavior transitions occurred between but not within epochs. As such, each robot behavior extended for the length of an epoch (1.5 min in duration) to have the participant fully exposed to the impact of that behavior.

For the affect-sensitive robot behavior adaptation phase of this study, once the affective state of the participant was determined, we defined the state, state transition, action and reward for the robot so that the robot could learn which actions to take given a certain affective state to maximize enjoyment of the participant. The overall goal was to increase satisfaction of the participant via increasing the robot's internal reward for selecting the correct action at a given affective state.

The QV-learning algorithm, which is a variant of the standard reinforcement learning algorithm called Q-learning (Wiering 2005) was applied to achieve this goal. It has two utility functions, i.e., the Q-function and the V-function. The Q-function keeps track of utility value for every possible pair of state and action whereas the V-function stores the utility for each state separately. Each of the six participants took part in two robot basketball sessions (RBB1 and RBB2). In RBB1 (non-affect-based), the robot selected its behavior randomly (i.e., without any regard to the liking information of the participant), and the presentation of each type of behavior was evenly distributed. This session was designed for two purposes: (1) to explore the state space and action space of the QV-learning algorithm used in RBB2 for behavior adaptation, and (2) to validate that the different robot behaviors have distinguishable impact on the child's level of liking. In RBB2 (liking-based), the robot continues to learn the child's individual preference and selects the desirable behavior based on interaction experiences (i.e., records of robot behavior and the consequent liking level of a participant predicted by the affective model). The idea is to investigate whether the robot can automatically choose the most liked behavior of each participant as observed from RBB1 by means of physiology-based affective model and QV-learning.

Each basketball session (RBB1 or RBB2) was approximately 1-h long and included 27 min of active HRI (i.e., 18 epochs of 1.5 min each). The remaining time was spent attaching sensors, guiding a short practice, taking a baseline recording, collecting subjective reports, and pausing for scheduled breaks. During the experiment, the participant was asked to take a break after every four epochs and the participant could request a break whenever he/she desired one. Each epoch was followed by subjective reports that took 30–60 s to collect. The subjective assessment procedure was the same as the protocol used in the affective modeling tasks prior to the RBB tasks. After the subjective report was complete, the next epoch would begin. To prevent habituation, a time interval of at least seven days between any two RBB sessions was enforced.

QV-Learning Based Affect-Sensitive Behavior Adaptation

We defined the state, action, state transition, and reward functions so that the affect-sensitive robot behavior adaptation problem could be solved using the QV-learning algorithm, as described in Wiering (2005). The set of states consisted of three robot behaviors, as described in Table II. In every state, the robot has three possible actions (1/2/3) that correspond to choosing behavior 1, 2, or 3, respectively, for the next time step (i.e., next epoch). Each robot behavior persists for one full epoch and the state/behavior transition occurs only at the end of an epoch. The detection of consequent affective cues (i.e., the real-time prediction of the liking level for the next epoch) was used to evaluate the desirability of a certain action. To have the robot adapt to a child's individual preference, a reward function was defined based on the predicted liking level. If the consequent liking level was recognized as high, the contributing action was interpreted as positive and a reward was granted ($r = 1$); otherwise the robot received a punishment ($r = -1$). QV-learning uses this reward function to have the robot learn how to select the behavior that was expected to result in a high liking level, and therefore, positively influenced the actual affective (e.g., liking) experience of the child. RBB1 enables state and action exploration where the behavior-switching actions are chosen randomly, with the number of visits to each state evenly distributed. After RBB1, the subjective reports are analyzed to examine the impacts of different behaviors on each participant's preference. In RBB2, the robot starts from a non-preferred behavior/state and continues the learning process. A greedy action selection mechanism is used to choose the behavior-switching action with the highest— value. The details of the learning algorithm employed in this study can be found in our earlier work (Liu et al. 2005; Rani et al. 2006).

Results

The results described here are based on the RBB1 (non-affect-based) and RBB2 (liking-based) tasks. First, we present results to validate that different behaviors of the robot had distinguishable impacts on the liking level of the children with ASD. To reduce the bias of validation, in RBB1, the robot selects behaviors randomly and the occurrence of each behavior is evenly distributed. To validate differences among different behaviors selected by the robot in RBB1, we ran a two-way ANOVA analysis on the robot behavior (i.e., most preferred, moderately preferred, and least preferred behavior) and participant, and it was found that the differences of reported liking for different behaviors were statistically significant ($p < 0.05$). No significant effect due to different participants was observed. Thus this analysis indicated that there were distinguishable differences between the behaviors that the robot selected, and the behaviors were individual specific. Furthermore, it was also observed that different children with ASD may have different preferences for the robot's behaviors. These results demonstrated that it is important to have a robot learn the individual's preference and adapt to it automatically, which may allow a more tailored and affect-sensitive interaction between children with ASD and the robot. For example, when a robot learns that a certain behavior is liked more by a particular child, it can choose that behavior as his/her "social feedback" or "reinforcement" in robot-assisted autism intervention. This is important because ASD intervention literature suggests that individualized and enjoyable interaction is the key to effective intervention. Further, we computed predictive accuracies of the affect recognizers as compared to the subjective rating of the affective states by a therapist. The therapist labelled the participants perceived affective state subjectively during the sessions and those subjective ratings were used as ground truth to compute predictive accuracies of the recognizers. The average predictive accuracy of liking across all the participants in comparison against the subjective report of a therapist was approximately 81.1 %. The predictive accuracy describes how closely the real-time physiology-based quantitative measures of liking, as obtained from affective models developed in Phase I, matched with that of the subjective rating of liking made by the therapist during Phase II.

Table 7.3 shows the percentages of three different behaviors that were chosen in the RBB2 session for each participant. The robot learned the individual's preference and selected the most preferred behavior with high probability for all the participants. Averaged across all participants, the most preferred, moderately preferred, and least preferred behaviors were chosen to be 72.5, 16.7, and 10.8 % of the time, respectively.

Table 7.3 Proportion of different behaviours performed in RBB2

Child ID	Most-liked behavior		Moderate-liked behavior		Least-liked behavior	
	ID	Proportion (%)	ID	Proportion (%)	ID	Proportion (%)
A	2	82.4	3	11.8	1	5.8
B	1	70.6	2	17.7	3	11.7
C	2	58.8	3	23.5	1	17.7
D	2	76.5	3	11.8	1	11.7
E	2	76.5	3	17.6	1	5.9
F	2	70.6	1	17.7	3	11.7

Discussion, Conclusion and Ongoing Work

We have shown that it is possible for a robot to detect human psychological states such as anxiety and liking in real-time through psychophysiological feedback as well as appropriately respond to it during an interaction task. We have designed a new HRI task, called robot-based basketball (RBB) task, and developed an experimental system for real-time implementation and verification. Experiments with 14 participants demonstrated that the robot could influence (lower) human anxiety for 11 of these participants during the course of task execution. Moreover, we have found that such anxiety-based game led to higher improvement of performance for 9 of these participants. It suggests that the implicit affective communication could be useful in HRI.

Results of the HRI study indicated that while physiology can be integrated with other modalities of affect-recognition such as facial expressions, vocal intonation, gestures and postures, it could also be employed independently to give reliable affect information. Physiology has distinct advantages over other modalities, as it is involuntary and continuously available. Wearing various sensors might be a limiting factor for now. However, with the advancement of wireless and miniaturized sensor technology such limitation can be mitigated to a large extent in the future (Viventi et al. 2010). Note that none of the participants in both studies had any objection to wearing the physiological sensors.

There is an increasing consensus in the autism community that development of assistive tools that exploit advanced technology will likely make the application of intensive intervention for children with ASD more readily accessible. In recent years, robotic technology has been investigated in order to facilitate and/or partially automate the existing behavioral intervention that addresses specific deficits associated with autism. However, the current robot-assisted intervention tools for children with ASD do not possess the ability to decipher affective cues from the children, which could be critical given that the affective factors of children with ASD have significant impacts on the intervention practice.

In our psychophysiology based social assistive robotics (SAR) work, we proposed a novel framework for affect-sensitive SAR where the robot can implicitly detect the affective states of the children with ASD as discerned by the therapist and respond to it accordingly. The presented affective modeling methodology could allow the recognition of affective states of children with ASD from physiological signals in real time and provide the basis for future robot-assisted affect-sensitive interactive autism intervention. The real-time prediction of liking level of the children with ASD was accomplished with an average accuracy of 81.1 %. The robot learned individual preferences of the children with ASD over time based on the interaction experience and the predicted liking level, and hence, automatically selected the most preferred behavior, on average, 72.5 % of the time. We have observed that such affect-sensitive robot behavior adaptation has led to an increase in reported liking level of the children with ASD.

Current Ongoing Psychophysiology Work

Currently, our group is investigating the use psychophysiological signals in the context of virtual reality (VR) based social and adaptive interaction tasks for children with Autism (Lahiri et al. 2012; Welch et al. 2009). Lessons learned from previous HRI and physiology based affect recognition tasks have been applied to the VR-based tasks.

Future Directions

We are currently expanding the range of application areas, tasks and contexts to which this framework can be applied to and increasing the reliability and robustness of the affect recognition system. Increasing the range of affective states that are detected simultaneously by the system and discerning between each affective state when they co-occur is a part of the future plan. We would also plan to incorporate a facially expressive social robot, surrounding smart interactive room, other affect detection modalities such as facial expressions detection together with physiology based affect recognition to develop more socially embodied and able agents that can help in variety of therapeutic tasks such as ASD intervention. We will investigate fast and robust learning mechanisms that would permit a robot's adaptive response in more complex HRI tasks, learn from their actual interaction experiences and allow the affect-sensitive robot to be adopted in the future clinical autism intervention and diagnosis.

Acknowledgements This work was supported in part by a Marino Autism Research Institute (MARI) grant, an Autism Speaks Foundation Pilot grant, the National Science Foundation Grant [award number 0967170], and the National Institute of Health Grant [award number 1R01MH091102-01A1]. We would like to thank all colleagues that helped in this research and give special thanks to all subjects and their families.

References

Agrawal P, Liu C, Sarkar N (2008) Interaction between human and robot an affect-inspired approach. Interact Stud 9(2):230–257

Bethel CL, Burke JL, Murphy RR, Salomon K (2007) Psychophysiological experimental design for use in human-robot interaction studies. In: International Symposium on Collaborative Technologies and Systems, 2007. CTS 2007. IEEE, pp 99–105

Bethel CL, Salomon K, Murphy RR (2009) Preliminary results: humans find emotive non-anthropomorphic robots more calming. In: 4th ACM/IEEE International Conference on Human-Robot Interaction (HRI), 2009. IEEE, pp 291–292

Bien ZZ, Lee HE (2007) Effective learning system techniques for human–robot interaction in service environment. Knowl-Based Syst 20(5):439–456

Cacioppo JT, Tassinary LG, Berntson G (2007) Handbook of psychophysiology. Cambridge University Press, Cambridge

Calvo RA, D'Mello S (2010) Affect detection: an interdisciplinary review of models, methods, and their applications. IEEE Trans Affect Comput 1(1):18–37

Conn K, Liu C, Sarkar N, Stone W, Warren Z (2010) Towards affect-sensitive assistive intervention technologies for children with autism. In Jimmy OR (ed) Affective computing: focus on emotion expression, synthesis and recognition. ARS/I-Tech Education and Publishing, Austria, pp 365–390

Cowie R, Douglas-Cowie E, Tsapatsoulis N, Votsis G, Kollias S, Fellenz W, Taylor JG (2001) Emotion recognition in human-computer interaction. Sig Process Mag IEEE 18(1):32–80

Croft DKEA (2003) Estimating intent for human-robot interaction. In: IEEE International Conference on Advanced Robotics, 2003. pp 810–815

D'Mello SK, Graesser A (2010) Multimodal semi-automated affect detection from conversational cues, gross body language, and facial features. User Model User-Adap Inter 20(2):147–187

Dawson ME, Schell AM, Filion DL (2007) The Electrodermal System. In: Cacioppo JT, Tassinary LG, Berntson GG (eds) Handbook of psychophysiology. Cambridge University Press, New York, p 159

Diehl JJ, Schmitt LM, Villano M, Crowell CR (2012) The clinical use of robots for individuals with autism spectrum disorders: A critical review. Res Autism Spectrum Disord 6(1):249–262

Dunn L, Williams KT, Wang JJ, Booklets N (1997) Peabody picture vocabulary test, (PPVT-III): Form IIA. American Guidance Service Inc, Circle Pines

Fairclough SH (2009) Fundamentals of physiological computing. Interact Comput 21(1):133–145

Feil-Seifer D, Mataric M (2011) Automated detection and classification of positive vs. negative robot interactions with children with autism using distance-based features. In: Proceedings of the 6th international conference on Human-robot interaction, 2011. ACM, pp 323–330

Feil-Seifer D, Mataric MJ (2005) A multi-modal approach to selective interaction in assistive domains. In: IEEE International Workshop on Robot and Human Interactive Communication, 2005. ROMAN 2005. IEEE, pp 416–421

Fong T, Nourbakhsh I, Dautenhahn K (2003) A survey of socially interactive robots. Robot Auton Syst 42(3):143–166

Goodrich MA, Schultz AC (2007) Human-robot interaction: a survey. Found Trends Hum Comput Interact 1(3):203–275

Hussain M, AlZoubi O, Calvo R, D'Mello S (2011) Affect detection from multichannel physiology during learning sessions with AutoTutor. In: Artificial intelligence in education. Springer, Berlin, pp 131–138

Hussain M, Monkaresi H, Calvo R (2012) Categorical vs. dimensional representations in multimodal affect detection during learning. In: Intelligent tutoring systems. Springer, Berlin, pp 78–83

Iani C, Gopher D, Lavie P (2004) Effects of task difficulty and invested mental effort on peripheral vasoconstriction. Psychophysiology 41(5):789–798

Jerritta S, Murugappan M, Nagarajan R, Wan K (2011) Physiological signals based human emotion recognition: a review. In: IEEE 7th International Colloquium on Signal Processing and its Applications (CSPA), 2011. IEEE, pp 410–415

Kim J, André E (2008) Emotion recognition based on physiological changes in music listening. IEEE Trans Pattern Anal Mach Intell 30(12):2067–2083

Koenig A, Novak D, Omlin X, Pulfer M, Perreault E, Zimmerli L, Mihelj M, Riener R (2011) Real-time closed-loop control of cognitive load in neurological patients during robot-assisted gait training. IEEE Trans Neural Syst Rehabil Eng 19(4):453–464

Kubicek W, Karnegis J, Patterson R, Witsoe D, Mattson R (1966) Development and evaluation of an impedance cardiac output system. Aerosp Med 37(12):1208

Kulic D, Croft E (2005) Anxiety detection during human-robot interaction. In: 2005 IEEE/RSJ International Conference on Intelligent Robots and Systems, 2005.(IROS 2005). IEEE, pp 616–621

Kulić D, Croft E (2007a) Pre-collision safety strategies for human-robot interaction. Auton Robots 22(2):149–164

Kulic D, Croft EA (2007b) Affective state estimation for human–robot interaction. IEEE Trans Robot 23(5):991–1000

Kwakkel G, Kollen BJ, Krebs HI (2008) Effects of robot-assisted therapy on upper limb recovery after stroke: a systematic review. Neurorehabil Neural Repair 22(2):111–121

Lacey JI, Lacey BC (1958) Verification and extension of the principle of autonomic response-stereotypy. The Am J Psychol 71(1):50–73

Lahiri U, Welch KC, Sarkar M (2012) Psychophysiological response in virtual reality based human-computer interaction in adolescents with ASD. In: Imaging and signal processing in health care and technology/772: human-computer interaction/773: communication, internet and information technology. ACTA Press, USA

Leon E, Clarke G, Callaghan V, Sepulveda F (2007) A user-independent real-time emotion recognition system for software agents in domestic environments. Eng Appl Artif Intell 20(3):337–345

Liu C, Conn K, Sarkar N, Stone W (2007) Affect recognition in robot assisted rehabilitation of children with autism spectrum disorder. In: IEEE International Conference on Robotics and Automation, 2007. IEEE, pp 1755–1760

Liu C, Conn K, Sarkar N, Stone W (2008a) Online affect detection and robot behavior adaptation for intervention of children with autism. IEEE Trans Robot 24(4):883–896

Liu C, Conn K, Sarkar N, Stone W (2008b) Physiology-based affect recognition for computer-assisted intervention of children with Autism Spectrum Disorder. Int J Hum Comput Stud 66(9):662–677

Liu C, Rani P, Sarkar N (2005) An empirical study of machine learning techniques for affect recognition in human-robot interaction. In: 2005 IEEE/RSJ International Conference on Intelligent Robots and Systems, (IROS 2005). IEEE, pp 2662–2667

Liu C, Rani P, Sarkar N (2006) Affective state recognition and adaptation in human-robot interaction: A design approach. In: 2006 IEEE/RSJ International Conference on Intelligent Robots and Systems 2006. IEEE, pp 3099–3106

Murphy RR (2004) Human-robot interaction in rescue robotics. IEEE Trans Syst Man Cybern Part C Appl Rev 34(2):138–153

Nourbakhsh IR, Sycara K, Koes M, Yong M, Lewis M, Burion S (2005) Human-robot teaming for search and rescue. IEEE Pervasive Comput 4(1):72–79

Pantic M, Pentland A, Nijholt A, Huang T (2007) Human computing and machine understanding of human behavior: A survey. Artifical intelligence for human computing. Springer, Berlin, pp 47–71

Papillo J, Shapiro D (1990) The cardiovascular system. In: Principles of psychophysiology: physical, social and inferential elements. Cambridge University Press, Cambridge

Pecchinenda A (1996) The affective significance of skin conductance activity during a difficult problem-solving task. Cogn Emot 10(5):481–504

Picard R (1997) Affective computing. MIT Press, Cambridge

Picard RW (1999) Affective computing for HCI. In: Proceedings of HCI International (the 8th International Conference on Human-Computer Interaction) on Human-Computer Interaction: Ergonomics and User Interfaces, 1999. pp 829–833

Rani P, Liu C, Sarkar N, Vanman E (2006) An empirical study of machine learning techniques for affect recognition in human–robot interaction. Pattern Anal Appl 9(1):58–69

Rani P, Sarkar N (2005) Making robots emotion-sensitive-preliminary experiments and results. In: IEEE International Workshop on Robot and Human Interactive Communication, 2005. ROMAN 2005. IEEE, pp 1–6

Rani P, Sarkar N, Smith CA, Kirby LD (2004) Anxiety detecting robotic system-towards implicit human-robot collaboration. Robotica 22(1):85–95

Rani P, Sims J, Brackin R, Sarkar N (2002) Online stress detection using psychophysiological signals for implicit human-robot cooperation. Robotica 20(06):673–685

Sarkar N (2002) Psychophysiological control architecture for human-robot coordination-concepts and initial experiments. In: Proceedings of the ICRA'02 IEEE International Conference on Robotics and Automation, 2002. IEEE, pp 3719–3724

Scassellati B, Admoni H, Mataric M (2012) Robots for use in autism research. Annu Rev Biomed Eng 14:275–294

Severinson-Eklundh K, Green A, Hüttenrauch H (2003) Social and collaborative aspects of interaction with a service robot. Robot Auton Syst 42(3):223–234

Tao J, Tan T (2005) Affective computing: A review. Affective computing and intelligent interaction. Springer, Heidelberg, pp 981–995

Tapus A, Mataric M (2008) Socially assistive robots: The link between personality, empathy, physiological signals, and task performance. In: AAAI Spring, 2008. pp 3–4

Thrun S (2004) Toward a framework for human-robot interaction. Hum Comput Interact 19(1–2):9–24

Vansteelandt K, Van Mechelen I, Nezlek JB (2005) The co-occurrence of emotions in daily life: A multilevel approach. J Res Pers 39(3):325–335

Viventi J, Kim D-H, Moss JD, Kim Y-S, Blanco JA, Annetta N, Hicks A, Xiao J, Huang Y, Callans DJ (2010) A conformal, bio-interfaced class of silicon electronics for mapping cardiac electrophysiology. Sci Transl Med 2(24):24ra22

Wagner J, Kim J, André E (2005) From physiological signals to emotions: Implementing and comparing selected methods for feature extraction and classification. In: IEEE International Conference on Multimedia and Expo, 2005 ICME 2005. IEEE, pp 940–943

Welch K, Lahiri U, Liu C, Weller R, Sarkar N, Warren Z (2009) An affect-sensitive social interaction paradigm utilizing virtual reality environments for autism intervention. Human-Computer Interaction Ambient, Ubiquitous and Intelligent Interaction, pp 703–712

Wiering MA (2005) QV (lambda)-learning: A new on-policy reinforcement learning algorithm. Proceedings of the 7th European Workshop on Reinforcement Learning

Chapter 8
The Drive to Explore: Physiological Computing in a Cultural Heritage Context

Alexander J. Karran and Ute Kreplin

Abstract Contemporary heritage institutions model installations and artefacts around a passive receivership where content is consumed but not influenced by visitors. Increasingly, heritage institutions are incorporating ubiquitous technologies to provide visitors with experiences that not only transfer knowledge but also entertain. This poses the challenge of how to incorporate technologies into exhibits to make them more approachable and memorable, whilst preserving cultural salience. We present work towards an adaptive interface which responds to a museum visitor's level of interest, in order to deliver a personalised experience through adaptive curation within a cultural heritage installation. The interface is realised through the use of psychophysiological measures, physiological computing and a machine learning algorithm. We present studies which serve to illustrate how entertainment, education, aesthetic experience and immersion, identified as four factors of visitor experience, can be operationalised through a psychological construct of "interest". Two studies are reported which take a subject-dependent experimental approach to record and classify psychophysiological signals using mobile physiological sensors and a machine learning algorithm. The results show that it is possible to reliably infer a state of interest from cultural heritage material, informing future work for the development of a real-time physiological computing system for use within an adaptive cultural heritage experience. We propose a framework for a potential adaptive system for cultural heritage based upon story telling principles and an operationalised model of the "knowledge emotion" interest.

A. J. Karran (✉) · U. Kreplin
School of Natural Science and Psychology, Liverpool John Moores University,
Liverpool, UK
e-mail: a.j.karran@ljmu.ac.uk

U. Kreplin
e-mail: U.Kreplin@2011.ljmu.ac.uk

S. H. Fairclough and K. Gilleade (eds.), *Advances in Physiological Computing*,
Human–Computer Interaction Series, DOI: 10.1007/978-1-4471-6392-3_8,
© Springer-Verlag London 2014

The Changing Face of Cultural Heritage

Cultural heritage (CH) is changing, contemporary museums and galleries are increasingly motivated to keep abreast of display and information technologies in order to create better experience and encourage increased visitors to exhibits. The introduction of technology into CH institutions to provide information about exhibits can be traced back to the early 1900s. Rapid industrialisation, urbanisation and immigration during this period created a shift in the demographic of the CH visitor, which until then consisted of the educated upper class (McLean 1993). This shift required CH institutions to provide wider and more varied information to overcome the lack of prior knowledge about installations and exhibits. During this period efforts were made to make museums more accessible through the use of new visual technologies and display techniques. The quest to make museums more accessible via the use of technology has continued to contemporary institutions. Today's CH institutions strive to fulfil visitor expectations, by providing a "total experience" that includes aspects of leisure, culture and social interaction where mental and emotional stimulation combine to create a distinctive, significant and more "memorable" experience (Tung and Richie 2011).

Recent advances in ubiquitous information technologies such as smart phones, tablet computers and augmented reality are changing the way CH institutions portray exhibits and present information. Surveys of institutions have demonstrated that use of these technologies within heritage installations is set to increase in the near future and beyond (Liew 2005). Ubiquitous technologies can be used both on-site, e.g. quick response codes (QR) and mobile guided tours, and off-site e.g. using web technologies to create heritage websites replicating in part existing CH installations. QR codes involve encoding information about an exhibit into a matrix barcode that is scanned by and then presented through a mobile device, offering a way for the museum visitor to self-curate information about an exhibit. Mobile device guided tours provide a navigation path through heritage installations, serving multimedia content about exhibits as they are viewed. Both of these technologies can act as standalone experience or as tools to augment the traditional museum-provided human expert tour. For example, the Louvre in Paris (Louvre 2013), France, has deployed a virtual museum application, available through mobile devices, that utilises QR codes, WiFi and multi-lingual media for exhibits available in the museum. However, these technologies are opaque to the visitor's physiological and psychological states and ignore what could potentially be the most important source of data about the cultural heritage experience, the visitors themselves.

This chapter concerns technology that monitors a visitor's psychophysiological state in real-time and adapts information regarding exhibits according to the interests of the visitor. This chapter will draw from research in the fields of museology, neuroaesthetics and physiological computing to describe how the visitors experience is modelled by CH institutes. We discuss how interest is modelled within psychology and posit our own interest model describing how to operationalise a visitor's experience through the use of psychophysiology. Furthermore, we describe an adaptive system which uses our interest model and discuss issues surrounding the application of adaptive systems in CH environments.

Background

Cultural Heritage Experiences

Visitors' experiences in cultural heritage environments are often measured in terms of satisfaction which hinges on the fulfilment of positive expectations of the individual (Tung and Richie 2011). The visitor's satisfaction with the exhibit and the formation of memorable experiences is guided by expressive and instrumental attributes of the exhibit; instrumental attributes act as facilitators of the experience, e.g. the museum environment, whereas expressive attributes refer to the experience itself (Tung and Richie 2011; Uysal and Noe 2003). The personal importance of the experience can be improved by creating a cognitive and emotional resonance by encoding the cultural heritage experience with personal meanings for the visitor. For example, an exhibit about an eighteenth century Valencian kitchen can be enriched by means of instrumental attributes such as introducing smells of chocolate (a common food amongst the upper classes of the time), kitchen noises or personal anecdotes of the people that inhabited the house. The engagement with the exhibit through all senses allows the visitor to make a personal connection to the artefact. A memorable experience is formed when the visitor has been engaged on a cognitive, emotional, physical or even spiritual level. Memorable experiences are highly individual because of the interaction between the information provided and the individual's cultural history, educational background and frame of mind (Pine and Gilmore 1998; Wang 1999). It is important for technology to support the creation of total or memorable experiences, but these terms are too broadly defined to be operationalised in a meaningful way.

Pine and Gilmore (1998) suggested that there are four crucial factors to facilitating memorable experiences in CH environments. These factors can be organised along the two dimensions: participation and connectivity. Participation is defined by the active or passive involvement in the exhibit by the visitor. A symphony-goer, for example, experiences the event as an observer without playing an active part in the performance, whereas the lead violinist would be an active participant. The second dimension describes the connectivity, or environmental relationship that unites the visitor with the artefact or event. At one end of this spectrum lies absorption at the other immersion. People viewing the Grand Prix through their television set absorb the event, whereas people attending the event in person will be immersed in the smells, sights and sounds that surround them. What differentiates these two states is the environmental relationship between the spectator and the event. Immersion becomes important for CH experiences, particularly when using technology to engage and engross the visitor in a specific artefact.

The four factors that facilitate memorable experiences, suggested by Pine and Gilmore (1998), are entertainment, education, aesthetics and immersion. Entertainment, either through leisure such as attending a concert or through narrative such as watching a movie, refers to the capacity of cultural heritage artefacts to engage the visitor in a cognitive and affective manner. The visitor is primarily entertained by cognitive information, which may be formatted in a manner to create an affective response. Listening to factual information about the production of chocolate in eighteenth century Valencia may, for example, create a feeling of pleasure because knowledge has been enhanced and personal associations to chocolate have been triggered. Education represents the process of knowledge transfer by which the visitor is informed about artefacts. The information provided may take the form of names and dates that engage the cognitive facilities of the visitor, i.e. perception, attention, memory. However, the purpose of knowledge transfer is to deepen a cognitive appreciation of the artefact. These first two factors combine to create a form of "infotainment", where information is provided through entertainment, which is the primary driver behind "memorable experience" in a cultural heritage context. The third factor is the aesthetic element. Aesthetic experiences of cultural heritage installations are often associated with the perception of beauty and the pursuit of pleasure; however the affective range evoked in response to artefacts may be more extensive. This aspect is perhaps the most difficult to understand because CH exhibits are capable of evoking a range of aesthetic responses such as awe, wonder or disgust. Previous definitions of aesthetic experience have emphasised both information processing and emotional responses (Leder et al. 2004), defining the aesthetic experience as a cognitive process that is accompanied by an emotional state. For example, an aesthetic response may be experienced during the cognitive processing of factual information about chocolate in the Valencian kitchen that is accompanied by the emotional associations of the chocolate. This resonance between cognitive and emotional appreciation underpins the sense of authenticity of the artefact or exhibit experienced by the visitor (McIntosh and Prentice 1999). It is speculated that artefacts experienced as particularly authentic will be associated with high magnitude changes in positive and negative valence.

The fourth and last factor is escapism. The escapist dimension is associated with the degree to which the visitor is immersed with the experience of the artefact. There are said to be three levels of immersion (ranging from low to high): (1) engagement (lack of awareness of time) (2) engrossment (lack of awareness of the real world), and (3) total immersion (Jennett et al. 2008). Like the aesthetic aspect, immersion is provoked by cognitive stimulation working in conjunction with changing emotional states. The combination of factual information and emotional association with chocolate in the Valencian kitchen enables the visitor to be immersed in the experience of eighteenth century Valencia to a degree that awareness about the environment and time is lost. The presentation of only factual information would benefit knowledge transfer, but would lack the emotional resonance that is needed to reach a state of total immersion. The escapist dimension has clear implications for creating memorable experiences in CH settings, particularly using technology to engage and engross the visitor.

Cultural heritage exhibits can encompass the four features described by Pine and Gilmore (1998) to enable memorable experiences and aid knowledge gain. Entertainment, education, aesthetics and escapist are organised along the two dimensions; participation (ranging from passive to active along the x-axis) and connectivity (ranging from immersion to absorption along the y-axis). Entertainment is associated with more passive participation and absorbing activities such as watching TV or going to a concert. Exhibits, or activities within exhibits aimed to include educational features are seen as more active rather than passive, but participants are still more outside the event, absorbing what is happening around them without being fully immersed. Escapist events, such as playing a musical instrument or acting in a play, can enhance knowledge as much as educational events through active participation, but are more immersive. Aesthetic experiences on the other hand are characterised by passive participation of the visitor with high factors of immersion. A visitor, for example, may be immersed in viewing the Mona Lisa without actively participating. Memorable experiences are defined by cognitive engagement resulting in knowledge gain, and emotional engagement creates personal relevance and authenticity of the exhibit. Both cognitive stimulation and emotional engagement interact in order to yield the escapist or immersive factors of the experience and provide supporting roles in the other factors.

An essential tool already in use by museums (Johnsson and Adeler 2006) to integrate cognitive and emotional stimulation to create interest in exhibits or artefacts is storytelling. Storytelling is a technique for knowledge transfer that is culturally significant, provides "infotainment" and reduces information overload. The study, formalisation, and effective use of narrative concepts used in storytelling has its roots with Aristotle's Poetic (c. 335 BCE) and can be seen more recently in the work of Campbell (1999). Aristotle conceived the notion that a well-designed narrative is a key element to reach the recipient and touch his inner feelings. Campbell proposed the "monomythos", as a narrative structure consisting of 3 major phases: separation, initiation and return. These three phases could be used to create memorable experiences. The phases give a narrative flow to information that allows the visitor to acquire new knowledge and become involved cognitively and emotionally with the subject matter. A good narrative would encompass elements of entertainment, education, aesthetics and escapism to foster a sense of interest, curiosity and possibly wonder. Thus, the four factor model by Pine and Gilmore (1998) parallels the psychological concept of interest as an emotion within a CH setting because both emphasise a combination of cognitive and emotional process which can generate greater engagement with an object or exhibit and lead to the creation of memorable experiences. The latter may be created by a technological system that is sensitive to those psychological dimensions underpinning interest as a psychological concept.

"Interest": The Knowledge Emotion

The concept of interest as a psychological entity was described by Berlyne (1960) as an exploratory drive within cultural heritage settings. "Interest" as an emotion fosters curiosity and the drive to explore the object or situation at hand. Berlyne (1960) explained that interest is experienced through increased arousal and sensation seeking, i.e. objects inspire curiosity via novelty and emotional conflict. This concept was expanded by Silvia (2008, 2010) to incorporate a cognitive dimension, whereby interest is driven by stimulus complexity. However, the cognitive appraisal of interest by Berlyne (1960) as well as Silvia (2008) does not take into account the influence of emotional resonances on the cultural heritage experience per se. An object may create interest as a result of its novelty or complexity, but the emotional states that accompany curiosity or interest also represent an important component of the process. For example, a visitor may be repulsed by a painting which leads to a sudden interest in the object. The experience of interest is followed by a sense of positive emotion derived from intellectual engagement; positive emotions experienced as a result of interest can therefore occur even during engagement with negative material (Hidi and Renninger 2006). Visitors' experiences of cultural heritage may therefore be enhanced by material that seeks to evoke the interest and curiosity of the visitor.

Emotions and cognitions are important parts of the conceptualisation of interest within cultural heritage settings because interest towards CH installations is experienced if the visitor is cognitively engaged by the exhibit, but also experiences an emotional resonance or connectivity to the piece. However, the emotional and cognitive domains of interest are not entirely separable as they share a common link through the arousal/activation domain. Arousal was described by Berlyne (1960) as an important aspect of the cognitive concept of interest, and activation by Russell (1980) as one dimension of the circumplex model of emotions. The psychological conceptualisation of emotions falls into two distinct camps. Theories of basic emotions, e.g. happiness and fear, argue that emotional experience may be divided into discrete and independent categories (Ekman 1992). This model contrasts with the circumplex model that represents emotional experience within a two-dimensional space consisting of arousal/activation (alert—tired) and valence (happy—sad) (Russell 1980). Unlike the basic emotion theory, the circumplex model emphasises the association between different categories of emotional experience via common dimensions of activation and valence.

In the following section we discuss how a sense of interest can be formalised as a psychological construct and operationalised for use as input into a physiological computing system that utilises modern media and sensor technologies to create a more dynamic and personalised cultural heritage experience using the visitor themselves as a kind of hidden narrator of a story written purely for their benefit.

Conceptualising a Model of "Interest" for Cultural Heritage

As discussed in the previous section a conceptual model of interest representing visitors' experiences within a cultural heritage environment needs to include cognitive components as well as emotional components. We therefore developed a model that consisted of six sub-components; three cognitive in nature and three emotional in nature. The model includes components of both cognition and emotion which are believed to underpin interest and memorable experiences in museums and galleries. The cognitive factors are derived from the work of Berlyne (1960) and Silvia (2008, 2010), whereas the emotional components are taken from the circumplex model of emotion (Russell 1980) with the added dimension of attraction. The cognitive sub-components consisted of:

- *Comprehension*: whether the representation/function of the object was clearly understood.
- *Complexity*: whether the perceptual complexity of the object is high or low.
- *Novelty*: how familiar or unusual the object was.

The emotional components consisted of:

- *Activation/Arousal*: whether consideration of the object was stimulating or not.
- *Valence*: whether viewing the object made the person feel happy or sad.
- *Attractiveness*: how attractive the object was.

The cognitive and emotional aspects of the interest model were explored via an online survey where participants (n = 1043) rated sixty artworks on all six dimensions. Each dimension was rated on a visually represented 9-point Likert scale (see Fig. 8.1a for an example). The results revealed a high degree of association (80 %) between the cognitive dimensions of Complexity, Novelty and Comprehension, i.e. novel objects were more complex and consequently hard to understand. It was also found that Attraction was positively related to Valence, i.e. attractive objects made people happy. As a group the cognitive components showed a weaker relationship to emotional factors, indicating that a degree of independence between cognitive and emotional facets of interest. In other words, images that were novel and hard to comprehend could be either positive or negative with respect to emotional valence. The interest model was therefore reduced to one cognitive component (representing a high/low cognitive response to the complexity/ease of comprehension associated with the stimulus), and two emotional factors; activation (high/low stimulation) and valence (positive/negative affect) creating a three-factor model of interest (Fig. 8.1b).

The three-factor interest model derived from the survey can be used to represent the visitor experience of interest in a CH setting. The three factors therefore serve an interactive role within the CH environment, distilling the four factors (entertainment, education, aesthetic and escapist) described by Pine and Gilmore (1998).

Fig. 8.1 a An example of the visually represented Likert scales used in the survey. **b** The three factor model of interest, with one cognitive (complexity/comprehension) factor and two emotional (valence and activation) factors

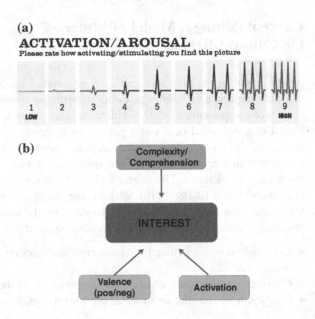

It is assumed that artefacts that are stimulating, in both cognitive and emotional aspects, will increase the activation level of the visitor. The precise effects on valence of the aesthetic domain will be shaped by content (i.e. representation, purpose) as well as the context of the presentation (i.e. personal relevance). It is speculated that particularly memorable artefacts will be associated with high magnitude changes in positive and negative valence that is related to physiological changes.

Operationalising the "Interest" Model

Operationalising the interest model for use with CH material involves deriving psychological variables from psychophysiological measures, such that an inference of interest can be established. Inference in this context concerns the creation of a one-to-many relationship in which two or more physiological elements are associated with one psychological element. Understanding the underlying neural pathways, and their connections to psychophysiological states, during aesthetic experiences in CH environments is therefore important to the development of accurate classification and real-time adaptation systems. Cognitive engagement can be quantified using Electroencephalography (EEG), particularly using alpha waves which have been associated with changes in cognitive load, i.e. a higher cognitive load is indicative of greater cognitive engagement (Goldman et al. 2002). Furthermore, although neuroaesthetic research is in its infancy, recent studies have used functional magnetic resonance imaging (fMRI), functional near infrared spectroscopy (fNIRS) and EEG to investigate the relationship between brain activity and cultural heritage experiences, in particular the perception of beauty and aesthetics (Nadal and Pearce 2011). Research within neuroaesthetics contends that the prefrontal cortex (PFC), in particular Brodman's area (BA) 10 located in the dorsal PFC, plays an important part in the evaluation of artworks through attentional top-down feedback that is the interpretation of sensory processing through cognitive engagement with the stimuli (e.g. Cupchik et al. 2009; Vessel et al. 2012; Hahn et al. 2006 for a review).

Psychological and neurological research using fMRI, fNIRS and EEG technology are almost always conducted in the laboratory because these devices are too intrusive to permit data capture in the field. These technologies allow for a detailed insight into activation within the brain during aesthetic experience but they lack ecological validity. Operationalising the interest model in an ecologically valid environment is a key step in the development of a cultural heritage physiological computing system. The development of mobile EEG sensors provides the possibility to capture cognitive engagement through sensors placed over the PFC, although with a loss of spatial accuracy compared to fMRI or fNIRS sensors. Advances in neuroaesthetics using EEG showed that stylistic information within art in the prefrontal cortex is processed on a different temporal basis to everyday object recognition (Augustin et al. 2011). For example, the shape of an apple is recognised faster than stylistic properties, such as pigment, colour or the medium to a surface, in an artwork. It has also been noted that alpha activation in the PFC is reduced during aesthetic experiences,[1] particularly during the judgment of beauty (Cela-Conde et al. 2004), making EEG an appropriate measure to encapsulate cognitive engagement in cultural heritage settings. Cognitive engagement can therefore be captured and quantified using spontaneous EEG measures of electrocortical activation in CH contexts. Additionally, the aspect of arousal or activation described by Berlyne (1960) and Russell (1980) can be captured through changes in the visitor's psychophysiology. Thus, cognitive engagement can be quantified through changes in psychophysiology and brain activation.

Wearing sensors connected to the facial skin or mobile eye-tracking devices may be perceived as uncomfortable, embarrassing and destructing from the experience of the exhibit. A monitoring system that captures the authenticity of the experience requires a multi–modal approach; however, such an approach requires more intrusive sensor technologies. It is important to understand the requirements and wishes of museum visitors as well as the psychological components of the experience and the technological requirements to build and implement a functional system. As we have seen above, EEG can be used as a mobile and relatively non-intrusive measure to capture the cognitive component of the CH experience. The activation component of interest can be captured via the level of skin conductance (SC) and supplemented by the measurement of heart rate (HR); SC is highly

---

[1] EEG alpha activation has a converse relationship with brain activity (Goldman et al. 2002), i.e. higher alpha activity is associated with reduced brain activation.

Table 8.1 Operationalised interest model: derived features for each measure

Interest model	Measure
Activation	Heart rate
	Skin conductance level
Cognition	EEG *ratio β/α*
	FP1,FP2,F3,F4,FPz
Valence	EEG *frontal asymmetry*
	$\alpha \ln(FP2) - (FP1)$
	$\alpha \ln(F4 - F3)$

sensitive to sympathetic activity (Boucsein 1992) and HR captures both sympathetic and parasympathetic components of the autonomic nervous system. SC and HR have been found to be appropriate measures to be used in CH environments (Tschacher et al. 2011). Valence is generally measured using facial electromyography (fEMG) (Cacioppo et al. 1990), but this measure requires electrodes to be worn on the face. Wearing visible sensors on the face may be seen as intrusive and embarrassing for the visitor in a public space and would therefore not be suitable for a classification system. Valence can also be captured through EEG frontal asymmetry. It has been hypothesised that greater activation of the left hemisphere of the PFC is associated with positive emotions whereas greater activation of the right hemisphere is linked to negative emotions (see Coan and Allen 2004 for a review).

Although SC and HR have been used before to map visitor experiences within a CH context, the question of sensor suitability is largely unanswered. Additionally this raises the question, to what extent will the CH visitor be prepared to wear sensor hardware? Ergonomics and social factors become major factors in system design when attempting to operationalise psychological constructs for use in the field. EEG for example can provide a wealth of new information about a visitor's psychological state. However, EEG sensor hardware is far from being ergonomically transparent, even with modern advances in commercially available technology such as the Neurosky and Emotiv mobile EEG headsets a certain amount of social stigma may be generated. The same cannot be said for skin conductance and heart rate measurement technologies, which have seen significant advances, to the point where these sensor technologies can be purchased commercially for sports, sleep monitoring or recreational purposes and packaged in a less intrusive format e.g. a wrist watch. The novelty of wearing a full sensor package for use in cultural heritage settings may offset the intrusiveness and stigma involved in their use. However, until research is completed to ascertain how acceptable sensor technologies are in various contexts, this question will remain unanswered. Table 8.1 summarises the array of physiological measures designed to deliver a multidimensional representation of the psychological state of interest, to quantify the interest level of an individual in a dynamic fashion.

In the following section we will discuss the use of physiological computing in a CH context to operationalise a system that enhances the visitor experience using psychophysiology. We will highlight aspects related to user agency during the use of a fully automated system and ethical considerations regarding data collection, however, a full discussion of these aspects is beyond the scope of this chapter.

Physiological Computing in a CH Context

Psychophysiology, physiological computing and machine learning can provide a unique way to operationalise the covert psychological experience of cultural heritage by measuring, analysing and classifying psychophysiological responses. Physiological computing systems monitor the physiology of the user and use these data as input to a computing system (Fairclough 2009). The passive monitoring of spontaneous changes in physiology indicative of cognition, emotion or motivation is used to adapt software in real time. These systems are constructed around a biocybernetic loop (Fairclough and Gilleade 2012) that handles the translation of raw physiological data into control input at the interface. Passive monitoring of user psychophysiology can be used to inform intelligent adaptation, thus permitting software to respond to the context of the user state in a personalised fashion.

A physiological computing system could be created to monitor CH experiences in real-time by quantifying the state of the visitor and using these data to personalize the provision of information via a process of "adaptive curation". For example, content for a museum audio guide could be selected based on the listener's psychophysiological responses to topical keywords. Whenever the listener responded with interest to a topic an adaptive guide pushes new content based on this theme. If the listener responded with no interest the system would skip this topic. To perform this act of personalisation, the physiological computing system must be sensitive to the psychological dimensions of the interest model. Our interest model proposed that activation, cognition and valence serve an interactive role in the CH experience.

One of the challenges in the creation of a physiological computing system is finding a reliable method of automatically classifying psychophysiological responses. To overcome this challenge, researchers have incorporated machine learning algorithms into experimental approaches, these algorithms apply various mathematical approaches to learn from existing data in order to generalise and predict the class of new or incoming data. A number of research studies have focused on combined multivariate physiological measures, such as HR, respiration (RSP), EEG and SC data (Picard 2000; Picard and Klein 2002; Mandryk and Atkins 2007; Wilhelm and Grossman 2010; Petrantonakis and Hadjileontiadis 2010), applying machine learning approaches to classify psychophysiological responses and map them onto psychological states. For example, Mandryk and Atkins (2007) applied fuzzy logic models to transform and transpose physiological responses into levels of arousal and valence, while Rani et al. (2005) and Villon and Lisetti (2007) used a series of regression decision trees (RDTs) to determine affective states from HR and SC. Other machine learning techniques used within psychophysiological research utilise more advanced algorithms, such as Support Vector Machines (SVM) and Artificial Neural Networks (ANN). Sakr et al. (2010) used an SVM to partition incoming signals in order to detect and classify levels of physiological activation, as a measure of agitation transition for monitoring the onset of epileptic episodes, whereas (Lee et al. 2005) applied ANN's to monitor indices of variance in the autonomic nervous system (ANS) when participants were presented with emotional stimuli.

These studies serve to illustrate how current research utilises a multidisciplinary approach towards solving physiological computing problems. When applied in a cultural heritage context psychophysiology and neuroaesthetics offer methods to measure, record, and infer information about a visitor's psychophysiological states as they interact with exhibits. Machine learning can provide a means to classify those responses, and a physiological computing system can utilise these classifications in order to provide a more memorable experience. This memorable experience could conceivably be achieved in real-time using unobtrusive sensor technologies and adaptive content delivery. To serve as a demonstration of a real-time physiological computing system in development, we present two completed studies which embrace the multidisciplinary approach and demonstrate the applicability of physiological computing within a cultural heritage setting.

The goal of the two studies was to operationalise the psychological construct of interest, as a psychophysiological measure consisting of the previously identified components (activation, cognition and valence). The cognitive component of interest was inferred from activation of the rostral prefrontal cortex; this variable was captured using spontaneous EEG measures of electrocortical activation. The activation component was captured via skin conductance level (SCL) and supplemented by measuring heart rate (HR); Valence was captured by measuring EEG frontal asymmetry. As previously discussed, greater left activation of the prefrontal cortex is associated with positive affect whereas greater right side activation is linked to negative affect (Davidson 2004). This array of psychophysiological measures was designed to deliver a multidimensional representation of interest to be used to quantify the interest level of an individual in a dynamic fashion, with the potential to inform a process of adaptive curation in near-real time.

Psychophysiological Measurement and Classification of Interest Using Cultural Heritage Material

To test the operationalisation of our interest model experimental studies were designed to record and classify psychophysiological responses to CH material developed by the Foundation for Art and Creative Technology (FACT, Liverpool) and the Museo Nacional de Artes Decorativas (Madrid). The approach we took combined our interest model with psychophysiological data and a machine learning algorithm in order to distinguish between stimuli that are high or low with respect to the level of interest provoked in the viewer.

For each study, interest was recorded using measures of variance in skin conductance, heart rate and electro-encephalic activity; a Mind Media Nexus X Mk II (sampled at 512 Hz) was used to record HR and SCL and for EEG a Enobio (StarLab, Inc) wireless sensor (sampled at 250 Hz). The studies were designed to fulfil the following goals:

- To measure and classify psychophysiological reactivity in response to CH content presented as visual and audio stimuli.
- To define psychophysiological reactivity in terms of two categories of interest (high and low) consisting of three dimensions: activation, cognition and valence.
- To evaluate the performance of the Support Vector Machine (SVM) classification algorithm (Burges 1998; Platt 1999) for real-time application and the precision of a SVM classifier trained to subjective responses to CH material.

Study One: A Virtual Heritage Installation

This study (Karran et al. 2013) set out to create a virtual heritage installation that replicated in part, a late eighteenth century Valencia kitchen mosaic installed at the Museo Nacional de Artes Decorativas in Madrid. In this study 10 participants, 8 female (aged 19–75) took part. Participants were asked to simultaneously view a visual representation of the Valencian kitchen and listen to four discrete pieces of narration. Participants also watched two control video clips. The stimuli were displayed upon a 2 by 3 meter projection screen in a light controlled room. The audio commentary was divided into four 'stories' consisting of three discrete 'facts'. The four stories were composed around elements in a still image featured on the wall, these were: the refreshments, the Lady of the House, the ceramics and the dog. To draw the gaze of the viewer specific fragments of the mosaic were highlighted (see Fig. 8.2). Participants were asked to stand in a natural relaxed manner whilst viewing a visual representation of the mosaic and to listen to an audio narration salient to the highlighted parts of the representation. Participants were asked to answer post hoc questions relating to interest level per auditory segment.

Feature Derivatives

Autonomic measures (activation) of heart rate and skin conductance level (SCL) were collected. A three-lead electrode connected to the chest was used to capture an ECG signal, which was filtered using a band-pass of 0.5–35 Hz. The SCL signal was collected from the intermediate phalanges of two fingers on the non-dominant hand and low-pass filtered at 35 Hz. Heart rate was captured as the mean and standard deviation of the inter-beat interval (IBI); the same descriptive statistics were used to represent SCL.

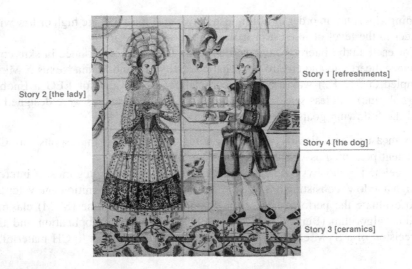

Fig. 8.2 The stimulus image used in the experiment, highlighted sections correspond to the audio narration. (Image courtesy of the Museo Nacional de Artes Decorativas, Madrid)

EEG data was collected using four EEG channels. Dry electrodes (i.e. no electro-conductive gel) were placed at Fp1 and Fp2 on the forehead. Electrodes were also placed at F3 and F4 using a small amount of electro-conductive gel and an electrode designed to make contact through hair. The resulting EEG signals from all four channels were band-pass filtered at 0.05 and 35 Hz. These data were subjected to a power spectral density analysis to yield power in the alpha (8–12 Hz) and beta (13–30 Hz) frequency bands. Cognition was measured using the ratio of the total power in the beta to alpha band for each electrode site i.e. 4 ratios.

$$\text{Cognition} = \text{total power in beta band}/\text{total power in alpha band}$$

Valence was measured using the natural logs of the total power in the alpha band of the right and left hemispheres, subtracted away from each other. This was calculated for the following pairs of electrode sites: Fp2 − Fp1 and F4 − F3.

$$\text{Valence} = \ln(\text{total alpha power right hemisphere}) - \ln(\text{total alpha power left hemisphere})$$

Positive values, indicative of left hemisphere dominance, as alpha power is inversely proportional to cortical activation, have been associated with negative affect and vice versa. All features were extracted from a stimulus epoch that equated to the length of each of the three facts related to each story (approx. 20 s per fact), these feature derivatives represent continuous values and not traditional change score from baseline, this approach was purposeful to be more representative of a real-time environment.

Training Data

The 10 feature derivatives described above i.e. 2 IBI, 2 SCL, 6 EEG, were used to create a classification vector representing the viewer's level of 'interest'. This feature vector was created for each of the 14 stimulus events (4 stories, 3 facts per story, plus 2 control events). These features were also subdivided to create classification vectors representing each component of the operationalised interest model, comprising features of activation (2 IBI, 2 SCL), cognition (4 EEG) and valence (2 EEG). Vectors were labelled based upon the participants' subjective assessment of each story. Participants were asked to select the 2 most interesting stories of the presented 4. All facts associated with these stories were labelled as 'high interest' along with their associated classification vectors. The remainder were labelled as 'low interest'. Psychophysiological responses to the relaxing and exciting movie segments were used to provide 'control' classification vectors, such that labels were applied to the physiological responses for each as low and high interest respectively.

Study Two: Liverpool FACT Study

The second study was undertaken in situ at the Foundation for Art and Creative Technology (FACT), a media arts centre based in Liverpool (UK). Eight participants, 3 female (aged 20-40), were asked to view a series of multimedia stimulus segments lasting 30 s related to an artist associated with the CH institute. A total of 15 stimulus segments were used in this study; all content was created by the CH institution. After each stimulus presentation, participants completed a questionnaire comprising self-ratings of physiological activation, cognitive engagement and emotional valence.

Feature Derivatives

For this study, 10 features were derived from physiological signals, filtered in the same manner as study one; for measures of activation the mean, maximum and standard deviation of IBI and SCL were derived. For cognition, the ratio of beta to alpha power at electrode sites Fp1, Fp2 and FpZ were derived. Valence was expressed as the natural log of total alpha power in the right hemisphere subtracted from the alpha power in the left hemisphere for the electrode pair Fp2–Fp1. Features derivatives were calculated every 2 s for the period of the stimulus exposure. Each stimulus was associated was all the features calculated during the exposure window.

Training Data

The 10 feature derivatives described above i.e. 3 IBI, 3 SCL, 4 EEG, were used to create a classification vector representing the participant's level of 'interest'. The feature vectors were created every 2 s for a stimulus epoch of 30 s for 15 multimedia stimulus events (3 artists, average 5 events per artist). These features were also subdivided to create classification vectors representing each component of the operationalised interest model, comprising features of activation (3 IBI, 3 SCL), cognition (3 EEG) and valence (1 EEG). Vectors were labelled based upon the participant's subjective assessment of each story. Participants were asked to complete a questionnaire consisting of three Likert scales ranked 1–10. These aligned to the 3 dimensions of the interest model; Activation: tired/passive 0 to activated/alert 10; Valence: sad/angry 0 to happy/cheerful 10; Cognition: low 0 to high 10. To derive the binary class labels from the Likert scaled scores; the scores for each participant were normalised in the form of:

$$y^i = \sum_{i=3} x_i \left(\frac{x_i - \min C}{\max C - \min C} \right)$$

where x_i is the sum of subjective scores for each dimension of the model (activation, cognition and valence) combined, $\min C$ and $\max C$ are the minima and maxima of the population of scores for each stimulus segment. The result y^i is a population of normalised scores. To set the threshold for class assignation, the median of this population was calculated. Above the median was labelled as high interest and below as low interest. The result from this process is a class label (either high or low interest), that represents a single subjective judgement score for each stimulus segment, which is then associated with the psychophysiological data for that stimulus segment to become the feature vector used to train the classifier.

Classification of the Psychophysiological Response

The feature data derived from both studies were analysed separately and features grouped according to the three components of the interest model, such that each feature set created a unique feature vector for an SVM classifier. Each component of the interest model has corresponding psychophysiological measures. These are: for activation features of heart rate and skin conductance, for cognition features of EEG and for valence features of EEG hemispheric asymmetry. This approach has a number of advantages. Firstly, each feature vector is identified as a separate component of the model; secondly feature sets can be combined as a fusion of features; and thirdly the effect of each feature set or fusion of features on classifier class recall can thusly be evaluated. Recall accuracy in the context of classification is determined by first validating the SVM model over the training data, the training data has both the classification vector (observation) and its associated label, and then by testing the SVM model over novel instances of test data. In a laboratory context, the labels associated with the test observations are known to the experimenter but unknown to the SVM model, thus recall accuracy is calculated by comparing SVM model classification output (in terms of class) and comparing those to the known labels, the result is how well the SVM model recalled the class of the observation.

Each participant's data was analysed separately to determine the recall accuracy of the SVM classifier for individual participant responses. The SVM classifier is a supervised pattern recognition algorithm, requiring an n dimensional vector (observation) and an associated label (class) for training. This training set is then used as the basis for classifying new instances of data into its respective class. For both studies the classification analysis was performed using the SVM routines from Matlab's Bioinformatics Toolbox. For study one, each feature set tested using 5-fold (k-fold) cross-validation. In k-fold cross-validation, k-1 folds are used for training and the last fold is used for evaluation. This process is repeated k times, leaving one different fold for evaluation each time.

Additionally, for the second study the "hold-out" cross-validation method was chosen; the hold-out method partitions the data into two parts, by randomly assigning data to either a training or testing set, ensuring that the classifier is trained and tested with novel data and is analogous to a real world task. The hold-out method of cross-validation has been shown to provide a more accurate assessment of classifier performance, compared to k-fold cross-validation when applied to small datasets, such as those gained from real-time applications (Isaksson et al. 2008).

In both studies, the class labels used to train the classifier were obtained from the subjective data taken during the experimental task. For study one, based on the subjective assessment of the participant six facts (two stories) were classified as 'high interest', i.e. they were associated with the psychophysiological data from the two stories assessed to be of most interest for that particular participant and two control labels (car chase high and sea life low interest) were used as class labels. For study two, only a composite "interest" score was used as class labels when classifying the individual components of the interest model e.g. investigating to what extent each component of the interest model contributed to the classification of the interest state.

Results

The results obtained from the first study are summarised in Table 8.2 below, and represent the classifier recall accuracies from the subject-dependent classification of the feature data. The feature sets (*activation*, *cognition* and *valence*) were classified alone and in combination, to determine which permutation of features provided the best class recall accuracy over all participants. We found that the fusion of activation and cognition features resulted in a mean class recall accuracy

Table 8.2 Study 1. Classification recall accuracy across individuals and feature sets (Activation (A), Cognition (C), Valence (V), Participant (P))

Feature(s)	P1	P2	P3	P4	P5	P6	P7	P8	P9	P10	Mean recall (%)
A	44	72	80	83	90	80	63	89	67	90	76
A,C	100	70	66	90	77	87	60	80	90	100	80
A,V	66	62	66	100	90	78	45	88	66	100	76
A,C,V	81	62	70	90	80	67	60	80	70	100	76
C,V	100	66	66	50	66	77	80	77	81	100	76
C	87	90	72	55	50	44	80	70	87	100	74
V	75	55	60	54	83	60	50	87	100	80	70

across all participants of 80 % (range 66–100 %). This result, which is significantly above chance, offers strong evidence that the combination of activation and cognition features affords an effective method, from which to ascertain a visitor's level of interest in a cultural heritage setting. However, the influence of individual differences in physiological responses towards the heritage material can be seen as variation in the recall rates for each individual.

Comparing the classifier recall accuracies from other feature sets, we found that the features of activation alone are only 4 % less accurate overall than those of the combined activation and cognitive feature sets; with a maximum of 76 % mean recall accuracy. Furthermore, we found that no clear benefit was gained by combining the features of activation with valence, or cognition with valence, highlighting a possible lack of emotional response to the material used in the study. These positive findings formed the basis from which to develop the methodology and analysis framework for the second in situ study, informing further improvement of the subject-dependent classifier approach and testing of the interest model.

Turning now to the experimental results from the second study conducted at FACT. Table 8.3 summarises the classifier recall accuracies for all feature sets. Analogous with the previous study, feature sets were classified alone and in combination to determine which permutation of features provided the best class recall accuracy over all participants. The working hypothesis, that features of activation and cognition would provide the best classification rates and thus a more positive determination of visitor interest, does not hold true for these data. However, a mean recall accuracy of 77.25 % (range 62.3–95.2 %) is significantly above chance and consistent with study one results. The classification results for these data indicate that, in this instance, the features of activation alone (87.25 %, range 73.77–95.5 %) and the combination of activation and valence features (84.67 %, range 62.3–95.2 %) provide the most accurate classifier recall rates. This highlights possible effects with the mixed media stimuli, such that the material was subjectively rated more stimulating and emotionally engaging when compared against stimuli from the previous study. However, a closer examination of the intra-participants recall rates shows the features of activation alone

Table 8.3 Study 2. Classification recall accuracy across individuals and feature sets (Activation (A), Cognition (C), Valence (V), Participant (P))

Participant	1	2	3	4	5	6	7	8	Mean recall (%)
A	92.49	93.55	95.5	80	87	73.77	84.2	88	87.25
A,C	73.68	88.71	95.2	69	68	62.3	79.0	82	77.25
A,V	92.98	91.94	95.2	69	68	62.30	79.0	84	84.67
A,C,V	71.93	88.37	93.6	69	68	60.66	80.7	84	77.02
C,V	68.42	62.9	64.5	67	68	62.3	71.9	70	66.62
C	66.67	69.35	67.7	67	70	60.66	73.7	72	68.38
V	61.4	66.13	66.1	67	62	62.3	68.4	63	64.63

presented the most stable classifier in this instance. Interestingly, comparing the mean classification recall accuracies for the combined feature set (representative of the full three dimensional interest model) between study one and two, we found a high degree of similarity, the intra-subject classification variation became less pronounced, and mean recall accuracies remained largely unaffected at 76 and 77.2 %, for studies one and two respectively.

These findings indicate, that for study two, participants possibly responded more "viscerally" to the emotional context and prosody embedded in the source CH material. This effect may have expressed itself as a stronger response in the measures of autonomic activity and hemispheric asymmetry and thus reflected in the subjective ratings of the material. Certainly this effect is mirrored by the high classification rates for these features (Table 8.3).

The results from both studies provide evidence that the combination of activation, cognition and valence features, coupled with a SVM classifier and a subject-dependent classification approach, can reliably infer the knowledge emotion "interest" within a cultural heritage context. This finding should be assessed in the context of a physiological computing system which adapts information to users' physiological responses; greater classification accuracy and less intra-personal variation between classification accuracies should equate to a more stable system. Stability here, equates to a system less prone to classification error when trained and applied to multiple users.

The next step is to integrate these findings into a real-time "adaptive curation" system, which responds to psychophysiological measures of interest in order to tailor the provision of information to sustain the interest of the visitor and create a memorable experience in the gallery or museum. The results from these studies indicate that the proposed operationalised model of interest can be classified with a reasonable degree of accuracy and could, therefore, be a candidate for use in systems that incorporate a user's interest state into a bio-cybernetic loop to drive adaptions. A challenge to designing such a system is how to increase the provision of information about the heritage installation without diluting the cultural significance via information overload.

The "Adaptive Curator": Proposing a Framework for an Adaptive Memorable CH Experience

To illustrate how an "adaptive curation" system, that adapts information based on a visitor's level of interest, could be constructed we propose the "INTREST framework" shown in Fig. 8.3. The proposed framework is based loosely around the narrative structure of Campbell (1999) *monomythos* in which the narrative elements separation, initiation and return are used as top level design structures. These structures denote the purpose and placement of the CH content (narrative arcs) used to drive psychophysiological responses. In this instance the physiological measurement and classification adaptive feedback mechanism is one of full automation, in that no decision is required from the user in order for the system to make adaptions. However, the framework can be adapted to fit other automation models. The INTREST framework is separated into five phases: narrative structure, adaptive story elements, physiological measurement, classification and narrative path. Each phase represents a requirement or process needed to form the system and can be summarised as: INput, sTimulus, REsponse, claSsification, ouTput.

Phase one is concerned with the conceptual narrative structure, each block representing one element of the narrative 'arc'. Phase two consists of the adaptive story elements or information blocks created to fit in within the narrative structure, such as semantically linked multimedia content about the exhibit or installation (the journey so to speak). Phase three is focused on operationalising the psychophysiological construct "interest" to record and measure physiological variance in response to story elements. In this case features of HR, SCL and EEG are indicated. In phase four the classification of the level of interest is completed, outputting either high or low interest in response to story elements. This output is then used in the final phase to pull new content from the adaptive story elements, to create the narrative path of adapted information. When applied the INTREST framework could potentially offer many distinct narrative pathways through a store of information. A starting point is chosen by the system; the psychophysiological response to this content is then evaluated; if visitor interest is high then the system continues to draw content from the store for that narrative arc; if visitor interest is low, new content is drawn first from the same store, or if responses still indicate low then from the store of content from another narrative arc in an attempt to elicit the more favourable high response.

Within this scenario the narrative arcs represent elements of the same "story" but with different content databases. For example, consider a Han dynasty vase (Circa 202 BC). The story starts with information about the vase and its provenance, interest is classified as low, new information is provided from further ahead in the story, however the response to this content is still classified as low interest. The system then adapts to these responses by drawing content from a concurrent narrative arc, this time the content is about how the vase is made and the ceramic processes of the period, this elicits a high response, after a number of content

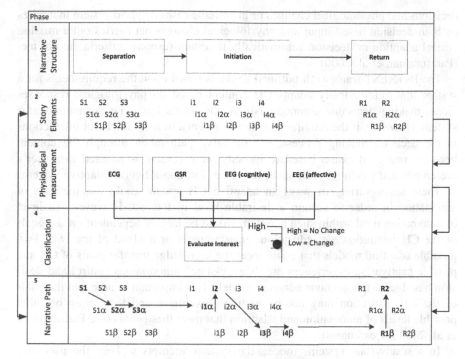

Fig. 8.3 INTREST a cultural heritage "digital curator" framework

blocks are displayed the response is still high and remains that way until the content is exhausted. From this information the system can ascertain, that for this user of the system, content that explains how artefacts are created is of interest. When the user then moves to a different artefact the system utilises this information as the new start point for further content provision, if responses remain high, then the system adapts to give only this type of content. When responses drop to low interest, the entire process begins again.

System Autonomy in Adaptive Systems

In a physiological computing context, adaptive systems can be divided into two categories, autonomous systems where physiological input alone is used to drive adaptions and manual, user-driven systems, where user decisions in conjunction with physiological input, is used to inform adaptions. Broadly speaking, the amount of automation provided by autonomous or hybrid user-driven adaptive systems can differ in both type and complexity, ranging from the simple organisation and provision of information in response to physiological changes, to multi-layered response adaptions at key stages in a process in response to both user decisions and physiological changes or in extreme cases a hybrid system that relies on both decision based input and physiological changes but carries out a mission critical adaption or decision automatically if certain response criteria are not met (Parasuraman et al. 2000).

The INTREST framework outlined above is based upon the requirements for a system that automatically adapts CH content based on physiological responses alone, making decisions autonomously of the user's input, i.e. an autonomous system. However, if the requirements are broadened to include visitor interactions in the decision making process, the narrative path taken through the content becomes one of decision based reciprocity were content is adapted to a user's preference and psychophysiological response, forming a hybrid adaptive system.

There are a variety of ways an adaptive CH system could use methods of automation in order to sustain a desirable level of interest. However, the level of automation used within such a system would be largely dependent on the goals of the CH institution e.g. education, entertainment or a blend of the two. Two possible adaption models that could meet the knowledge transfer goals of CH and provide captivating experiences are "steady-state" autonomous control and decision based semi-autonomous adaption models. It is important to note that the goals of the CH institution may not be mutually exclusive and there may be other possible levels of automation and adaption that meet these goals (see Parasuraman et al. 2000 for examples).

In a steady-state systems model, the system attempts to keep the user in a continuous (desirable) state of interest, which allows the user to experience constant engagement with the exhibit. However, conscious choices are never given to the user and all information is adapted based on physiological response alone. This creates a fully automated, implicit dynamic bio-cybernetic loop, in which, content, unconscious psychophysiological responses, and the user's conscious experience of interest form a seamless "total experience". This steady state systems model which uses a bio-cybernetic loop to sustain engagement has been demonstrated in the context of computer games (Rani et al. 2005). However, in the context of CH, it may not always be desirable to enforce a steady state of interest, which may cause overstimulation or interfere with knowledge transfer goals. It may therefore be better to tailor CH experiences to allow for lulls in content provision allowing users time for reflection. The second adaptation model is a decision based semi-autonomous model in which the system advises the user through an interface that certain types of information best meet their needs, or could enhance their experience and the user then actively choses the content. This style of system utilises unconscious physiological responses and user interactive decisions as input to create an explicit decision based loop. In both of these system models, the adaption process drives the delivery of context dependant information to augment visitor perception, cognition and engagement while concurrently providing inputs for the next series of adaptions.

For example, in a hybrid psychophysiology user-decision adaptive system, a list of content choices is offered to the visitor. The decisions taken by the visitor nearly always produce a physiological response indicative of low interest. These choices are stored and weighted internally then associated with the physiological response to the content. The system evaluates the weighted physiological responses and during use the system prunes the pallet of new content choices offered to the visitor to create a more favourable high interest response. As the number of high responses increases, these choices are stored and used as a basis for the next round of content adaptions; this can be likened to an allosteric logic "see-saw" which attempts to cultivate positive psychophysiological interest responses by drawing on information from previous interactions to inhibit or activate adaption choices. Serbedzija and Fairclough (2009) classify this form of short term adaption as a "pervasive adjustment". These authors identify emotional states as non-rigid phenomena which require an adaptive system to monitor and control the success of its own actions as a two part reflexive process. In the first instance the user state is monitored to create adaptions (or choices) when required which naturally leads to a second order of monitoring which evaluates the effectiveness of those adaptions in terms of favourable responses from the first stage. Positive and negative responses are then held in storage to tailor future system behaviours over the course of use.

When designing an adaptive system for cultural heritage that encourages a steady state of information gain and potentiates a "memorable experience", the decision as to what level of automation is required is of paramount importance and should be taken at the outset. The choice of autonomous or hybrid semi-autonomous system design can create adaptive system experiences ranging from a "fairground ride" to a deeper more meaningful self-created narrative learning experience. Too much automation creates a risk that visitors feel alienated with no control as information is pushed at them, too little and the experience provided appears bland and requires too much effort to complete.

Adaptive Systems and the Memorable Experience

Creating memorable experiences in heritage installations is becoming more and more important with higher visitor expectations and greater competition between installations, creating an experience economy (Pine and Gilmore 1998; De Rojas and Cameron 2008). Previous evaluations of visitors' satisfaction with exhibits took a purely cognitive approach by investigating visitors' cognitive state evaluated through knowledge gain, product satisfaction (the exhibit in this case) or product use. However, a visitor's satisfaction is not only related to perceived quality and satisfied expectations, but also to emotional reactions (De Rojas and Cameron, 2008).

Adaptive physiological computing systems may therefore satisfy more than one dimension of the CH experience. They have the potential to provide experiences that draw on either or both, the cognitive and emotional factors related to Pine and Gilmore (1998) total experience model or be separated from this by providing either cognitive or emotional experiences. A visitor's experience can, for example be enhanced through learning about cognitive aspects of an exhibit, such as the period the piece was created in or aspects about the materials/ways it was made. Alternatively, the visitor may be presented with audio content that is aimed at evoking relevant emotional reactions towards the exhibit without adding cognitive content. Music, for example, may be used to either reflect the mood of the exhibit or influence the visitor's emotions in order to create a change in perception towards the exhibit. Although a multisensory approach would most likely work best in the cultural heritage context, the problem lies in finding the correct balance between immersion, storytelling and information gain (even if these are the goals of the system).

There is a dichotomy within cultural heritage between the visitor's and the institutional needs. Institutions aim to transfer knowledge, accurate facts and authenticity about the exhibit, and the visitors aim to have a memorable experience (Pine and Gilmore 1998). An adaptive system may provide the ideal medium to address these needs by providing environment specific systems that can be: either autonomously or manually controlled, driven by the emotional òr cognitive aspects of knowledge transfer, and in addition, provide the opportunity to collect user metrics specific to the context it is used in. For example, an autonomous system may be applied in an environment that is aiming to provide a traditional learning experience about an exhibit. The system can be used to guide the visitor through the experience whilst adapting the content to their levels of interest without interruption or the need to make a choice to what content is preferred over another. Manual decision based systems, on the other hand, can be used to give the visitor more agency by introducing interactive elements where content is selected upon recommendation.

The visitors' psychophysiology can also be used in other ways in a cultural heritage environment. For example it could be used as input control to an interactive art installation, allowing the visitor to manipulate an artwork through their psychophysiological reactions (e.g. the Sound Glove: Graugaard 2005). These can be referred to as adaptive artworks. Adaptive artworks could change, for example, the colour within a painting according to the visitor's heart-rate, or a heat-map next to the painting could show average heart rates from all visitors who have seen the picture. Data collected by the adaptive system may also be of great interest to the institution, either as feedback on their performance or in the use of new exhibits. However, adaptive systems, and in particular adaptive artworks, raise important ethical questions pertaining to data mining and the privacy of the user (see Boehle et al. 2013).

Concluding Remarks

The cultural heritage model by Pine and Gilmore (1998) and the psychological interest model described in this chapter can be viewed as parallel concepts that describe the visitor's engagement with cultural heritage exhibits. Within the context of developing adaptive systems the psychological interest model helps to embody the four factors of Pine and Gilmore (1998) within the physiological domain. This allows for measurement of psychophysiological parameters that permit the operationalisation of aspects of the cultural heritage experience for use in adaptive systems.

Physiologically adaptive information systems created for cultural heritage settings can provide new ways to create memorable experiences for the visitor, and the ability for institutions to adapt their content to meet the needs of a fast growing knowledge economy. Adaptive systems, created using psychophysiological and HCI principles, coupled with narrative structures may allow institutions to develop user experiences that are tailored to their individual needs. Thus, neither fully automated nor manually driven systems can be regarded as the better approach, but each individual institution will need to decide what their requirements are. These requirements will dictate the type of system that is chosen, or employed.

We envision many possible applications of this approach within the context of cultural heritage. Additionally user metrics could be used for "interest" profiling which would involve the implicit tagging of heritage material to build up heat maps that use levels of interest towards information or exhibits to inform future content development and build cultural heritage installations that imbue artefacts with a sense of modernity, whilst at the same time preserving any cultural and historical significance.

Acknowledgements This work was supported by EU FP7 project No.270318 (ARtSENSE).

References

Augustin MD, Defranceschi B, Fuchs HK, Carbon CC, Hutzler F (2011) The neural time course of art perception: an ERP study on the processing of style versus content in art. Neuropsychologia 49(7):2071–2081

Berlyne DE (1960) Conflict, arousal, and curiosity. McGraw-Hill Book Company, London

Boucsein W (1992) Electrodermal activity. Plenum Press, New York

Boehle K, Coenen C, Decker M, Rader M (2013) Biocybernetic adaptation and privacy. Innov: Eur J Soc Sci Res 26(1–2)

Burges CJC (1998) A tutorial on support vector machines for pattern recognition. Knowl Disc Data Min 2(2):121–167

Cacioppo JT, Bush LK, Tassinary LG (1990) Microexpressive facial actions as a function of affective stimuli: replication and extension. Pers Soc Psychol Bull 18:515–526

Campell J (1999) Der Heros in tausend Gestalten. Insel Verlag, Frankfurt am Main und Leipzig

Cela-Conde CJ, Marty G, Maestú F, Ortiz T, Munar E, Fernández A, Roca M, Rosselló J, Quesney F (2004) Activation of the prefrontal cortex in the human visual aesthetic perception. Proc Natl Acad Sci USA 101(16):6321–6325

Coan JA, Allen JJB (2004) Frontal EEG asymmetry as a moderator and mediator of emotion. Biol Psychol 67(1–2):7–49

Cupchik GC, Vartanian O, Crawley A, Mikulis DJ (2009) Viewing artworks: contributions of cognitive control and perceptual facilitation to aesthetic experience. Brain Cogn 70(1):84–91

Davidson RJ (2004) What does the prefrontal cortex "do" in affect: perspectives in frontal EEG asymmetry research. Biol Psychol 67:219–234

De Rojas C, Camarero C (2008) Visitors' experience, mood and satisfaction in a heritage context: evidence from an interpretation center. Tour Manag 29:525–537

Ekman P (1992) An argument for basic emotions. Cogn Emot 6:169–200

Fairclough SH (2009) Fundamentals of physiological computing. Interact Comput 21:133–145

Fairclough SH, Gilleade K (2012) Construction of the biocybernetic loop: a case study. In: Proceedings of the 14th ACM international conference on multimodal interaction, Santa Monica

Goldman RI, Stern JM, Engel J Jr, Cohen MS (2002) Simultaneous EEG and fMRI of the alpha rhythm. NeuroReport 13:2487–2494

Graugaard L (2005) The SoundGlove II: using sEMG data for intuitive audio and video affecting in real-time. In: Proceedings of the 3rd annual conference in computer game design and technology, Liverpool, pp 119–128

Hahn B, Ross TJ, Stein EA (2006) Neuroanatomical dissociation between bottom-up and top-down processes of visuospatial selective attention. Neuroimage 32:842–853

Hidi S, Renninger KA (2006) The four-phase model of interest development. Educ Psychol 41(2):111–127

Isaksson A, Wallman M, Göransson H, Gustafsson MG (2008) Cross-validation and bootstrapping are unreliable in small sample classification. Pattern Recogn Lett 29(14):1960–1965

Jennett C, Cox AL, Cairns P, Dhoparee S, Epps A, Tijs T, Walton A (2008) Measuring and defining the experience of immersion in games. Int J Hum Comput Stud 66:641–661

Johnsson E, Adler C (2006) A guide to developing effective storytelling programmes for museums. London Museums Hub

Karran AJ, Fairclough SH, Gilleade K (2013) Towards an adaptive cultural heritage experience using physiological computing. In Proceeding of: CHI 2013 "changing perspectives", Extended Abstracts, Paris, April 27–May 2, 2013

Leder H, Belke B, Oeberst A, Augustin D (2004) A model of aesthetic appreciation and aesthetic judgments. Br J Psychol 95(Pt 4):489–508

Lee CK, Yoo SK, Park YJ (2005) Using neural network to recognize human emotions from heart rate variability and skin resistance. In: 27th annual international conference of the engineering in medicine and biology society (IEEE-EMBS 2005), pp 5523–5525, 17–18 Jan 2006

Liew CL (2005) Online cultural heritage exhibitions: a survey of information retrieval features. Program Electron Libr Inf Syst 39(1):4–24

Louvre Paris (2013) http://www.louvre.fr/en/media-en-ligne?criteria-keywords=&criteria-year= &tab=1153#tabs; Accessed 5 Sept 2013

Mandryk R, Atkins M (2007) A fuzzy physiological approach for continuously modeling emotion during interaction with play technologies. Int J Hum Comput Stud 65(4):329–347

McIntosh A, Prentice R (1999) Affirming authenticity: consuming cultural heritage. Ann Tour Res 26(3):589–612

McLean K (1993) Planning for people in museum exhibitions. Association of Science-Technology Centres, Michigan

Nadal M, Pearce MT (2011) The Copenhagen neuroaesthetics conference: prospects and pitfalls for an emerging field. Brain Cogn 76:172–183

Parasuraman R, Sheridan TB, Wickens C (2000) A model for types and levels of human interaction with automation. IEEE Trans Syst Man Cybern Part A Syst Humans 30(3):273–285

Petrantonakis PC, Hadjileontiadis LJ (2010) Emotion recognition from EEG using higher order crossings. IEEE Trans Inf Technol Biomed. A publication of the IEEE engineering in medicine and biology society 14(2):186–197

Picard RW (2000) Toward computers that recognize and respond to user emotion. IBM Syst J 39(3 and 4):705–719

Picard RW, Klein J (2002) Computers that recognise and respond to user emotion: theoretical and practical implications. Interact Comput 14(2):141–169

Pine B, Gilmore J (1998) Welcome to the experience economy. Harvard Bus Rev 76(4):97–105

Platt JC (1999) Fast training of support vector machines using sequential minimal optimization. In: Schlkopf B, Burges CJC, Smola AJ (eds) Advances in kernel methods, MIT Press, Cambridge, pp 185–208

Rani P, Sarkar N, Liu C, (2005) Maintaining optimal challenge in computer games through realtime physiological feedback. In: Proceedings of the 11th international conference on human computer interaction, pp 184–192

Russell JA (1980) A circumplex model of affect. Pers Soc Psychol 39:1161–1178

Sakr GE, Elhajj IH, Huijer HA-S (2010) Support vector machines to define and detect agitation transition. IEEE Trans Affect Comput 1(2):98–108

Serbedzija N, Fairclough SH (2009) Biocybernetic loop: from awareness to evolution. In: IEEE congress on evolutionary computation, Trondheim, May 2009

Silvia PJ (2008) Interest—the curious emotion. Curr Dir Psychol Sci 17(1):57–60

Silvia PJ (2010) Confusion and interest: the role of knowledge emotions in aesthetic experience. Psychol Aesthet Creativity Arts 4(2):75–80

Tschacher W, Greenwood S, Kirchberg V, Wintzerith S, van den Berg K, Trondle M (2011) Physiological correlates of aesthetic perception of artworks in a museum. Psychol Aesthet Creativity Arts 6(1):96–103

Tung VWS, Ritchie JRB (2011) Exploring the essence of memorable tourism experiences. Ann Tour Res 38(4):1367–1386

Uysal M, Noe F (2003) Satisfaction in outdoor recreation and tourism settings. In: Laws E (ed) Case studies in tourism marketing. Continuum Publisher, London, pp 140–158

Vessel EA, Starr GG, Rubin N (2012) The brain on art: intense aesthetic experience activates the default mode network. Frontiers in Hum Neurosci 6:66

Villon O, Lisetti C (2007) toward recognizing individual's subjective emotion from physiological signals in practical application. In: 20th IEEE international symposium on computer-based medical systems (CBMS'07), pp 357–362

Wang N (1999) Rethinking authenticity in tourism experience. Ann Tour Res 2(1):349–370

Wilhelm FH, Grossman P (2010) Emotions beyond the laboratory: theoretical fundaments, study design, and analytic strategies for advanced ambulatory assessment. Biol Psychol 84:552–569

Chapter 9
The Vitality Bracelet: Bringing Balance to Your Life with Psychophysiological Measurements

Joyce Westerink, William van Beek, Elke Daemen, Joris Janssen,
Gert-Jan de Vries and Martin Ouwerkerk

Abstract We present the concept of the Vitality Bracelet, a wrist-worn device that helps users in bringing more balance in their daily life, especially a balance between stressful and relaxing situations. On the one hand, the Vitality Bracelet comprises the measurement of your skin conductance, reflecting the current level of arousal of your autonomic nervous system. These skin conductance measurements are analyzed in real-time to give an indication of upcoming tension, but they could also be recorded and visualized to present an overview of the daily or weekly tension patterns. On the other hand, the Vitality Bracelet offers paced breathing exercises, supporting instant relaxation as well as general health and vitality on the long run. This chapter describes the design, development and a first evaluation of the Vitality Bracelet concept.

Introduction

Stress is a common word in our everyday society, reflecting the fact that a majority of us consider our lives to be stressful in some (negative) way. In the Western world, as well as in Asia, employees indicate they feel stressed because of increased workload, competition, and job instability (APA 2010; China Daily 2010). Also in the personal domain many causes of stress accumulate, for instance in caring for one's children or other loved ones. As a consequence, stress is a topic of psychological and physiological research, in which the reflection of mental stress in bodily signals is studied (McEwen 1998). This link between mental and bodily aspects of stress management is also present in the increased interest in the western world in oriental spiritual techniques like yoga, paced breathing and mindfulness (Parati et al. 2008; Kabat-Zinn 2003).

J. Westerink (✉) · W. van Beek · E. Daemen · J. Janssen · G.-J. de Vries · M. Ouwerkerk
Philips Research Europe, Eindhoven, The Netherlands

S. H. Fairclough and K. Gilleade (eds.), *Advances in Physiological Computing*, 197
Human–Computer Interaction Series, DOI: 10.1007/978-1-4471-6392-3_9,
© Springer-Verlag London 2014

Combining these fields, we set out to make a device that would help users to maintain an adequate balance between stress and relaxation in their lives. One part of our objectives was to support the users in the recognition and interpretation of their bodily signals indicating stress. Many people these days have grown alienated to some extent from bodily reactions (Rouse et al. 1988; Dunn et al. 2007), and an objective measurement of such signals might bring renewed awareness. In addition, we had the objective to also present the users with a means to actively manage relaxation. We hoped that the combination of these components would enhance their individual effects. For reasons that will become clear later in this chapter, we called our concept the Vitality Bracelet. In the next sections we present the Vitality Bracelet. We will explain its design and technology in more detail, present some physiological data measured while using the device, as well as describe the results of an initial experience study.

Design

Internal pilot investigations had indicated that especially women between 30 and 60 years recognize that it takes effort to balance the many roles in their lives (mother, partner, caregiver, colleague, friend), and are open to accept technological support for this. So from the beginning we focused on designing this device for females.

In order to enhance their awareness of bodily stress-related signals we considered the measurement of skin conductance. It is a good candidate for this job, since it is known to reflect arousal and tension (Boucsein 1992), and thus most likely is related to stress. Also the Affective Health system (Kosmack Vaara et al. 2009) has the goal of helping users to reflect on their emotional state and presents the continuously measured skin conductance signal to the users as one of their relevant parameters. Even though other bodily signals can be related to arousal to some extent as well, for instance the alpha frequency range of the electroencephalogram (EEG) or the heart rate variability (HRV), skin conductance is specifically acceptable for use in daily life, since recently a wrist-based means of measuring skin conductance has become available (Westerink et al. 2009). A continuous analysis of the skin conductance measurements allows real-time interpretation of the signal and instantaneous feedback on arousal levels. The device should detect instances in which the arousal rapidly increases, and present these warnings as so-called 'mindfulness moments' to the user, assuming this will motivate the user to start to relax when that is most needed.

As a means to offer instant relaxation, we considered the yoga-based technique of paced breathing. It offers the user guidance to breathe slowly, and the slow breathing rhythm triggers activity of the vagus nerve, which, in turn, has restorative and relaxing effects (Porges 2007; Lehrer et al. 2000). An extra reason to offer paced breathing is that it is also beneficial for one's general health and vitality (hence the name Vitality Bracelet): a daily 15 min of paced breathing is

Fig. 9.1 First sketch of the Vitality Bracelet

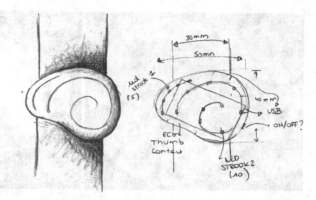

known to lower blood pressure (Grossman et al. 2001) and reduce depression and anxiety (Clark and Hirschman 1990). But it is not always easy to adhere to the strict regime of 15 min/day (Janakiramaiah 2000). We anticipated that awareness brought by the skin conductance measurements would also help the user get motivated to perform the paced breathing exercises on a daily basis.

Because of the skin conductance measurements, the Vitality Bracelet had to be a wrist-based device. Since the device was to be worn on the body, we avoided shapes with sharp edges, such as a box shape or a cube shape, due to their increased chance of being noticed by the wearer. Keeping the female target group in mind the bracelet was designed to have an organic and female shape (Fig. 9.1). In addition, we chose to make the bracelet purple, since that was a fashionable color for females that winter. Another design decision was to offer the paced breathing guidance by means of an array of LEDs, sequentially turning on and off.

Most other design decisions were directly related to the requirements of the electronics and sensors, such as its dimensions, weight, sensor contacts, processing means, communication means, and power supply.

Sensing Electronics

The sensor electronics of the Vitality Bracelet were designed and built in-house on the basis of an existing emotion sensing platform (Ouwerkerk 2011). Electronics from of the skin conductance module of the emotion sensing platform was combined with modules for paced breathing guidance on a single printed circuit board (See Fig. 9.2).

The skin conductance is sensed by a small (less than 1 μA) DC current from two electrodes placed on the inside of the wristband at the bottom of the wrist. A stable 1.2 V reference voltage source provides this current, which passes a reference resistor, a safety resistor, and the skin. The software can choose between a 330 kΩ and a 3.3 MΩ reference resistor to enable precise measurements over a

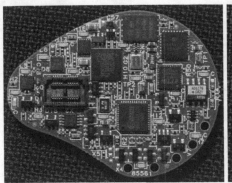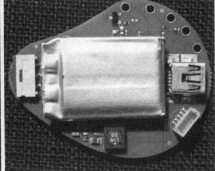

Fig. 9.2 Electronics module of the Vitality Bracelet

wide range of skin conductance. The voltage over the reference resistor is amplified 2.8-fold, and digitized by a 12 bit analog-to-digital converter. A stable 3.0 V voltage is as a reference for the analog-to-digital converter.

The analog noise level of the skin conductance sensor output was less than the least significant bit of the analog-to-digital converter. The skin conductance signal is stored in flash memory with 0.5 s intervals. When the wrist strap was fastened in a firm but comfortable manner little motion artifacts were present in the skin conductance data. Compared to the skin conductance sensor on the emotion sensing platform, the signal level was significantly higher due to the use of a water impermeable wristband material, which inhibited the evaporation of emotion induced sweat. The decay of the skin conductance peaks was therefore elongated up to about 30 min (as can be seen in Fig. 9.5), whereas it is only ~10 s for traditional skin conductance measurements at the palm of the hand (Boucsein 1992). This long decay causes the skin conductance level to rise to much higher levels in periods with a large number of skin conductance responses. Therefore such periods are easy to spot in a skin conductance graph.

In addition to the sensing electronics, also other components were added to the printed circuit board to support the paced breathing (and other) functionalities of the Vitality Bracelet. LEDs were needed for communication of the breathing guidance, for the time elapsed in exercise, and for a charger indication. A vibration motor allows discrete tactile stimulation, for instance when a mindfulness moment occurs. A means for connecting to a PC was provided for the offloading of stored data and the recharging of the battery.

Mindfulness Moments Algorithm

We intended to use the skin conductance sensors to measure, what we call, mindfulness moments. As outlined in De Waele et al. (2009), biosignal processing in daily life requires different approaches from the biomedical field. Our main

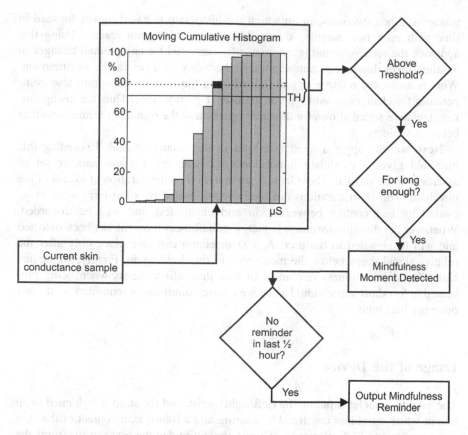

Fig. 9.3 Schematic overview of the algorithm for detecting mindfulness moments. The *black* mark indicates that the relative value of the current sample is 80 %

measurement modality, skin conductance, is not only influenced by the mental and bodily effects related to daily life stress, but also by a number of other factors such as temperature, air humidity, and movement. Hence, we used adaptive methods that provide robustness to these noise factors, yet retain the signal properties containing stress information. Figure 9.3 displays the outlines of our algorithm for the detection of mindfulness moments; the following provides a more detailed description.

The basis of our robust method for the detection of mindfulness moments is formed by a normalization procedure performed by referencing the current signal to a histogram of recent samples. This histogram takes into account the samples measured in a fixed timespan up to the current sample, but not the older samples outside the chosen timespan. Referencing the current sample against the histogram transforms the absolute signal into a relative signal that reflects signal values relative to measurements taken in the last period of time, e.g. indicating that the current sample ranks among the 35 % highest values measured in the last timespan. Since the timespan on which the histogram is based moves forward in time with each new sample, a so-called moving histogram results. Using this approach the relative signal is automatically corrected for any gradual changes in baseline level due to e.g. temperature or humidity changes in the environment. What is more, the relative signal derived from the moving histogram also compensates for changes in skin type of the user (e.g., dry skin). Thus the histogram-based relative signal allows for direct comparison of the signal over time as well as between subjects.

Next, we can apply a fixed threshold to this relative signal. Exceeding this threshold gives a candidate mindfulness moment and triggers another set of assertions to be verified. These include an assertion on the duration of excess of the threshold. Too short durations are likely to be caused by short-term noise (e.g., caused by bad contact between skin and electrodes) and will be discarded. Whenever the duration-assertion is met, a mindfulness moment has been detected and will be signaled to the user. A next detection can take place only after the relative signal drops below the measurement threshold again. Finally, we empirically found mindfulness reminders to lose their effectiveness when being presented in too short succession. Hence we restrict mindfulness reminders to at most once per half hour.

Usage of the Device

The vitality bracelet is put on the (left/right) wrist, and the strap is tightened to an extent which combines comfortable wearing and a robust skin contact of the skin conductance and ECG electrodes. During the entire day the bracelet measures the skin conductance at the bottom of the wrist, and stores the data in flash memory. The skin conductance signal is processed in real-time to generate mindfulness moments, and then a vibration motor causes a tactile stimulation (buzz).

A breathing guidance exercise can be started at any moment, and also when a mindfulness buzz has just occurred. The exercise is started (and stopped) with a dedicated button. The breathing guidance is presented through a number of LEDs visible on the top of the bracelet (Fig. 9.4). When the green lights spiral inwards, one is supposed to breathe in, and when then they spiral outwards, this is an indication that one has to breathe out. For the first 15 min of the exercise, the time spent so far is shown via a number of blue LEDs visible on the top of the bracelet (1 blue LED for each 3 min). The breathing guidance exercise offers a breathing pacer which in the first 5 min gradually slows down from 10 breaths per minute (bpm) at the start to 6 bpm for the remainder of the exercise.

At the end of the day the device can be connected to a PC for offloading of stored data and recharging of the battery.

Fig. 9.4 Final prototype of the vitality bracelet with all paced-breathing related LEDs turned on

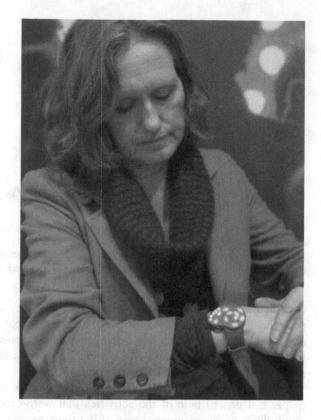

Physiological Measurements of the Vitality Bracelet

Figure 9.5 gives an example skin conductance measurement as done by the Vitality Bracelet over a time interval extending from early afternoon till late in the evening. On the vertical axis the data had a maximum value of roughly 10 μSiemens. At first sight, the shape of the peaks in the graph is reminiscent of the well-known skin conductance responses. However, it should not be forgotten that the present time scale is completely different from that encountered in traditional psychophysiological experiments. In fact, as already discussed before, the main variation observed in Fig. 9.5 stems from relatively slow variations in skin conductance, on which the traditional skin conductance responses (lasting only a certain number of seconds) are superimposed, and they appear as the 'noise' on the main curve.

In purple vertical lines in Fig. 9.5 we indicated the instances on which our mindfulness moments algorithm detected a sharp increase in arousal, and on which a warning buzz was given to the wearer. One can see that during this recording the thresholds were set to generate a relatively high number of buzzes. Most of these buzzes seem indeed to be related to (relatively) high peaks in the signal. It is also

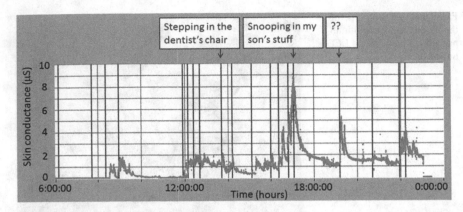

Fig. 9.5 Example skin conductance measurement by the Vitality Bracelet. In green the skin conductance signal as measured on one particular day. The *purple vertical lines* depict the 'mindfulness moments' as calculated by our algorithm and given by the buzzer. Some of the activities being carried out at the moment of a mindfulness buzz are indicated in boxes

clear that some candidate peaks are skipped since they appear too quickly after a peak that did get a buzz, for example the very first real peak of the trace. On the other hand, there are also a few buzzes that do not appear to be relevant, like the first three buzzes of the day, which were based on a histogram of a very small range of near-zero skin conductance values.

The person wearing the Vitality Bracelet during the recording in Fig. 9.5 made (paper and pencil) note of the activities that were carried out at the moment a mindfulness buzz was given. Some of the more emotional activities are indicated in Fig. 9.5, like stepping into the dentist's chair (the person claims to be afraid of the dentist), and snooping in their teenage son's stuff. Afterwards the person commented that it was very instructive to see the relative height of these two peaks, and deriving from it that the dentist was less stressful than the internal voice of conscience commenting on the objectionable snooping activity. With this in mind, the person became increasingly curious about the activity connected to the second highest peak, which had not been noticed or noted down (even though a mindfulness buzz was given). This curiosity underlines the usefulness of the skin conductance overview in 'getting to know oneself'.

Results of an Initial Experience Evaluation

With the Vitality Bracelet prototypes we set up a small experience evaluation involving 15 female participants. All were employees of Philips Research and signed a consent form. At the start of the experiment we held an intake session with each of the participants. They were told how to use the device and were given a short written manual. Especially two functions of the device were explained: the paced breathing guidance and the mindfulness buzzes. They were also advised to do a paced breathing exercise once per day for 15 min. A short questionnaire was administered probing their initial impression of the device. By way of measuring a lab baseline of their physiology, they then did a 15-min paced breathing exercise using the Vitality Bracelet for paced breathing guidance, preceded by an 8-min baseline of viewing a neutral movie while sitting still. During both periods their ECG and skin conductance were measured with a Nexus 10 device (MindMedia). The ECG was taken with electrodes in standard Lead II placement. The skin conductance electrodes were placed at the upper phalanxes of the index and ring fingers of the non-dominant hand. During the baseline, also their blood pressure was measured with an MH 901i digital blood pressure meter (Innovative Business Promotion). After the intake session the participants entered into a 3-week period of use, in which the experiment leader exchanged devices and improved or updated software when needed. After 3 weeks there was an outtake session, in which again physiological measurements were taken during baseline and paced breathing, in a similar way as in the intake session. In addition, there was an extensive interview, including a standardized questionnaire asking for their experience with the Vitality Bracelet and their suggestions for improvements. Participants were never shown data similar to that given in Fig. 9.5, although in the outtake interview they were asked whether they would have liked to see their measurement data.

Figure 9.6 presents the results of the physiology measurement during the intake sessions. For each minute of the baseline and paced breathing activities the average skin conductance was calculated separately and corrected for the average baseline level. It is seen to rise at the start of the paced breathing exercise, but then to decline during the activity in a similar way as during the baseline. The data thus indicate that though paced breathing is exciting to some extent in the beginning, during the exercise the SCL is decreasing to more or less the same extent as when sitting still and viewing a neutral movie, thus indicating relative relaxation. The ECG data were used to extract the inter beat intervals (IBIs) between heart beats, and from their spectral power density the heart rate variability was calculated, focusing on a high frequency (HF) component for 0.15–0.4 Hz and a low frequency (LF) component for 0.05–0.15 Hz separately. Again both components were corrected for the average value measured during baseline. While during baseline both components are low (Fig. 9.6), it is clear that paced breathing does change the heart rate variability as expected. There is a build-up of the HRV-LF component and a decline of the HRV-HF component over time, which is related to the gradual lowering of the frequency of the paced breathing guidance of the Vitality Bracelet from 10 bpm (0.16 Hz) at the very start to roughly 6 bpm (0.1 Hz) after a few minutes. As expected, similar results were found for the paced breathing exercise during the outtake session. It shows that as expected, low-frequency heart rate variability is exercised during a paced breathing session.

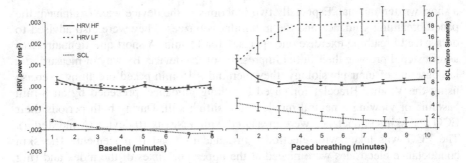

Fig. 9.6 Average skin conductance (*SCL*) and heart rate variability (*HRV*) as measured during the intake session. Both measurement during the baseline (*left*) and the paced breathing activity (*right*) are presented. Of the heart rate variability both the high frequency (*HF*) and low frequency (*LF*) components are presented, and the related vertical axis is presented on the *left*. For skin conductance the related vertical axis is presented on the *right*. All three parameters have been corrected for the average baseline value

As far as blood pressure is concerned, we found a significant difference in systolic blood pressure (SBP) measured between intake and outtake sessions: While the average SBP at intake was 123.9 mmHg, it had dropped to 119.7 mmHg at outtake ($p < 0.05$). This drop is in line with expectations, although it cannot be understood as proof for the benefit of paced breathing for lack of a control group in the evaluation.

From the interview and questionnaire at the intake session it became clear that the participants thought they understood the device, and that the majority could imagine a device like this could be beneficial to someone's vitality. On the down side, there was consensus that they did not like the design of the device, and they could not image wearing something like this all day. Instead, they would have liked a more jewel-like design, or something that would not attract attention at all. At the outtake interview, 50 % of the participants stated they could see themselves using a device like the Vitality Bracelet in the future. A majority (65 %) indicated they would find it appealing to see their body signs information presented in a clear way. While 20 % found the mindfulness buzzes annoying, 57 % found them useful, mainly as a way to bring awareness. However, for none of the participants did the mindfulness buzzes guide the start of the paced breathing exercises. Instead, the participants initiated the paced breathings exercises at a convenient moment, usually in the evening at home (83 %), and mostly once per day as advised (57 %), but never more often. Half of the participants indicated it was easy to follow the guiding breathing rhythm, whereas the others were equally divided between finding it too slow or too fast. A big majority (77 %) agreed that 15 min of paced breathing exercise was too long. In addition, many (43 %) indicated they would have liked a breathing guidance that would allow them to follow the rhythm with their eyes closed.

Discussion and Conclusion

We described the design, development and initial evaluation of the Vitality Bracelet, a wearable device that intends to help you manage the balance between stress and relaxation. The device consists of a measurement part (skin conductance) and an actionable part (paced breathing) and we'll discuss both separately.

The measurement component of the Vitality bracelet samples skin conductance unobtrusively and on a continuous basis in real life. In this respect it is similar to Affectiva's Q-sensor (Picard 2011). We have shown example data (Fig. 9.5) that demonstrate how such skin conductance traces can help individuals to gain more awareness of their stressful and relaxed moments. Indeed, our evaluation study participants generally found it appealing to see their body signs presented in an informative manner. Also the mindfulness buzzes were considered to bring awareness, even though it is obvious that not all of them are spot-on. Maybe a high accuracy is not that critical, as long as really stressful moments do get identified. We should be clear, though, that we have not been able to explore whether such awareness-bringing information will indeed help a user to decide and try to make changes to the daily activities underlying it.

The actionable component of the Vitality Bracelet involved paced breathing guidance. Measurements in the intake session showed that indeed a paced breathing exercise does bring relaxation (reducing SCL). Additionally, paced breathing brings enhanced heart rate variability (HRV), which is usually interpreted as a sign of activity of the parasympathic nervous system (Chapleau and Sabharwal 2011), again indicating relaxation. Both thus suggest that paced breathing is a good exercise to do when one wants to calm down at a stressful moment. However, it appeared that none of our participants ever started a paced breathing exercise after a mindfulness buzz had made them aware of heightened tension. Apparently the routine of daily activities is not easily interrupted on the fly and often people prefer to finish the tasks they have set out to do. It is known that it is difficult to adhere to a regime of 15 min of paced breathing per day (Janaki-ramaiah et al. 2000), and we find the same. The fact that none of our participants ever started a paced breathing exercise in reaction to a mindfulness buzz also suggests that the mindfulness buzz is not instrumental in enhancing adherence in a direct way. Possibly however, the mindfulness buzz does help in an indirect way through bringing awareness of the many stressful moments in a day. Indeed, our participants preferred to do their paced breathing exercise at the end of the day, but even for the short evaluation period of 3 weeks, not all of them found the motivation to spend a daily 15 min. Thus, the link between the measurement (mindfulness buzz) and actionable (paced breathing) components in the Vitality Bracelet apparently is not strong enough to motivate full paced breathing adherence. Maybe if the users are given a clear presentation of their measurement data, like they indicated they were interested in, for instance as done in the Affective Health system (Kosmack Vaara et al. 2009) this would bring enhanced awareness, and through that increased adherence to the paced breathing exercise schedule.

All in all, we conclude that with the Vitality Bracelet we have presented a concept that is appealing and functional in bringing awareness about the stressful and relaxing moments in our daily routines. And this awareness could help users to maintain a good balance between them. In addition, the paced breathing exercises are instantly beneficial for relaxation. It still remains unclear to what extent the enhanced awareness of stressors in one's life is instrumental in motivating the beneficial daily 15 min of paced breathing.

Acknowledgement We would like to thank David Browning for the inspiration and support of this work.

References

APA, American Psychological Association (2010) Stress in America findings. Available via http://www.stressinamerica.org

Boucsein W (1992) Electrodermal activity, 1st edn. Plenum Press, NewYork

Chapleau MW, Sabharwal R (2011) Methods of assessing vagus nerve activity and reflexes. Heart Fail Rev 16:109–127

China Daily (2010) Entrepreneurs experience heavy work stress study

Clark M, Hirschman R (1990) Effects of paced respiration on anxiety reduction in a clinical population. Biofeedback Self Regul 15:273–284

De Waele S, De Vries G-J, Jäger M (2009) Experiences with adaptive statistical models for biosignals in daily life. In: Proceedings of the international conference on affective computing and intelligent interaction, vol 1. (pp 710–715)

Dunn BD, Dalgleish T, Ogilvie AD, Lawrence AD (2007) Heartbeat perception in depression. Behav Res Ther 45:1921–1930

Grossman E, Grossman A, Schein MH, Zimlichman R, Gavish B (2001) Breathing-control lowers blood pressure. J Hum Hypertens 15(4):263–269

Janakiramaiah N, Gangadhar BN, Naga Venkatesha Murthy PJ, et al (2000) Antidepressant efficacy of Sudarshan Kriya Yoga (SKY) in melancholia: A randomized comparison with electroconvulsive therapy (ECT) and imipramine. J Affect Disord 57:255–259

Kabat-Zinn J (2003) Mindfulness-based interventions in context: past, present, and future. Clin Psychol Sci Pract 10:144–156. doi:10.1093/clipsy.bpg016

Kosmack Vaara E, Höök K, Tholander J (2009) Mirroring bodily experiences over time. In: Proceedings CHI EA'09 CHI'09 extended abstracts on human factors in computing systems, pp 4471–4476, ACM New York, NY, USA ©2009, ISBN: 978-1-60558-247-4

Lehrer PM, Vaschillo E, Vaschillo B (2000) Resonant frequency biofeedback training to increase cardiac variability: rationale and manual for training. Appl Psychophysiol Biofeedback 25(3):177–191

McEwen BS (1998) Stress, adaptation, and disease: allostasis and allostatic load. Ann N Y Acad Sci 840:33–44. doi:10.1111/j.1749-6632.1998.tb09546.x

Ouwerkerk M (2011) Unobtrusive emotions sensing in daily life. In: Westerink J, Krans M, Ouwerkerk M (eds) Sensing emotions—the impact of context on experience measurements, Philips Resarch Book Series vol 12. Springer, Heidelberg, p 21–40

Parati G, Malfatto G, Boarin S, Branzi G, Caldara G, Giglio A, Bilo G, Ongaro G, Alter A, Gavish B, Mancia G (2008) Device-guided paced breathing in the home setting: effects on exercise capacity, pulmonary and ventricular function in patients with chronic heart failure: a pilot study. Circ Heart Fail 1(3):178–183

Picard RW (2011) Measuring affect in the wild. In: Proceedings of the 4th international conference on affective computing and intelligent interaction ACII'11–volume Part I. Springer, Heidelberg, p 3-3, ISBN: 978-3-642-24599-2

Porges SW (2007) The polyvagal perspective. Biol Psychol 74:116–143

Rouse CH, Jones GE, Jones KR (1988) The effect of body composition and gender on cardiac awareness. Psychophysiology 25(4):400–407

Westerink J, Ouwerkerk M, De Vries GJ, De Waele S, Van den Eerenbeemd J, Van Boven M (2009) Emotion measurement platform for daily life situations. In: Proceedings 2009 international conference on affective computing and intelligent interaction, ACII 2009, Sep10–12, 2009, vol 1. Amsterdam, The Netherlands, pp 217–222

Chapter 10
Capturing Human Digital Memories for Assisting Memory Recall

Chelsea Dobbins, Madjid Merabti, Paul Fergus
and David Llewellyn-Jones

Abstract As the life expectancy of adults is increasing, so is the occurrence of illness, disability and the demand on hospitals. The probability of becoming cognitively impaired increases with age, with one side effect of increasing life expectancy being the emerging number of dementia patients. In order to enable people to live more independently the use of digital technologies, as an artificial memory aid, is gaining momentum. The area of Human Digital Memories (HDMs) provides such an outlet where users can interact with their data, with the use of visual lifelogs, which can help sufferers relive life experiences. Computing devices are, nowadays, capable of storing a lifetime's worth of data and capturing our every move, interactions and physiological signals. As a result of living in such a data-rich society, a greater number of data sources are available, which can be incorporated into building more vivid HDMs. This chapter explores the area of human digital memories. More specifically, focusing on wearable systems and physiological devices, the methods that are used to capture human digital memory data are presented. Once it has been established how data can be collected, a more in-depth look at how digital memories are created is also explored. The chapter is then concluded with a summary of the key challenges of the area.

Introduction

The turn of the twenty-first century has seen a fundamental advancement in technology. Computing devices are, nowadays, capable of storing a lifetime's worth of data and capturing our every move, interactions and physiological signals. We are now living in a data rich society, where the ability to generate and

C. Dobbins (✉) · M. Merabti · P. Fergus · D. Llewellyn-Jones
School of Computing and Mathematical Sciences, Liverpool John Moores University,
Byrom Street, Liverpool L3 3AF, UK
e-mail: C.M.Dobbins@ljmu.ac.uk

S. H. Fairclough and K. Gilleade (eds.), *Advances in Physiological Computing*,
Human–Computer Interaction Series, DOI: 10.1007/978-1-4471-6392-3_10,
© Springer-Verlag London 2014

access a number of different data sources is feasible. Any object, embedded with a sensor, is capable of providing us with information. This phenomenon is known as pervasive computing and can be defined as the, *"Integration of computing power (micro-processors) and sensing (sensors) into anything, including not only traditional computers, personal digital assistants (PDAs), printers,* etc. *but also everyday objects like white goods, toys, houses, furniture, or even paint ("smart dust")"* (Korhonen and Bardram 2004). These machines now fit seamlessly into our world, instead of forcing users to enter their environment, a concept first envisioned by Weiser (1999). As these devices become more prevalent, people are developing a greater interest in enhancing their knowledge about their bodies, and in becoming more involved in self-management (Cruickshank et al. 2013). Over a lifetime, people will interact with many devices and applications, which produce a lot of information (Lee et al. 2010). An entire lifetime can be reconstructed from these collected digital artefacts. However, with all of this data readily available, harnessing it into an accurate description of a person's life, which can be used to enhance the user's wellbeing, is a significant challenge.

As the life expectancy of adults is increasing, so is the occurrence of illness, disability and the demand on hospitals (Office for National Statistics 2010). Since the probability of becoming cognitively impaired increases with age (roughly 10 % of over 65 years old), one side-effect of increasing life expectancy is the emerging number of dementia patients (Huang et al. 2012). Dementia is a progressive and irreversible chronic disease, with varying degrees of stages (early, middle and late), that causes a mental deterioration, thus affecting the brain (Davies et al. 2009). People with dementia face a decline of their cognitive functions, including memory impairment, difficulties performing familiar tasks and diminished judgement (Vogt et al. 2012). It is a syndrome with different causes, of which Alzheimer's disease (AD) is the most common type (Vogt et al. 2012). Worldwide, there is a new case of dementia every 7 s (Alzheimer's Research UK 2012). Currently, there are over 820,000 people living with dementia in the UK today and more than 35 million people worldwide (Alzheimer's Research UK 2012). The financial impact on the economy is also quite severe. Dementia costs the UK £23 billion per year, which is twice that of cancer, three times the impact of heart disease and four times that of strokes (Alzheimer's Research UK 2012). As a result, there is a very strong need to support ambient assistive living technologies, which promotes independent living, in the home (Lee et al. 2011a). The strain placed on these health resources is apparent, and clearly, a user-centric approach is needed. As such, the area of dementia has been identified as one which would benefit from the introduction of innovative technological solutions (Davies et al. 2009).

The area of Human Digital Memories (HDMs) is seen as a way to address these issues. Persons with dementia often rely on external memory aids, such as calendars, diaries, alarms, whiteboards, notebooks, and timers, to help them compensate for their memory deficits and to maintain an account of their daily life (Kikhia et al. 2010). As such, the platform of HDMs enables a digital record of our lives to be recorded by allowing us to capture, from a variety of data sources, rich information about the surrounding environment and ourselves, which can be viewed at a later time. The practice of obtaining this information is known as 'lifelogging' and refers to the process of automatically recording aspects of one's life in digital form (Doherty et al. 2011a). HDMs are the result of lifelogging and, as defined by Kelly (Kelly 2007), are *"A combination of many types of media, audio, video, images, and many texts of textual content"*. They are a digital representation of ourselves that evolve and grow alongside us and are seen as a window into our past. Such an interest has been gained from people wanting to store, search and interpret their HDMs that this has led to *"Memories for Life: Managing Information over a Human Lifetime"* being declared a grand challenge in computing research (Fitzgibbon and Reiter 2005). These vast digital archives of one's personal life experiences are constructed from a wide range of data sources, across various media types (Kelly and Jones 2007; Gurrin et al. 2008). For example, content recorded from someone's life might include all documents read, written, and downloaded; photographs taken; videos seen; music listened to; details of places visited; details of people met etc. (Kelly and Jones 2007).

Taking this concept further, the inclusion of physiological data enables another dimension of ourselves that can be included in these digital records. This is reiterated by Gilleade and Fairclough (2010) who states, *"Quantifying how we change over time is a powerful tool, for it allows us to better understand the impact of events and our behavior on our psychological and physiological wellbeing"*. The development of smaller sensing devices and wireless communications is revolutionising the way in which this data can be obtained, ubiquitously (Pantelopoulos and Bourbakis 2010b). However, these devices are primarily used within wearable health-monitoring systems (WHMS). As Pantelopoulos and Bourbakis (2010a) observe, *"These systems represent the new generation of healthcare by providing real-time, unobtrusive, monitoring of patients' physiological parameters, through the deployment of several on-body and even intra-body biosensors"*. As well as monitoring our health and wellbeing, the data generated from WHMS can also be used to enhance a HDM, by providing us with physiological data, which can be reasoned upon. The evolution in short-range communication technology, such as ultra-wideband radio technology (Hirt 2003), Bluetooth (Haartsen 1998) and ZigBee (Wang and Wang 2010) have allowed these systems to become more sophisticated (Bonato 2010). WHMS, composed of a number of different sensors, can measure a variety of parameters, including electrocardiogram (ECG), blood pressure, respiration, body and/or skin temperature etc. (Pantelopoulos and Bourbakis 2010b). Incorporating this multitude of data, into a HDM, allows memories to become more dynamic and personal to the user and enables a richer understanding about ourselves to emerge.

This chapter explores the area of HDMs. More specifically, focusing on wearable systems and physiological devices, the methods that are used to capture HDM data are presented. Once it has been established how data can be collected, a more in-depth look at how digital memories are created is also explored. The chapter is then concluded with a summary of the key challenges of the area.

Background

Memories shape our existence, influence every aspect of our lives and link our past with our future. Remembering the past helps people to re-examine their lives, recalling previous activities and accomplishments, and seek personal validation (Kikhia et al. 2010). Supporting our memory, through cave paintings, storytelling, books and personal diaries, has been done for thousands of years and has been a way to preserve memories over a lifetime (Doherty 2005). However, losing the ability to recollect memories is not only disadvantageous, but can prove quite detrimental, particularly to many older people (McCarthy et al. 2007). As such, retaining every aspect of our lives, for example, how we felt or what we did on a specific day is virtually impossible, especially if we are recollecting events from 10 years ago. As people get older, the ability to remember this information declines (Prull et al. 2006). However, recent advances in technology can alleviate this problem, to a certain extent. Devices are now capable of capturing an enormous amount of personal information. This has led to people creating extensive digital collections and reflection of those items has become an active part of people's lives (Kalnikaitė and Whittaker 2011).

Capturing Human Digital Memory Data

Research into capturing and creating HDMs has received a great deal of attention, from researchers, over the last few decades. The idea was first proposed in 1945 by Vannevar Bush who foresaw this challenge and invented the *Memex*, a *"device in which an individual stores all his books, records, and communications, and which is mechanized so that it may be consulted with exceeding speed and flexibility. It is an enlarged intimate supplement to his memory"* (Bush 1945). Since the *Memex* (Bush 1945) in 1945, research into how aspects of our lives can be captured and organised, have been investigated. Over time, this vision of storing accumulated items has evolved into digitally capturing information about our environment and ourselves. The culmination of this practise has been to continually capture content, with the aid of wearable systems (lifelogging). Since the 1980s, Steve Mann has been the pioneer of such systems (Doherty et al. 2011a). Mann's *EyeTap* device (Mann 1997, 2004; Mann et al. 2005) has evolved over the last 30 years, and, with the progression of smaller components, has *"become more feasible for commercialisation and mass production"* (Mann 2004). The system consists of eyeglasses, with a camera, display and diverter, and enables precise lifetime personal experiences to be captured (Mann et al. 2005).

Mann paved the way for wearable lifelogging systems. Many other projects have taken this vision further, to produce their own implementations. For instance, Healey and Picard's (Healey and Picard 1998) *StartleCam*, uses a wearable camera and a skin conductivity sensor (GSR) to *"Capture events that are likely to get the user's attention and to be remembered"*. Whilst, Dickie et al. (2004a) *eyeBlog* consists of *ECSGlasses*, which are a pair of glasses augmented with a wireless eye contact and glyph sensing camera, and a web application that visualizes the video from the camera as chronologically delineated blog entries (Dickie et al. 2004a, b). The device captures video streams based on eye contact with the user.

A revolutionary device, which has dominated the area of lifelogging, in the last few years, has been Microsoft's *SenseCam* (Hodges et al. 2006)—a small wearable digital camera, with built-in sensors, that is designed to take photographs automatically, without user intervention (Hodges et al. 2006). Between May 06–Dec 08, this device has been worn continuously, by Cathal Gurrin (Doherty et al. 2009; Gurrin 2012). During this time, he recorded 2,579,455 images (3,080/ day) = 29,301 events (35/day). The device was worn for an average duration of 14 h 22 min per day and managed to capture 846 days (90.2 %) worth of information; 92 days had missing data (9.8 %) due to missing sensor files (Doherty et al. 2009).

These technical developments have opened the possibility for users to passively capture and store comprehensive representations of their personal experiences (Crete-Nishihata et al. 2012). Continuous lifelogging is slowly becoming socially acceptable and, as Mann et al. (2005) observes, *"Recent prototypes have been gaining acceptance in social situations. This can be attributed partly to miniaturized smaller units, but also to dramatic changes in the attitude toward personal electronics"*. As these devices become smaller, lifelogging will only increase.

Wearable Lifelogging Systems

Microsoft's *SenseCam* (Hodges et al. 2006), as stated above, is a revolutionary lifelogging device, which is capable of storing up to 30,000 images, in total (Hodges et al. 2006). By default, photos are captured and stored every 30 s, usually resulting in 1,500–2,500 photos per day (Lee et al. 2008). The device contains a digital camera, with a fisheye lens, and multiple sensors, including sensors to detect changes in light levels and a passive infrared sensor to detect the presence of people (Hodges et al. 2006). A log file also gets created that records the data from the sensors every few seconds and the reason for taking each photograph (e.g., manual shutter press, timed capture, or significant change in sensor readings) (Hodges et al. 2011). Each day, the photos can be uploaded, via Universal Serial Bus (USB), onto a computer (Hodges et al. 2011) and viewed using Microsoft's simple viewer application (Microsoft Research 2011).

Since 2010, over 50 research institutions and labs worldwide have used the *SenseCam* in their research (Hodges et al. 2011). The device was originally developed as a retrospective memory aid (Hodges et al. 2006) and various studies have used it as a memory aid device and to monitor behaviour (Sellen et al. 2007; Berry et al. 2007; Lee et al. 2008; Byrne and Jones 2008; Hallberg and Kikhia 2009; Kikhia et al. 2009, 2010; Davies et al. 2009; Lindley et al. 2009; Kalnikaite et al. 2010; Piasek et al. 2011; Kelly et al. 2011, 2012; De Leo et al. 2011; Karaman et al. 2011;

Qiu et al. 2011; Doherty et al. 2011a, b; Brindley et al. 2011; Browne et al. 2011; Hodges et al. 2011; Pauly-Takacs et al. 2011; Crete-Nishihata et al. 2012; Huang et al. 2012; Wang and Smeaton 2013). In particular, the results from (Hodges et al. 2006, 2011; Berry et al. 2007) illustrate that *"Through the use of SenseCam, a markedly amnesic patient was consistently able to remember aspects of several events. Recall was maintained almost a year after some of the events took place, and without any review of those events for up to 3 months"* (Hodges et al. 2006). Furthermore, the patient reported that *"Seeing the beginning of a clip brought memories "flooding back" without necessarily having to view further images"* (Berry et al. 2007). This suggests that she was remembering the event itself rather than the images, which was confirmed by her husband, who said that his wife was able to recall details of events not contained in the images (Berry et al. 2007). It also suggests that the visual images themselves provided a potent cue to recall (Berry et al. 2007).

Furthermore, Browne et al. (2011) study further highlights its effectiveness as a memory aid tool. In this investigation, the *SenseCam* was used to generate images for rehearsal, promoting consolidation and retrieval of memories for significant events in a patient with memory retrieval deficits (Browne et al. 2011). The results indicated that regularly reviewing the *SenseCam* images resulted in superior recall of recent events, compared to reviewing a written diary, and this effect was maintained in the long term (Browne et al. 2011). This study also supports Crete-Nishihata et al. (2012) work that used the device with patients that had Alzheimer's or mild cognitive impairment. The results, from this work, suggest that reviewing *SenseCam* images, of personal events, can support episodic recollection of the experiences over time (Crete-Nishihata et al. 2012). Whether it's used for private reflection or as a memory-aid device repeated viewings of *SenseCam* images play an important role in the long-term retention of personally experienced events (Pauly-Takacs et al. 2011).

Whilst the technologies and methods discussed are a useful starting point, within the area of lifelogging, novel solutions are needed that include much richer data capturing capabilities and require a less obtrusive and expensive, approach. Whilst the *SenseCam* has produced exciting results, for the use of lifelogs in aiding autobiographical memory, there are limitations. As reported in (Berry et al. 2007), the time taken to upload, access and combine particular image segments is cumbersome. *SenseCam* images have to be downloaded periodically, which can be very time-consuming and mundane for the user. Furthermore, the absence of sound information and that the viewing software runs on a standard desktop or laptop PC, which may be unfamiliar or anxiety-provoking for some people, have also been identified as further limitations (Berry et al. 2007). Another drawback is that the data that is captured is limited, as only photos and a very small amount of sensor data are recorded. Whilst photos are a good place to start, memories are made up of so much more than that. Factors such as temperature, location and physiological readings, to name but a few, also contribute to the composition of memories. These important features need to be considered when creating an accurate HDM. The device is also expensive, which limits its availability. Exploiting the services of devices, already present within our environment, is a far less expensive approach.

In addition to capturing photos, physiological devices can also record a range of information about ourselves, and coupled with other collected data items, can offer a way to see how we were feeling at any point in our lives. Utilizing the information that these devices provide adds another dimension to our HDMs. These devices are capable of providing us with a range of information, as we shall see in the next section.

Physiological Devices

In terms of obtaining other types of, more personal, information sensor-based systems are emerging as a new way to capture our every move and to monitor our health and wellbeing. The development of smaller sensing devices, and wireless communications, is revolutionising the way in which a subject can be ubiquitously observed (Pantelopoulos and Bourbakis 2010b). These devices offer a new generation of inexpensive, unobtrusive wearable/implanted devices (Pantelopoulos and Bourbakis 2010a), which are capable of capturing content over a lifetime. As well as monitoring the wellbeing of the wearer, this data can also be used to enhance HDMs. These systems provide highly personalized data and are another source of information, which can be reasoned upon. In order to add more depth and detail to HDMs incorporating this technology is essential.

One such system is Lee et al. (2011b) real-time single tri-axial accelerometer-based personal life log (PLL) system. The system is capable of recognizing human activity and generating exercise information. It recognizes the occurrence of activities, based on the statistical and spectral features of the accelerometer signals. Once an activity is recognized the system further estimates exercise information that includes energy expenditure based on metabolic equivalents, stride length, step count, walking distance, and walking speed (Lee et al. 2011b). The system has been tested against six daily activities (lying, standing, walking, going-upstairs, going-downstairs, and driving), via subject-independent and subject-dependent recognition, on a total of twenty subjects, achieving an average recognition accuracy of 94.43 and 96.61 %, respectively (Lee et al. 2011b). This study is quite interesting due to the level of accuracy that has been achieved. The study uses voice annotation as a method to ascertain the subject's true activities (Lee et al. 2011b). However, as a method of determining the subject's true activities the use of visual diaries would have provided a better depiction of such times. These items would have been more useful to help validate the classifiers accuracy, rather than vocal descriptions. Furthermore, the collection of this data can occur automatically, through the use of a wearable camera, which is more convenient for the user.

Wearable systems (Paradiso et al. 2005; Pacelli et al. 2006; Langereis et al. 2007; Matthews et al. 2007; Pandian et al. 2008; Figueiredo et al. 2010; Coyle et al. 2010; Curone et al. 2010; Pantelopoulos and Bourbakis 2010a; López et al. 2010; Taraldsen et al. 2011) have also been designed to measure a user's biological signals. One such approach has been Matthews et al. (2007) "*Physiological Sensor Suite (PSS)*", which gathers electrocardiogram (ECG), electromyogram (EMG), electrooculogram (EOG) and through-hair electroencephalogram (EEG) data. The information is then communicated, wirelessly, to a data logger, which the user is wearing. In terms of gathering information, this suite is particularly interesting because the sensors are quite small and *"no modification of the skin's outer layer is required"* (Matthews et al. 2007). In other words, the user does not have to prepare their skin with special gel (as is common practise amongst other systems). In other works, the *BIOTEX* project (Coyle et al. 2010) consists of a textile-based system that collects and analyses sweat, by using a textile-based sensor capable of performing chemical measurements. The system monitors a number of physiological parameters, together with sweat composition, in real-time (Coyle et al. 2010). This work is interesting because the components are quite small; a 1×3 cm piece of superabsorbent (Absorbtex) has been used to collect the sweat. Furthermore, monitoring a number of physiological parameters together with sweat composition in real time is beneficial. For example, in the case of athletes who partake in endurance sports, analysis of sweat can give information on hydration levels (Coyle et al. 2010). However, since the system has been designed to analyse sweat, the analysis of non-strenuous physiological signals, e.g. sitting or lying down would not be possible. Therefore monitoring is limited to specific activities and would be unsuitable for daily activity data collection.

Whilst these systems can gather a range of information they are quite cumbersome to wear for a lengthy period of time. Integrating sensors into everyday clothing, using *"smart fabrics and interactive textiles (SFIT)"* (Lymberis and Paradiso 2008), is a more practical solution. Sensors don't have to be placed on the body by a professional; therefore, the user can be monitored at any time (Lymberis and Paradiso 2008). One such approach, in this area, has been López et al. (2010) *LOBIN* project. A combination of e-textile and wireless sensor networks have been used to provide an efficient way to support non-invasive and pervasive services (López et al. 2010). The system consists of a set of *"smart shirts"* that monitor heart rate, angle of inclination, activity index, and body temperature and a location tracking system, which monitors the patient's location (López et al. 2010). The information is then sent to the management subsystem, which processes and stores the data. This system is quite interesting due to the parameters that can be measured and the location system, particularly as patients are tracked indoors.

As it can be seen, many signals can be captured from the user. However, these methods are used in very separate fields and have rarely been combined. In order to form a more rounded snapshot of our lives these technologies need to work together. So that not only can a visual representation of experiences be recapped, but also the feelings and changes our bodies were experiencing when those events were occurring. A significant drawback is the ambiguity of physiological data, which can require extensive data analysis. However, by incorporating even more data, for instance, from smart objects and our environment, this ambiguity could be reduced. For example, a higher heart rate, than normal, and an increase in sweat production could be attributed to many things. Presenting only this information, as a memory, is insufficient. However, if it was known that it was a hot day, by incorporating a temperature reading and that a photo of the user doing physical activity was also obtained, then the context of the physiological data is known. Bringing together data, from separate sources, enables a finer level of detail to be achieved, as the range of accessible information is increased. In order to integrate this data into HDMs, advanced solutions are needed.

Organising Human Digital Memory Data

Capturing HDM data can be an easy and enjoyable activity. Nevertheless, searching and organising this information can take a considerable amount of time and is a task that is often neglected by the user. If data is not structured correctly, the risk of it becoming useless and unmanageable is greater. Whittaker et al. (2009) study on people's ability to retrieve photos, which were over a year old, reinforces the idea that without proper structure, data can be inaccessible. The study concluded that for many people, the ability to collect more digital information is not matched by a similar ability to organize and maintain such information (Whittaker et al. 2009). However, HDMs are not limited to photographs. The data sources that we have access to are increasing; therefore, lifelogs will not only be composed of photos but of a variety of assorted data, with physiological information being a particularly powerful source of information. This is reiterated by Teraoka (2011) who states, *"Interactive visual interfaces are essential for exploring heterogeneous data"*. It is important to structure this data into events, as this is how episodic memory functions, within our own mind (Tulving 1984, 1993). This is echoed by Doherty and Smeaton (Doherty and Smeaton 2010), who state, *"While there are many technologies, which can be used to generate lifelogs, perhaps the most important of the key dimensions for accessing lifelogs, is to structure our lives into events or happenings, corresponding to the happenings which occur in our lives"*. However, as the data within lifelogs increases, this remains a significant challenge.

Organizing Photographic Data

The use of timelines to organise visual data is not a new concept and has been the subject of many projects. Microsoft's *MyLifeBits* (Gemmell et al. 2002, 2004) is a *"system for storing a lifetime's worth of media, with a database at its heart"* and is seen as a 21st century interpretation of Bush's original *Memex* idea (Bush 1945). This system addresses a user's need to store all of their personal files more easily, as well as having effortless access to them. Sensor readings are displayed in a time series graph, with black dots situated on the graph line, which indicates that a picture has been taken at that time (Gemmell et al. 2004). *SenseCam* data is displayed based on time and text searches that have been performed (Gemmell et al. 2002). Fuller et al. (2008) argue that this is the best way to remember content, *"Standard forms of context data, such as time, date, number of accesses, etc. have proven beneficial in retrieval from various collections"*. Doherty et al. (2011b) also utilize the timeline concept in their *SenseCam browser* and structure the information as "events". They have created a technique *"to automatically structure and organise SenseCam data and later facilitate quick retrieval of desired events with a lower cognitive load on the user, through returning them fewer candidate events that are more relevant to the information they seek"* (Doherty et al. 2011b). Lee et al. (2008) also use the *SenseCam* to capture the user's daily routine and present the images in a timeline format, similar to the approach used in Microsoft's *MyLifeBits* (Gemmell et al. 2002) project.

Using timelines has become a very popular way to organize file systems. Picault et al. (2010) also present some interesting ideas on how to structure and arrange a user's personal information so that it is easily accessible and can be more effectively retrieved. Their work focuses on structuring data into a timeline format, as *"recalling a piece of information is easier when the user can remind themselves about events in time and space"* (Picault et al. 2010). In similar work, Gozali et al. (Gozali et al. 2012) have *"developed a photo browser called Chapters that helps users organize their event photos by automatically grouping photos in each event into smaller groups of photos"*. Using *Chapters*, they conducted an exploratory study involving 23 college students, with a total of 8,096 personal photos, from 92 events. This study was conducted in order to understand how different spatial organization strategies were used in performing storytelling, photo search and photo set interpretation tasks (Gozali et al. 2012). The results indicated that subjects valued the chronological order of the chapter's more than maximizing screen space usage, and that they valued chapter consistency more than the chronological order of the photos (Gozali et al. 2012).

The Centre for Digital Video Processing (DCU 2011) has also done extensive work in relation to searching lifelogs and creating systems to organise HDM data (O'Hare et al. 2006; Lalanne and van den Hoven 2007; Kelly 2007; Kelly and Jones 2007, 2009; Chen and J.F. Jones 2008; Lee et al. 2008; Byrne and Jones 2008, 2009; Chen and Jones 2009; O'Hare and Smeaton 2009; Chen and Jones 2010; Qiu et al. 2011; Wang and Smeaton 2012, 2013). In one such project, *MediAssist* (O'Hare et al. 2006), personal digital photo collections are organised based on *contextual information, such as time* and location. This information is then combined with content–based analysis such as face detection and other feature detectors. Time-based queries, corresponding to the users partial recall of the temporal context of a photo-capturing event, for example, all photos taken in the evening, at the weekend, during the summer, can be used to search the data (O'Hare et al. 2006). A timeline format is also used to display the information and semi-automatic annotation of the data is another feature that is possible. Meanwhile, the centre's *iCLIPS* project (Chen and Jones 2010) uses *SenseCam* data to index every computer activity and *SenseCam* image with time stamps and context data, including location, people, and weather. It then enables these files to be searched by textual content and the context data, such as location, people present, weather conditions and date/time (Chen and Jones 2010). The retrieved data is also presented in a timeline fashion.

Organizing Physiological Data

Whilst a timeline approach may be appropriate to organize photographic data, HDMs are composed of much more data than this. The inclusion of physiological data enables us to capture and understand ourselves in a more detailed manner. As stated by Fairclough (Fairclough 2009), *"Physiological computing has the potential to provide a new paradigm for human-computer interaction (HCI) by allowing a computer system to develop and access a dynamic representation of the cognitions, emotions and motivation of the user"*. This data is inherently personal to each individual and enables deeper reflection to occur, as we can see how our bodies react to certain situations/environments. However, it has been argued that the 'intelligence' exhibited by a physiological computing system is directly related to how the representation of the user is translated into an adaptive output (Fairclough 2009). This is a significant challenge, with recent developments, within the field, having attempted to address this issue.

One such approach is the *Affective Diary* (Lindström et al. 2006; Ståhl et al. 2009) system, which is a digital diary where *"users can scribble their notes, but that also allows for bodily memorabilia to be recorded from body sensors"* (Ståhl et al. 2009). The system uses colour and body postures to convey different levels of arousal and has been used to explore the emotional aspect to creating diaries and is designed to support self-reflection (Lindström et al. 2006; Machajdik et al. 2011). In terms of displaying physiological data in this manner Lindstrom et al. (2006) states, *"The experience of using these sensors showed that there is a real risk of creating a disembodied experience based on these data if represented using graphs. The body starts to live a life of its own, in a sense separated from our experiences of what was really going on…. Thus, moving away from those graph-like diagrammatic representations to the body postures and colours discussed above is seen to encourage a more holistic experience"*. Taking a similar approach, the *Body Blogger* also uses colour to illustrate the user's mood (Fairclough and Gilleade 2013). Heart rate data is periodically collected and, depending on the rate of beats per minute (bpm), is mapped to a mood colour on their website's interface (Fairclough and Gilleade 2013). For example, when the user's heart rate is low (<60 bpm) the website turns blue to indicate that the user is relaxed. This is an interesting approach; however, the context of those times is unknown, which is one of the main issues of representing physiological data for memory recall. For example a high heart rate can be attributed to many things, such as physical exercise or being frightened. Simply presenting this physiological data to the user doesn't provide enough detail into the circumstances surrounding that particular time. In terms of memory recall, a great level of associated data is required so that the user can see exactly where they were and what was occurring.

In other works, *AffectAura* (McDuff et al. 2012) is *"an emotional prosthetic that allows users to reflect on their emotional states over long periods of time"*. This system has been designed as a technology probe to explore the potential reflective power that might be offered by pairing affective data with knowledge of workers' information and data interaction artefacts (McDuff et al. 2012). Data is collected from a variety of devices, including a webcam, Kinect and microphone. Supervised machine learning was then used to develop an affect recognition engine, based on the sensed data. The data is displayed in a timeline format, which captured the ebb and flow of affects, represented by a series of bubbles (McDuff et al. 2012). The study was run over 4 days, using six participants. The results indicated that users were able to leverage cues from *AffectAura* to construct stories about their days, even after they had forgotten these particular incidents or their related emotional tones (McDuff et al. 2012). In terms of correctly classifying emotional states, an overall accuracy of 68 % across the states of valence (negative, neutral, positive), arousal (low, high) and engagement (low, high) was achieved (McDuff et al. 2012). This system is interesting, due to its focus on the emotional state of the user.

Taking an opposing approach, Harle et al. (2011) implementation uses an on-body sensor system for sprint training sessions. Sensors placed in the runner's shoes measured the application of force on the ground, whilst an on-body sensor node is used to collect, store and communicate the data to a laptop at the side of the track (Harle et al. 2011). The data is visualised as a set of time-based line graphs, with facilities to select sections of the run and scale the graphs to any desired level of detail (Harle et al. 2011). This method of organising the physiological data is interesting as it is clear when a high-energy activity has occurred, due to the amplitude of the lines.

Presenting physiological data, in a manner that can be interpreted, is a difficult challenge, due to the ambiguous nature of the data. Whilst current solutions offer interesting insights into how this data is able to be displayed, merging this data with other data sources poses a great challenge. Furthermore, interpreting this information so that its context can be associated with our memories is another difficulty. Nevertheless, Chowdhury et al. (2010) system, *MediAlly*, is a step closer to solving this problem. *MediAlly* uses a mobile device, to collect and store the subject's contextual states, whilst *Shimmer* sensors (Burns et al. 2010) collect physiological data. The system then produces a metadata stream that describes the related origins surrounding the physiological data collection (Chowdhury et al. 2010). Nonetheless, the devices only record location data, which is quite limited. More advanced solutions are needed that are able to merge this data with a number of different sources.

Research Challenges

The literature illustrates that the use of technology to aid in the recovery of memories in dementia patients is mostly positive. Nevertheless, it is reasonable to say that advanced solutions are needed, which include richer data sources. Data is being generated at a tremendous rate. The advent of smart environments, pervasive and mobile computing has enabled users, and their surroundings, to become active participants in generating information. However, this data is very disjointed. With all of this information surrounding us, bringing it together and creating HDMs, which span across diverse environments, enables more vivid HDMs to be created and is a significant challenge. The following is an overview of the key research challenges, which need to be addressed, in order to achieve this.

1. **Recreating any time of our lives:** The fundamental challenge of HDM research is to enable us to relive anytime of our lives, through our digital data. Information amassed over a lifetime needs to be efficiently searched and composed so that any moment of our lives can be extracted, recalled and replayed. In the case of those with Alzheimer's disease, this is fundamental as they can no longer rely upon their biological memory to consciously recollect and relive a past experience, thus making the future more difficult to anticipate (Bassett and Graham 2007). By providing a method of reliving personally experienced events, digitally, moments of recall can occur (Hodges et al. 2011). These periods are often referred to as a *"Proustian moment"* and are described as a moment of intense recollection when images of the past flood into consciousness, and the rememberer has a powerful experience of recollection (Loveday and Conway 2011). This is a significant challenge that raises many other secondary challenges, which are detailed below.

2. **The composition of a HDM:** Recent advances in technology have enabled a variety of information to be automatically captured. As stated above, the proliferation of pervasive devices has enabled any object, embedded with a sensor, to provide us with data. The culmination of this advancement is a world awash with sensing devices, which can record our every move and the environment around us. A human memory is not made up of a finite set of variables. However, it is safe to assume that the more information we can remember, the greater the level of detail, and the more vivid, a memory is. It is this idea that is of particular interest. Currently, devices, such as the *SenseCam* (Hodges et al. 2006), focus on only collecting specific information, such as photos. This method is limited because restricting the information that is being collected, results in a memory that is also limited. Instead of focusing on collecting a specific set of data items, the process of capturing HDM data needs to be flexible enough to adapt to the user's current situation (Dobbins et al. 2012b). Each environment that we occupy offers a different set of devices and information. These devices shape the memories. Devices present in one environment will differ to those of another, thus altering the information that is available. In this sense, the memories that are being created will never be the same. Therefore, as we move through different environments this will be reflected in the memories that are created. To form a more vivid memory, physiological sensors are able to record subconscious reactions to such situations/environments. Coupled with data from these different environments, we can see how certain situations and places make us feel. This is a very powerful tool to have. The integration of physiological data enables a deeper understanding of ourselves to emerge. An extensible and open platform is required to support the independent use of such sensors and through extended research, support for

interconnecting and internetworking services that support much richer compositions (Dobbins et al. 2012a). Harnessing this information into a HDM is a significant challenge and one that is currently being explored (Dobbins et al. 2013a, b, c).

3. **Searching a lifetime of data:** A key concern in human digital memory research relates to the amount of data that is generated, and stored. In particular, searching this set of big data is a key challenge. As previously stated, the vision of the *Memories for Life* grand challenge is to help people manage and use their digital memories across their entire lifetime (Fitzgibbon and Reiter 2005). Collecting data over this extensive period of time yields a phenomenal amount of information. When HDMs are created this massive amount of data needs to be intelligently searched and the associated information brought together. As stated by Ranpura (Ranpura 2000), *"Memories are rich because they are formed through associations. When we experience an event, our brains tie the sights, smells, sounds, and our own impressions together into a relationship. That relationship itself is the memory of the event"*. Whilst humans can do this type of processing, subconsciously, in a matter of nanoseconds, creating these associations, digitally, poses a greater challenge. HDM systems need to be able to cope with searching a vast pool of data so that relevant information can be extracted and visualised. Machine learning algorithms are seen as a way to alleviate this problem, as large datasets are capable of being processed (Dobbins et al. 2013c). As HDM vectors increase in size, it becomes progressively more difficult to keep track of accumulated data, especially from 10 or 20 years ago. Therefore, when defining explicit queries, it is easy to overlook pieces of information. However, using a matrix representation of the data, allows the searching of this information to be treated as a machine learning problem, based on the similarities in a vector object (Dobbins et al. 2013c). Consequently, a wider range of information can be included in the memory, as searching by similarity allows the desired information to be retrieved, as well as associated data that the user might not be aware of. This method enables much richer and more-detailed memories to be created, than previously seen. Memories created, in this way, are a "mash-up" of all the data of a specific time. This method allows us to obtain inferences of events that are impossible from a single data source, reduces data overload and allows a lot of data to be transformed into a smaller amount of more meaningful information. Searching massive amounts of user-generated data is already a problem; searching a lifetime's worth of information can therefore seem impossible.

4. **Structuring data into a representation of a digital memory:** As the data that we have access to, and are collecting, is growing so is the inability to effectively manage it. Current approaches are not flexible enough to deal with this highly heterogeneous data. The amount of data that can be collected over a lifetime is phenomenal. If these collections are to realize their potential, we need to focus on new tools that allow participants to filter, evaluate, maintain and share the huge digital collections that they are now accumulating (Whittaker et al. 2009). Structuring lifelogs is a major challenge in lifelogging systems, which need to

present these logs in a concise and meaningful way to the user (Kikhia et al. 2011). However, since a human memory is not a physical item, this challenge has no right, wrong or indeed, definitive answer. How can you re-create something that does not physically exist in front of you? However, we can draw upon past research into the elements of human memory to structure HDM data into a reasonable representation of a memory. Episodic memory relates to memories about personally experienced occasions. The information concerned is mainly about the subject's experiences of temporally dated episodes or events, and the temporal-spatial relations between them (Tulving 1984, 1993). This type of memory is concerned about happenings, in particular, places at particular times, or about *"what"*, *"where"*, and *"when"* (Tulving 2002). When an event or "episode" is remembered we usually answer these three points subconsciously. Primarily, we tend to remember where we were, the time of the event and what happened. This temporal episode, which has been brought to the forefront of our mind, can be imagined as a "box" of an event. All the information, from a specific time, is searched and grouped together in one place. In this context, a "memory box" is formed. It is this idea that is used, in current research, to structure HDM data as memory boxes of temporal human-life experiences (Dobbins et al. 2013a, b, c). In this sense, an interactive viewer is essential. By allowing users to "go into" their memories and to see numerous data items, such as temperature, location and emotions, they are able to reflect on their activities and also to see how their bodies are reacting. This is beneficial as the more detailed; a HDM is the more useful it is. In the case of elderly users, carers are able to work with them in order to recall any point in their life and to help them reflect and relive any moment in time.

5. **Integration of Physiological Information into a HDM:** Physiological data enables spontaneous and subconscious facets of a user's state to be captured (Fairclough 2009). Integrating this information into a HDM enables a whole new dimension of ourselves to emerge, along with a greater understanding of our subconscious. However, for the purpose of memory recall, organising and representing this data is challenging. Currently, graph-based solutions plot this data in a very clinical way. In contrast, as previously seen, colour-coding is an alternative to such methods (Lindström et al. 2006; Fairclough and Gilleade 2013). This is an interesting idea that would enable memory boxes to be colour-coded, depending on the physiological parameters of the user's data. In this instance, the user can see how they were feeling at certain times of their lives. For example, recalling a memory of a birthday party is generally seen as a happy event. When recalling this memory box all the data from that time (location, photos, videos etc.) would be brought together into a box. The processed physiological data would dictate the colour of the box. In this instance, the box could be blue to indicate that this event was a happy one. As described by Crozier (1999), *"Blue may lend itself to positive associations, particularly those which relate to "pleasantness""*. This information is imperative to enable memory boxes to be highly personal objects that can be used for memory recall.

6. **The longevity of HDMs:** As previously stated, the goal of the *Memories for Life* grand challenge is to help people manage and use their digital memories across their *entire* lifetime (Fitzgibbon and Reiter 2005). As new technologies emerge, data types become obsolete. Data needs to be accessible, regardless of time. This is an important challenge and one that Fitzgibbon and Reiter (2005) reiterate, *"How can we ensure that data is still accessible in 50 years time, despite inevitable changes in software, hardware and formats?"* The use of linked data, semantic web principles and the Resource Description Framework (RDF) is seen as a way to alleviate this difficulty (Dobbins et al. 2012c, 2013b). The use of RDF enables data to be incorporated into a memory, irrespective of its format. As time goes on and new devices and formats emerge they can, nevertheless, be incorporated into a HDM, using this method. This is reiterated by the W3C (2004), who comment that, *"RDF has features that facilitate data merging even if the underlying schemas differ, and it specifically supports the evolution of schemas over time without requiring all the data consumers to be changed"*. As new standards become available their data, as well as data collected 10 years ago, for instance, need to still be incorporated in a HDM.

7. **Privacy and Security:** In any system that records personal information, privacy becomes an issue. Whenever Memories for Life is discussed with the general public or the non-scientific media, privacy and security issues are the ones most frequently raised (Fitzgibbon and Reiter 2005). The European Network and Information Security Agency's (ENISA) report (2011) into the benefits and risks of lifelogging reiterates this point. In this report, they comment that, *"The top risk for individuals utilising life-logging devices and scenarios is the threat to privacy that accompany using them. Loss of control over this data might result in individuals being subjected to financial fraud or unauthorised access might result in reputational harm or discrimination and exclusion"* (European Network and Information Security Agency (ENISA) 2011). Fitzgibbon and Reiter (2005) also question, *"How should privacy be protected, especially when an individual is present in someone else's memory? For example, if Joe has a digital picture of Mary and he is holding hands, what rights does Mary have over the use and distribution of this picture?"* This is a very important point to consider, especially when photographic data is concerned, as inevitably, this type of information will contain the images of multiple users. Another point to consider is the security of physiological data, as this type of information is very personal. When an individual's data is combined with other sources, there are a number of issues to consider. Such issues include this data being aggregated with data streams from a variety of sources and other individuals and data being used in an unauthorised mash-up, which removes the user's control of the presentation of their data (Gilleade and Lee 2011). Furthermore, collecting a lifetime's worth of information undoubtedly produces a vast amount of data. Securing this collection becomes harder as it grows in size. Private areas need to be established where users can store their information and choose what memories to share with others. Another issue, regarding privacy, relates to identity theft. If devices are stolen, and false memories created, then this affects the user's entire HDM store.

Addressing the challenges, raised above, is important so that a more realistic representation of a memory can be constructed and content–based searches can be performed. Processes need to be developed in order to store and share memories in a more flexible way. These challenges have helped to formulate the reasoning that HDMs should not be "tied-down" to a fixed number of information sources; the more data that can be accessed the more detailed the memory will be (Dobbins et al. 2012b). Since this data is highly heterogeneous, an intelligent way of searching this information is also needed. As previously stated, machine learning is seen as a way to alleviate this problem (Dobbins et al. 2013c). Treating the searching of these documents as a machine learning problem also eliminates the need to produce complex and exact queries. This enables a wider range of information to be utilized in the creation HDMs and allows the system to learn about its user. For example, User A (who has Alzheimer's) and her husband are visiting the Eiffel Tower. They have visited this location before, however, on this occasion User A cannot recall that previous time. In this instance she, or her husband, can log into the system and ask it, *"Have I been here before, does this location make me happy?"* Using a learning approach, the system would have learnt the features of being happy and mapped this to their current location to return an answer of *"Yes"*. However, this alone is not enough to stimulate her memory. Working in conjunction with this aspect of the system, a memory box about their earlier visit to the Eiffel Tower is created, thus providing the visual stimulation that the user needs to actively recall her previous visit to this location. In this instance, all of the data that the system has from that time is clustered together and displayed in the memory box. User A can now see all of the information that has been previously captured (e.g. photos, videos, temperature, etc.). Using her archived physiological data the memory box is also blue (as this was a happy memory). There is also a key next to the memory box that displays the mood that each memory box colour is associated with. When User A sees all of the data from her previous visit she slowly starts to remember that she has been here before and starts to feel more at ease that she has remembered that time. This is extremely important as, *"The significance of one's personal past in making sense of the present is especially relevant for people with Alzheimer's disease"* (Programs et al. 2002). Dementia sufferers often feel a loss of self-identity, and reminiscing is seen as a particularly rich method of rediscovering themselves. Moreover, place-based recollection can be seen as a means for getting into associated memories of events and social interactions, etc. from the past, thus opening an avenue to other life experiences (Programs et al. 2002).

Interaction with our HDMs is fundamental and is what makes our work unique (Dobbins et al. 2012c, 2013b). By enabling users to be able to "go into" their memories and to see and understand various pieces of information, such as temperature, location and emotions, enables a greater level of detail to be retrieved (Dobbins et al. 2011, 2012a, c). This very interesting feature can be used to gain a better insight into ourselves. For instance, a particular location might provoke certain physiological responses, which we are unaware of having. By recording and questioning this information, a greater level of recall and understanding about ourselves is gained.

Summary

Dementia is a progressive and irreversible chronic disease (Davies et al. 2009). However, the use of external memory aids to help people to compensate for their memory deficits is thought to be one of the most valuable and effective ways to aid rehabilitation (Hodges et al. 2006). As it can be seen, a great deal of research has been undertaken within the area of HDMs. However, novel solutions are still needed that include much richer data capturing capabilities and can handle searching and organising a lifetime of information. Providing a secure platform that enables sufferers to recall events better and live more independently is essential. This view is reiterated by Davies et al. (2009) who state, *"Such solutions will offer people with mild dementia with the ability to increase their independence and quality of life and furthermore prolong the period of time that they can live within their home environment"*. HDMs are already offering promising results in aiding dementia patients in remembering the past (Hodges et al. 2006; Davies et al. 2009; Browne et al. 2011; Crete-Nishihata et al. 2012). Nevertheless, this technology has mainly focused on collecting and using *SenseCam* images in the task of recollecting such events. Whilst this is a good place to start, incorporating more data sources, such as from physiological sensors, enables a more vivid HDM to be created, and it is posited that a greater rate of recall can be achieved.

References

Alzheimer's Research UK (2012) Dementia statistics. pp 1–8

Bassett R, Graham JE (2007) Memorabilities: enduring relationships, memories and abilities in dementia. Ageing Soc 27:533–554. doi:10.1017/S0144686X07005971

Berry E, Kapur N, Williams L et al (2007) The use of a wearable camera, SenseCam, as a pictorial diary to improve autobiographical memory in a patient with limbic encephalitis: a preliminary report. Neuropsychol Rehabil 17:582–601. doi: 10.1080/09602010601029780, http://dx.doi.org/10.1080/09602010601029780

Bonato P (2010) Wearable sensors and systems. From enabling technology to clinical applications. IEEE Eng Med Biol Soc Mag 29:25–36. doi:10.1109/MEMB.2010.936554

Brindley R, Bateman A, Gracey F (2011) Exploration of use of SenseCam to support autobiographical memory retrieval within a cognitive-behavioural therapeutic intervention following acquired brain injury. Memory 19:745–757. doi:10.1080/09658211.2010.493893

Browne G, Berry E, Kapur N et al (2011) SenseCam improves memory for recent events and quality of life in a patient with memory retrieval difficulties. Memory 19:713–722. doi:10.1080/09658211.2011.614622

Burns A, Greene BR, McGrath MJ et al (2010) SHIMMER™: a wireless sensor platform for noninvasive biomedical research. IEEE Sens J 10:1527–1534. doi:10.1109/JSEN.2010.2045498

Bush V (1945) As we may think. Atl. Mon 176:101–108

Byrne D, Jones GJF (2008) Towards computational autobiographical narratives through human digital memories. In: Proceeding 2nd ACM international work story represent mechanism context—SRMC '08 9. doi: 10.1145/1462014.1462017

Byrne D, Jones GJF (2009) Exploring narrative presentation for large multimodal lifelog collections through card sorting. In: Iurgel IA, Zagalo N, Petta P (eds) Proceedings of the interactive storytelling, second joint international conference on interactive digital storytelling ICIDS 2009, Guimarães, Port, Berlin, Heidelberg, 9–11 Dec 2009, pp 92–97

Chen Y, Jones GJF (2008) Integrating memory context into personal information re-finding. In: 2nd BCS IRSG symposium on future directions in information access, pp 14–21

Chen Y, Jones GJF (2009) An event-based interface to support personal lifelog search. In: Proceedings of HCI international, San Diego, July 2009

Chen Y, Jones GJF (2010) Augmenting human memory using personal lifelogs. In: Proceedings of the 1st augmented human intelligence conference. doi: 10.1145/1785455.1785479

Chowdhury A, Falchuk B, Misra A (2010) MediAlly: a provenance-aware remote health monitoring middleware. IEEE Int Conf Pervasive Comput Commun 2010:125–134. doi:10.1109/PERCOM.2010.5466985

Coyle S, Lau K-T, Moyna N et al (2010) BIOTEX—biosensing textiles for personalised healthcare management. IEEE Trans Inf Technol Biomed 14:364–370. doi:10.1109/TITB.2009.2038484

Crete-Nishihata M, Baecker RM, Massimi M et al (2012) Reconstructing the past: personal memory technologies are not just personal and not just for memory. Human-Computer Interact 27:92–123. doi:10.1080/07370024.2012.656062

Crozier WR (1999) The meanings of colour: preferences among hues. Pigment Resin Technol 28:6–14. doi:10.1108/03699429910252315

Cruickshank J, Harding J, Paxman J, Morris C (2013) 2020health report making connections: a transatlantic exchange to support the adoption of digital health between the US VHA and England's NHS. Health Devices 41:1–90

Curone D, Secco EL, Tognetti A et al (2010) Smart garments for emergency operators: the ProeTEX project. IEEE Trans Inf Technol Biomed 14:694–701. doi:10.1109/TITB.2010.2045003

Davies RJ, Nugent CD, Donnelly MP et al (2009) A user driven approach to develop a cognitive prosthetic to address the unmet needs of people with mild dementia. Pervasive Mob Comput 5:253–267. doi:10.1016/j.pmcj.2008.07.002

DCU (2011) Centre for digital video processing. Dublin City University, Ireland. http://www.cdvp.dcu.ie/. Accessed 15 Nov 2012

Dickie C, Vertegaal R, Fono D et al (2004a) Augmenting and sharing memory with eyeBlog. In: Proceedings of the 1st ACM workshop on continuous archival and retrieval of personal experience—CARPE'04, ACM Press, New York, p 105

Dickie C, Vertegaal R, Shell JS et al (2004b) Eye contact sensing glasses for attention-sensitive wearable video blogging. In: Extended abstracts of the ACM conference on human factors in computing systems, CHI 2004, ACM Press, Vienna, pp 769–770

Dobbins C, Fergus P, Merabti M, Llewellyn-Jones D (2012a) Monitoring and measuring sedentary behaviour with the aid of human digital memories. In: Proceedings of the 9th annual IEEE consumer communications and networking conference, Las Vegas, pp 395–398

Dobbins C, Merabti M, Fergus P et al (2013a) Exploiting linked data to create rich human digital memories. Comput Commun 36:1639–1656. doi:10.1016/j.comcom.2013.06.008

Dobbins C, Merabti M, Fergus P, Llewellyn-Jones D (2012b) Capturing and sharing human digital memories with the aid of ubiquitous peer–to–peer mobile services. In: Proceedings of the 10th annual IEEE international conference on pervasive computing and communications, Lugano, pp 64–69

Dobbins C, Merabti M, Fergus P, Llewellyn-Jones D (2012c) Augmenting human digital memories with physiological data. In: Proceedings of the 3rd IEEE international conference on networked embedded systems for every application, Liverpool, pp 35–41

Dobbins C, Merabti M, Fergus P, Llewellyn-Jones D (2013b) Creating human digital memories for a Richer recall of life experiences. In: Proceedings of 10th IEEE international conference on networking, sensing and control, IEEE, Evry, pp 246–251

Dobbins C, Merabti M, Fergus P, Llewellyn-Jones D (2013c) Creating human digital memories with the aid of pervasive mobile devices. Pervasive Mob Comput (in Press). doi:10.1016/j.pmcj.2013.10.009

Dobbins C, Merabti M, Fergus P, Llewellyn-Jones D (2011) Towards a framework for capturing and distributing rich interactive human digital memories. In: Proceedings of the 12th annual postgraduate symposium on convergence of telecommunications, networking and broadcasting

Doherty AR (2005) Human digital memories. In: Health promotion. http://www.computing.dcu.ie/~cgurrin/ca168/seminar7.pdf. Accessed 1 Aug 2013

Doherty AR, Caprani N, Conaire CÓ et al (2011a) Passively recognising human activities through lifelogging. Comput Human Behav 27:1948–1958. doi:10.1016/j.chb.2011.05.002

Doherty AR, Moulin CJA, Smeaton AF (2011b) Automatically assisting human memory: a SenseCam browser. Memory 19:785–795. doi:10.1080/09658211.2010.509732

Doherty AR, Pauly-Takacs K, Gurrin C et al (2009) Three years of SenseCam images: observations on cued recall. In: Invited speech at: SenseCam 2009 symposium at the 39th annual meeting of the society for neuroscience: neuroscience 2009, Chicago, 16–17 October 2009

Doherty AR, Smeaton AF (2010) Automatically augmenting lifelog events using pervasively generated content from millions of people. Sensors 10:1423–1446. doi:10.3390/100301423

European Network and Information Security Agency (ENISA) (2011) To log or not to log? Risks and benefits of emerging life-logging applications. pp 1–100

Fairclough S, Gilleade K (2013) Physiological computing where brain and body drive technology. http://www.physiologicalcomputing.net/?page_id=461. Accessed 12 Nov 2013

Fairclough SH (2009) Fundamentals of physiological computing. Interact Comput 21:133–145. doi:10.1016/j.intcom.2008.10.011

Figueiredo CP, Becher K, Hoffmann KP, Mendes PM (2010) Low power wireless acquisition module for wearable health monitoring systems. 32nd annual international conference of the IEEE engineering in medicine and biology society, pp 704–707

Fitzgibbon A, Reiter E (2005) Grand challenges in computing research: GC3 memories for life: managing information over a human lifetime. In: Conference on geometric design and computing research, pp 13–16

Fuller M, Kelly L, Jones GJF (2008) Applying contextual memory cues for retrieval from personal information archives. Personal information management (PIM), conjunction with CHI 2008 Work

Gemmell J, Bell G, Lueder R et al (2002) MyLifeBits: fulfilling the Memex vision. In: Proceedings of the 10th ACM international conference on multimedia—multimedia '02, ACM Press, New York, pp 235–238

Gemmell J, Williams L, Wood K et al (2004) Passive capture and ensuing issues for a personal lifetime store. In: Proceedings of the 1st ACM workshop on continuous archival and retrieval of personal experiences—CARPE'04. ACM Press, New York, pp 48–55

Gilleade K, Fairclough SH (2010) Physiology as XP—body blogging to victory. Paper presented at BioS-Play workshop at fun and games, Leuven

Gilleade K, Lee K (2011) Issues inherent in controlling the interpretation of the physiological cloud. In: CHI 2011 workshops, Vancouver, pp 1–4

Gozali JP, Kan M-Y, Sundaram H (2012) How do people organize their photos in each event and how does it affect storytelling, searching and interpretation tasks?.In: Proceedings of the 12th ACM/IEEE-CS joint conference on digital libraries—JCDL 2012, ACM Press, New York, pp 315–324

Gurrin C (2012) Living with SenseCam: experiences, motivations and advances. In: Invited talk SenseCam 2012, Oxford, 3–4 April 2012

Gurrin C, Byrne D, O'Connor N et al (2008) Architecture and challenges of maintaining a large-scale, context-aware human digital memory. In: Proceedings of the 5th international conference on visual information engineering, pp 158–163

Haartsen J (1998) Bluetooth—the universal radio interface for ad hoc, wireless connectivity. Ericsson Rev 1:110–117

Hallberg J, Kikhia B (2009) Reminiscence process using life-log entities for persons with mild dementia'. Proceedings of the first international workshop on reminiscence systems, pp 16–21

Harle R, Taherian S, Pias M et al (2011) Towards real-time profiling of sprints using wearable pressure sensors. Comput Commun 35:650–660. doi:10.1016/j.comcom.2011.03.019

Healey J, Picard RW (1998) StartleCam: a cybernetic wearable camera. In: 2nd international symposium on wearable computers: digest of papers (Cat No98EX215), pp 42–49. doi: 10.1109/ISWC.1998.729528

Hirt W (2003) Ultra-wideband radio technology: overview and future research. Comput Commun 26:46–52. doi:10.1016/S1403-3664(02)00119-6

Hodges S, Berry E, Wood K (2011) SenseCam: a wearable camera that stimulates and rehabilitates autobiographical memory. Memory 19:685–696. doi:10.1080/09658211.2011.605591

Hodges S, Williams L, Berry E et al (2006) SenseCam: a retrospective memory aid. UbiComp 2006 Ubiquitous Comput 4206:177–193. doi: 10.1007/11853565

Huang H-H, Matsushita H, Kawagoe K et al (2012) Toward a memory assistant companion for the individuals with mild memory impairment. In: IEEE 11th international conference on cognitive informatics and cognitive computing, IEEE, pp 295–299

Kalnikaite V, Sellen A, Whittaker S, Kirk D (2010) Now let me see where i was: understanding how lifelogs mediate memory. In: Proceedings of the 28th international conference on human factors in computing systems—CHI 2010, ACM Press, New York, p 2045

Kalnikaitė V, Whittaker S (2011) A saunter down memory lane: digital reflection on personal mementos. Int J Hum Comput Stud 69:298–310. doi:10.1016/j.ijhcs.2010.12.004

Karaman S, Benois-Pineau J, Megret R et al (2011) Activities of daily living indexing by hierarchical HMM for dementia diagnostics. In: 9th international workshop on content-based multimedia indexing, IEEE, pp 79–84

Kelly L (2007) The information retrieval challenge of human digital memories. In: BCS IRSG symposium: future directions in information

Kelly L, Jones GJF (2007) Venturing into the labyrinth: the information retrieval challenge of human digital memories. In: Workshop supporting human memory with interactive system, Lancaster, pp 37–40

Kelly L, Jones GJF (2009) Examining the utility of affective response in search of personal lifelogs. In: 5th workshop on emotion in human-computer interaction, held at the 23rd BCS HCI group conference 2009, Cambridge, 1 Sept 2009

Kelly P, Doherty A, Berry E et al (2011) Can we use digital life-log images to investigate active and sedentary travel behaviour? results from a pilot study. Int J Behav Nutr Phys Act 8:44. doi:10.1186/1479-5868-8-44

Kelly P, Doherty AR, Hamilton A et al (2012) Evaluating the feasibility of measuring travel to school using a wearable camera. Am J Prev Med 43:546–550. doi:10.1016/j.amepre.2012.07.027

Kikhia B, Boytsov A, Hallberg J et al (2011) Structuring and presenting lifelogs based on location data. Image (IN) 4:5–24

Kikhia B, Hallberg J, Bengtsson JE et al (2010) Building digital life stories for memory support. Int J Comput Healthc 1:161–176

Kikhia B, Hallberg J, Synnes K, Sani Z ul H (2009) Context-aware life-logging for persons with mild dementia. In: Annual international conference of the IEEE engineering in medicine and biology society, pp 6183–6186

Korhonen I, Bardram JE (2004) Guest editorial introduction to the special section on pervasive healthcare. IEEE Trans Inf Technol Biomed 8:229–234

Lalanne D, van den Hoven E (2007) Supporting human memory with interactive systems. In: Workshop at the 2007 British HCI conference, Lancaster, 4 Sept 2007

Langereis G, de Voogd-Claessen L, Spaepen A et al (2007) ConText: contactless sensors for body monitoring incorporated in textiles. In: IEEE international conference on portable information devices. pp 1–5

Lee H, Smeaton AF, O'Connor NE et al (2008) Constructing a SenseCam visual diary as a media process. Multimed Syst 14:341–349. doi:10.1007/s00530-008-0129-x

Lee KM, Lunney TF, Curran KJ, Santos JA (2011a) Context-aware support for assistive systems and services. In: IET seminar on assisted living

Lee MW, Khan AM, Kim T-S (2011b) A single tri-axial accelerometer-based real-time personal life log system capable of human activity recognition and exercise information generation. Pers Ubiquitous Comput 15:887–898. doi:10.1007/s00779-011-0403-3

Lee S, Gong G, Lee S (2010) Entity-event lifelog ontology model (EELOM) for lifeLog ontology schema definition. In: 12th international Asia-Pacific web conference 2010 pp 344–346. doi: 10.1109/APWeb.2010.58

De Leo G, Brivio E, Sautter SW (2011) Supporting autobiographical memory in patients with Alzheimer's disease using smart phones. Appl Neuropsychol 18:69–76. doi:10.1080/09084282.2011.545730

Lindley SE, Randall D, Sharrock W et al (2009) Narrative, memory and practice: tensions and choices in the use of a digital artefact. In: Proceedings of the 23rd British HCI group annual conference on people and computers: celebrating people and technology, pp 1–9

Lindström M, Ståhl A, Höök K et al (2006) Affective diary—designing for bodily expressiveness and self-reflection. In: Proceedings of CHI '06: extended abstract on human factors in computing systems, ACM Press, New York, pp 1037–1042

López G, Custodio V, Moreno JI (2010) LOBIN: E-textile and wireless-sensor-network-based platform for healthcare monitoring in future hospital environments. IEEE Trans Inf Technol Biomed 14:1446–1458. doi:10.1109/TITB.2010.2058812

Loveday C, Conway MA (2011) Using SenseCam with an amnesic patient: accessing inaccessible everyday memories. Memory 19:697–704. doi:10.1080/09658211.2011.610803

Lymberis A, Paradiso R (2008) Smart fabrics and interactive textile enabling wearable personal applications: R&D state of the art and future challenges. In: 30th annual international conference of the IEEE engineering in medicine and biology society, pp 5270–5273

Machajdik J, Hanbury A, Garz A, Sablatnig R (2011) Affective computing for wearable diary and lifelogging systems: an overview. In: 35th annual workshop of the Austrian association for pattern recognition

Mann S (1997) Wearable computing: a first step toward personal imaging. Computer (Long Beach Calif) 30:25–32. doi:10.1109/2.566147

Mann S (2004) Continuous lifelong capture of personal experience with EyeTap. In: Proceedings of the 1st ACM workshop on continuous archival and retrieval of personal experience—CARPE'04, ACM Press, New York, pp 1–21

Mann S, Fung J, Aimone C et al (2005) Designing EyeTap digital eyeglasses for continuous lifelong capture and sharing of personal experiences. In: Proceedings of the CHI 2005 conference on human factors in computing systems

Matthews R, McDonald NJ, Hervieux P et al (2007) A wearable physiological sensor suite for unobtrusive monitoring of physiological and cognitive state. In: 29th annual international conference of the IEEE engineering in medicine and biology society, pp 5276–5281

McCarthy S, McKevitt P, McTear M, Sayers H (2007) MemoryLane: an intelligent mobile companion for elderly users. In: 7th information technology & telecommunications conference IT&T, Dublin, Ireland, pp 72–82

McDuff D, Karlson A, Kapoor A et al (2012) AffectAura: an intelligent system for emotional memory. In: Proceedings of 2012 ACM annual conference on human factors in computing systems—CHI '12. ACM Press, New York, USA, pp 849–858

Microsoft Research (2011) Reviewing and sharing SenseCam images. http://research.microsoft.com/en-us/um/cambridge/projects/sensecam/review.htm. Accessed 1 Jun 2013

O'Hare N, Lee H, Cooray S et al (2006) MediAssist: using content-based analysis and context to manage personal photo collections. Image Video Retr 4071:529–532. doi:10.1007/11788034

O'Hare N, Smeaton AF (2009) Context-aware person identification in personal photo collections. IEEE Trans Multimed 11:220–228. doi:10.1109/TMM.2008.2009679

Office for National Statistics (2010) Healthy life expectancy: living longer in poor health. http://www.statistics.gov.uk/cci/nugget.asp?id=2159. Accessed 1 June 2013

Pacelli M, Loriga G, Taccini N, Paradiso R (2006) Sensing fabrics for monitoring physiological and biomechanical variables: e-textile solutions. In: 3rd IEEE-EMBS international summer school and symposium on medical devices and biosensors, pp 1–4

Pandian PS, Mohanavelu K, Safeer KP et al (2008) Smart vest: wearable multi-parameter remote physiological monitoring system. Med Eng Phys 30:466–477. doi:10.1016/j.medengphy.2007.05.014

Pantelopoulos A, Bourbakis NG (2010a) Prognosis—a wearable health-monitoring system for people at risk: methodology and modeling. IEEE Trans Inf Technol Biomed 14:613–621. doi:10.1109/TITB.2010.2040085

Pantelopoulos A, Bourbakis NG (2010b) A survey on wearable sensor-based systems for health monitoring and prognosis. IEEE Trans Syst Man, Cybern Part C Appl Rev 40:1–12. doi: 10.1109/TSMCC.2009.2032660

Paradiso R, Loriga G, Taccini N (2005) A wearable health care system based on knitted integrated sensors. IEEE Trans Inf Technol Biomed 9:337–344. doi:10.1109/TITB.2005.854512

Pauly-Takacs K, Moulin CJA, Estlin EJ (2011) SenseCam as a rehabilitation tool in a child with anterograde amnesia. Memory 19:705–712. doi:10.1080/09658211.2010.494046

Piasek P, Irving K, Smeaton AF (2011) SenseCam intervention based on cognitive stimulation therapy framework for early-stage dementia. In: 5th international conference on pervasive computing technologies for healthcare, pp 522–525

Picault J, Ribière M, Senot C (2010) Beyond life streams: activities and intentions for managing personal digital memories. In: Proceedings of 1st international workshop on adaptive personality recommission Society Web (APRESW 2010) 25–32

Programs G, Fraser S, Columbia B (2002) Journey back home: recollecting past places by people with dementia. J Hous Elderly 16:85–106. doi:10.1300/J081v16n01

Prull MW, Dawes LLC, Martin AM et al (2006) Recollection and familiarity in recognition memory: adult age differences and neuropsychological test correlates. Psychol Aging 21:107–118. doi:10.1037/0882-7974.21.1.107

Qiu Z, Doherty AR, Gurrin C, Smeaton AF (2011) Mining user activity as a context source for search and retrieval. In: IEEE international conference on semantic technology and information retrieval, pp 162–166

Ranpura A (2000) How we remember, and why we forget. In: BrainConnection.com. http://brainconnection.positscience.com/how-we-remember-and-why-we-forget/

Sellen A, Fogg A, Aitken M et al (2007) Do life-logging technologies support memory for the past? an experimental study using SenseCam. In: Conference on human factors in computing systems CHI '07, Irvine, CA, pp 81–90

Ståhl A, Höök K, Svensson M et al (2009) Experiencing the affective diary. Pers Ubiquitous Comput 13:365–378. doi:10.1007/s00779-008-0202-7

Taraldsen K, Askim T, Sletvold O et al (2011) Evaluation of a body-worn sensor system to measure physical activity in older people with impaired function. Phys Ther J Am Phys Ther Assoc 91:277–285. doi:10.2522/ptj.20100159

Teraoka T (2011) Aggregation and exploration of heterogeneous data collected from diverse information sources. In: Proceedings of 1st international symposium on from digital footprints to society community Intelligence—SCI '11. ACM Press, New York, USA, pp 31–36

Tulving E (1984) Precis of elements of episodic memory. Behav Brain Sci 7:223–268

Tulving E (1993) What Is episodic memory? Curr Dir Psychol Sci 2:67–70

Tulving E (2002) Episodic memory: from mind to brain. Annu Rev Psychol 53:1–25. doi:10.1146/annurev.psych.53.100901.135114

Vogt J, Luyten K, Van den Bergh J et al (2012) Putting dementia into context. Lect Notes Comput Sci 7623:181–198. doi:10.1007/978-3-642-34347-6

W3C (2004) Resource description framework (RDF). http://www.w3.org/RDF/. Accessed 12 Aug 2013

Wang J-J, Wang S (2010) Wireless sensor networks for home appliance energy management based on ZigBee technology. In: IEEE international conference on machine learning and cybernetics, pp 1041–1046

Wang P, Smeaton AF (2013) Using visual lifelogs to automatically characterize everyday activities. Inf Sci (Ny) 230:147–161. doi:10.1016/j.ins.2012.12.028

Wang P, Smeaton AF (2012) Semantics-based selection of everyday concepts in visual lifelogging. Int J Multimed Inf Retr 1:87–101. doi:10.1007/s13735-012-0010-8

Weiser M (1999) The computer for the 21st century. ACM SIGMOBILE Mob Comput Commun Rev 3:3–11. doi:10.1145/329124.329126

Whittaker S, Bergman O, Clough P (2009) Easy on that trigger dad: a study of long term family photo retrieval. Pers Ubiquitous Comput 14:31–43. doi:10.1007/s00779-009-0218-7

Index

A

Accelerometers, 27
Active brain-computer interfaces, 22, 30, 71, 72, 75, 77–79
Adaptation, 2, 5, 9, 10, 13, 69, 76, 78, 85, 92, 99, 100, 121, 134–136, 142, 160, 161, 164, 176, 179, 189, 190, 191–194
Adaptive curator, 188
Adaptive gaming technologies, XIV, 10
Affectaura, 221, 222
Affective computing, 2, 4, 9, 27, 78
Affective diary, 11, 12, 221
Affective states, 9, 143–145, 148–151, 153, 158, 159, 162–164, 179
Alzheimer's disease, 212, 223
Ambulatory monitoring, 3, 4, 6, 51
Amyotrophic lateral sclerosis (ALS), 70
Anxiety, 4, 104, 143–145, 149–155, 158, 159, 163, 199
Artifacts, 19, 45, 79, 119, 120, 126, 200
Artificial neural network, 78, 180
Artwork, 175, 177, 192
Attention deficit hyperactivity disorder (ADHD), 94, 95, 98
Attentive intelligent tutoring systems, 58
Attentive user interfaces, 42, 53
Autism, 95, 141–143, 158, 162–164
Autonomic nervous system, 24, 26, 28, 33, 76, 110, 142, 178, 180, 197

B

Bayesian network, 28, 150
Biocybernetic adaptation, 2–6, 9, 10, 13–15, 92, 93, 97, 101, 106, 117, 121, 131, 133, 179
Biofeedback, 5, 92, 93, 95, 109
Biofeedback games, 96, 98, 101, 102
Biofeedback training, 91, 93–95, 101, 109, 111

C

Calibration, 46–50, 77, 85, 100, 133
Calmprix, 95
Circumplex model, 174, 175
Clinical biofeedback training, 93
Cognitive impairment, 216
Context awareness, 26–28, 33, 74
Corneal reflection, 42, 44, 57
Crew resource management, 108
Cultural heritage, 169–175, 177, 179, 180, 186, 187, 191–193
Cybernetics, 93

D

Data fusion algorithms, 28, 34
Dementia, 211, 212, 222, 227, 228
Depression, 199
Digital memories, 211, 213, 224, 226
Dimension reduction, 26
Driver fatigue monitoring, 30

E

Electrocardiography (ECG), 12, 21, 76, 143, 213, 217
Electroencephalography (EEG), 7, 18, 69, 101, 104, 120, 176, 177
Electromyography (EMG), 143, 145, 178, 217
Electrooculography (EOG), 3, 42, 45, 218

BIOTEX, 218

Blood pressure, 3, 4, 13, 94, 199, 205, 206
Body blogger, 6, 11, 12, 14, 221
Body schema, 2, 3, 5, 14
Brain-computer interface (BCI), 1–9, 22, 30, 67, 69–80, 83, 85, 97, 109, 119, 132
Brainput, 134, 136

S. H. Fairclough and K. Gilleade (eds.), *Advances in Physiological Computing*,
Human–Computer Interaction Series, DOI: 10.1007/978-1-4471-6392-3,
© Springer-Verlag London 2014

Printed in the United States
By Bookmasters